FAMILY BUILDING THROUGH EGG AND SPERM DONATION

Medical, Legal, and Ethical Issues

Edited by

Machelle M. Seibel, M.D.
Medical Director, Faulkner Center for Reproductive Medicine
Associate Clinical Professor of Gynecology, Harvard Medical School
Boston, MA

Susan L. Crockin, J.D.
Kassler & Feuer P.C.
Adjunct Professor, Northeastern University School of Law
Boston, MA

Jones and Bartlett Publishers
Sudbury, Massachusetts

Boston   London   Singapore

Editorial, Sales, and Customer Service Offices
Jones and Bartlett Publishers
40 Tall Pine Drive
Sudbury, MA 01776
1-800-832-0034
1-508-443-5000

Jones and Bartlett Publishers International
7 Melrose Terrace
London W6 7RL
England

Library of Congress Cataloging-in-Publication Data

Seibel, Machelle M.
    Family building through egg and sperm donation:
  medical, legal, and ethical issues; / Machelle M. Seibel, Susan L.
  Crockin.
        p.   cm.
      Includes bibliographical references and index.
      ISBN O-86720-483-4
      1. Artificial insemination. Human.   I. Crockin, Susan L.
    II. Title.
    RG134.S45   1996
    618.1'78—dc20   95-31221
                                                                 CIP

Acquisitions Editor: Joseph E. Burns
Production Editor: Nadine Fitzwilliam
Manufacturing Buyer: Dana L. Cerrito
Editorial Production: WordCrafters Editorial Services, Inc.
Typesetting: Publishers' Design and Production Services, Inc.
Cover Design: Marshall Henrichs
Printing and Binding: Hamilton Printing Company
Cover Printing: John P. Pow Company

Printed in the United States of America
99 98 97 96   10 9 8 7 6 5 4 3 2 1

Contents

9 Legal Issues in Egg Donation

144

John A. Robertson, J.D., Susan L. Crockin, J.D.

10 Egg Donation Consent Forms

158

Joan C. Stoddard, J.D., Janis Fox, M.D.

PART III   Social/Ethical Issues   217

Foreword

ELLIOT L. SAGALL, M.D.
Founder, the American Society of Law, Medicine & Ethics

Medically assisted human fertilization has from its beginning created a myriad of challenging and vexing medical, legal, ethical, moral, religious, societal, and governmental problems and concerns. The initial medical issues mainly involved sperm donor selection, semen preservation, and improving the techniques of artificial insemination. The initial legal actions consisted of occasional lawsuits alleging improper donor sperm selection, storage, and/or application; parental financial support and visitation rights of the donor father; inheritance and support rights of the conceived child as well as those of siblings; malpractice actions against health care providers and operators of sperm banks for untoward results; and even the specter of adultery charges against the artificially impregnated mother. Societal concerns primarily addressed the question of whether or not to impose governmental regulations on the physical and mental fitness of sperm donors and the maintenance of sperm banks. Ethical problems were limited primarily to the morality of "unnatural methods" of procreation and the extent of information to be imparted by parents and others to children conceived by donor insemination.

Today, rapidly evolving advances in reproductive technology have not only multiplied the number of problem areas but also greatly expanded the scope of potential legal actions in an almost geometric progression. Gamete donation in particular creates a myriad of potential issues. Critics worry about techniques that could potentially enable the conception of "designer babies." Sperm and egg bank storage allow progeny to be born long after their genetic parents' death. Intrafamily social, psychiatric, and economic problems arising from generation gaps created when childbearing occurs beyond usually accepted ages, and surrogate motherhood and contract enforcement are but a few additional areas in which divisive issues have already mushroomed to mind-boggling proportions. In addition, the ability to obtain eggs from aborted fetuses or corpses creates potential circumstances of unknown and almost unthinkable consequences.

Continuing breakthroughs on the frontiers of human reproduction promises a burgeoning of medical, legal, and social/ethical issues. A single-source multi-disciplined, multifaceted guide to fertility procedures and their application to real-life situations, although sorely needed, has not been readily available. *Understanding Family Building Through Egg and Sperm Donation: Medical, Legal, and Ethical Issues* fills this gap in a timely and topical manner. This treatise, a collection of chapters written by recognized authorities and edited by a hands-on practitioner and researcher and a practicing attorney in the field of reproductive law, covers in depth a practical approach to key medical, legal, and social/ethical issues that are faced daily by those concerned with gamete donation.

Elliot L. Sagall, M.D.

Prologue

MACHELLE M. SEIBEL

Traditionally, falling in love, getting married, and having a baby constitutes the basis of a family. Terms such as "mom" and "dad" require no definition, fertilization requires no assistance, and gestation requires no elaboration. However, with the widespread availability of in vitro fertilization and the growing acceptance of egg and sperm donation, third-party involvement in the reproductive process has become almost commonplace.

As a result of this participation, new terminology is necessary to clarify the participants and define the family. The rearing parents are the people who raise the child. They may or may not be the source of genetic material (genetic mother or father). Fertilization may occur in the body through intercourse, insemination, or gamete transfer or in a laboratory through in vitro fertilization. Once fertilization occurs, the subsequent pregnancy may not be carried by the rearing mother, thus separating completely conceiving, giving birth, and parenting.

The source of genetic material may come either from the rearing parent or from a donor. As such, the rearing father may contribute genetic material to either the rearing mother or a donor egg. Similarly, the rearing mother may receive genetic material from a donor woman, man, or both. Finally, in rare cases, neither the rearing mother nor the rearing father may contribute genetic material, using instead both donor eggs and donor sperm to create a donor embryo; this situation is similar to adoption but before conception. Therefore four combinations of genetic material exist.

Each of these four sets of conditions may achieve fertilization either in the body or in the lab, creating a total of eight combinations. Add to this the possibility that each of these eight combinations could gestate either in the rearing mother or in a surrogate/gestational carrier, and there become sixteen ways to have a baby (see figure).

While this seems at first glance to be a phenomenon exclusively in the domain of reproductive technology, one must at the same time acknowledge that nearly one in two marriages ends in divorce and much of the time children are involved. When these divorced individuals remarry, their traditionally conceived children will have two sets of parents and four sets of grandparents, each consisting of one genetically unrelated rearing parent and two genetically unrelated rearing grandparents. The situation is further amplified with adoption, in which the children have no genetic link to either parent or set of grandparents.

Upon reflection, the definition of the traditional family has clearly changed and its boundaries have expanded to include alternative arrangements for childbearing as well as parenting. Families that result from innovations in repro-

Sixteen Ways to Make a Baby

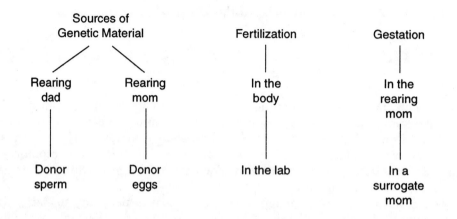

ductive technology, such as gamete donation, mirror society's changing norms rather than defining them. Like the "traditional" family examples cited above, they reflect the overwhelming desire to parent and create families where otherwise none would exist. Because of that desire, gamete donation is increasingly being sought out as a means of achieving parenthood. To gain insight into gamete donation, understanding its medical, legal, ethical and social aspects is required.

Machelle M. Seibel

Contributors

Judith Bernstein, R.N.C., M.S.N.
Brandeis University
Waltham, Massachusetts

J. R. Blatt, R.N., M.P.H.
Newton, Massachusetts

Andrea Mechanick Braverman, Ph.D.
Director of Psychological Services
Pennsylvania Reproductive Associates
Pennsylvania Hospital
Philadelphia, Pennsylvania

Mara Brill, M.D.
Director of Mental Health
Faulkner Centre for Reproductive Medicine
Assistant Clinical Professor of Psychiatry
Tufts New England Medical Centre
Boston, Massachusetts

Diane N. Clapp, B.S.N., R.N.
Counselor, National Resolve
Somerville, Massachusetts
Private Practice, Fertility Resources
Sudbury, Massachusetts

Susan L. Crockin, J.D.
Kassler & Feuer, P.C.
Northeastern University School of Law
Boston, Massachusetts

Janice H. Fox, M.D.
Department of Obstetrics and Gynecology
Brigham & Women's Hospital
Boston, Massachusetts

Paula A. Hindle, R.N., M.S.N., M.B.A.
Vice President
Nursing and Support Services
Alexandria Hospital
Alexandria, Virginia

Ami Jaeger, M.A., J.D.
Health Care Consultant
Washington, D.C.

Susan Levin, L.I.C.S.W.
Private Practice
Boston, Massachusetts

R. Tracy MacNab, Ph.D., C.G.T.
Staff Psychologist
Faulkner Centre for Reproductive Medicine
Director, Stress Reduction Program
Marino Centre for Progressive Health
Boston, Massachusetts

Mary Mahowald, Ph.D.
Professor, Department of Obstetrics and
    Gynecology and
Centre for Clinical Medical Ethics
University of Chicago
Chicago, Illinois

John Robertson, J.D.
Vinson and Elkins Chair
School of Law
University of Texas at Austin
Austin, Texas

Elliot L. Sagall, M.D.
Founder, the American Society of Law,
  Medicine, and Ethics
Assistant Clinical Professor of Medicine
Harvard Medical School
Boston, Massachusetts

Mark Sauer, M.D.
Professor of Obstetrics and Gynecology
Chief, Division of Reproductive Endocrinology
Columbia University
New York, New York

Joseph G. Schenker, M.D.
Professor and Chairman
Department of Obstetrics and Gynecology
Hadassah University Medical Center
Israel

Machelle M. Seibel, M.D.
Associate Clinical Professor of Surgery
  (Gynecology)
Harvard Medical School
Director
Faulkner Centre for Reproductive Medicine
Boston, Massachusetts

Mollie K. Sherry, M.S.W.
Clinical Coordinator, Young Parents Program
The Children's Hospital
Boston, Massachusetts

Norman Sherry, M.D.
Clinical Assistant Professor of Pediatrics
Harvard Medical School
Boston, Massachusetts

Joan C. Stoddard, J.D.
Associate General Counsel
Partners HealthCare Systems, Inc.
Boston, Massachusetts

Marion S. Verp, M.D.
Associate Professor
Department of Obstetrics and Gynecology
University of Chicago
Chicago, Illinois

Moshe Zilberstein, M.D.
Clinical Instructor of Surgery
Harvard Medical School
Director, Reproductive Genetics
Faulkner Centre for Reproductive Medicine
Boston, Massachusetts

PART I

MEDICAL ISSUES

The use of donor sperm to overcome male infertility has been described since biblical times. Recent advances in assisted reproductive technology (ART) have allowed egg donation to also become a standard method of family building. A woman of any age can now receive an oocyte from another woman of reproductive age, become pregnant, and deliver a baby. Obviously, the introduction of a third party into the reproductive process adds enormous complexity to having a child for the donor, the recipient, and the child.

This section explores the medical aspects of gamete donation. Chapter 1 reviews the many medical procedures and acronyms that have evolved in ART to provide the reader with a technical background for understanding the subsequent chapters. Chapter 2 describes the medical aspects of therapeutic donor insemination including practical and key issues in providing the service. This is followed by Chapter 3, which describes the psychologic concerns associated with therapeutic donor insemination. Chapter 4 describes the major issues in establishing an egg donation program, and Chapter 5 provides an approach for counseling and screening egg donors and recipients. The last chapter in this section, Chapter 6, explores the genetic issues that providers and patients must understand to involve themselves with gamete donation.

As medical technology advances, a substantially increasing number of patients will request egg and sperm donation. As such, there will be an increasing need for all parties involved to understand what they are about to experience medically, psychologically, and genetically.

Machelle M. Seibel, M.D.

1

Understanding the Medical Procedures and Terminology Surrounding Reproductive Technology

MACHELLE M. SEIBEL, M.D.

Assisted reproductive technology (ART) has become one of the most exciting areas in medicine, providing opportunities for family building that have never before been possible and creating in its wake complex medical, legal, social, and ethical issues for both medicine and society (Seibel MM, et al., 1993). A seemingly endless array of techniques and procedures has been developed, each a slight variation of another. However, confusion often results because each technique is usually referred to by a descriptive acronym (Table 1.1). This chapter is intended to explain the various procedures performed in reproductive technology. Because the majority of proce-

dures are based on either in vitro fertilization (IVF) or gamete intrafallopian transfer (GIFT), these two procedures will be described first.

IN VITRO FERTILIZATION (IVF)

In vitro fertilization involves the removal of one or more eggs, also called oocytes, from a woman's ovary just before ovulation. The egg is placed with sperm for 48–72 hours, during which time fertilization and division occur. The fertilized egg is then transferred into the woman's uterus using a thin catheter (Seibel MM, 1988).

There are several variations that can occur during an IVF cycle. The first has to do with whether or not medications are used to stimulate egg maturation. At the beginning of each menstrual cycle, approximately twenty or more eggs begin to mature. However, usually only one of those eggs is selected to ovulate. If the woman receives no medication during the first half of her IVF cycle, it is called a natural cycle, and only one mature egg can be anticipated from the retrieval. Success rates using one egg can rival those obtained in medicated cycles among women who are less than 35 years of age. With increasing age, however, results decrease. Natural cycles reduce the cost of the cycle by eliminating the need for medi-

TABLE 1.1. Common Acronyms in Reproductive Technology

ART	Assisted reproductive technology
IVF	In vitro fertilization
GIFT	Gamete intrafallopian transfer
PROST	Pronuclear stage tubal transfer
TET	Tubal embryo transfer
ZIFT	Zygote intrafallopian transfer
GUT	Gamete uterine transfer
POST	Peritoneal ovum and sperm transfer
AIH	Artificial insemination, husband
TDI	Therapeutic donor insemination
IUI	Intrauterine insemination
SUZI	Subzonal insemination
ICSI	Intracytoplasmic single sperm injection

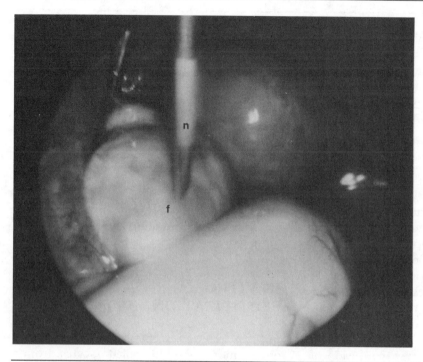

**FIGURE 1.1.
Laparoscopic Oocyte
Retrieval. The needle
(n) can be seen enter-
ing the follicle (f).**

cation. They also eliminate the risk of multiple births and the need for freezing "extra" fertilized eggs (Seibel MM, et al., 1995).

Medicated cycles use one or a combination of fertility drugs to increase the number of mature eggs available for retrieval (Seibel and Blackwell, 1994). The most commonly used drugs are human menopausal gonadotropins (HMG), which contain equal amounts of the pituitary hormones follicle-stimulating hormone (FSH) and luteinizing hormone (LH), and purified FSH, which is a purification of HMG. Both of these medications stimulate follicle growth. Many centers combine HMG and FSH with another type of medication called gonadotropin-releasing hormone (GnRH) agonists. The GnRH agonists help to control the rate of follicle development and prevent the woman from ovulating on her own.

Whether or not medications are used to stimulate follicle growth, a final injection of human chorionic gonadotropin (HCG) is given to complete the final stages of egg maturation and to time ovulation. The egg retrieval is usually performed approximately 34 hours after the HCG injection, a few hours before the egg would be released. The egg retrieval can be performed either by laparoscopy (Figure 1.1) or by ultrasound-guided retrieval. Because ultrasound retrievals can be performed under local anesthesia with mild sedation, they are generally the method of choice. Variations of ultrasound retrieval include transabdominal-transvesicle, transurethral-transvesicle (Figure 1.2), and transvaginal (Figure 1.3). The names describe the path the needle takes to reach the follicle; through the abdominal wall and bladder, through the urethra and bladder, and through the back wall of the vagina.

Once the egg is retrieved, the next step is fertilization. This occurs by preparing the sperm

FIGURE 1.2. Ultrasound-Guided Oocyte Retrieval (Transurethral-Transvesicle Approach). The needle can be seen penetrating the bladder and entering the follicle. (a) Ultrasound view; (b) laparoscopic view.

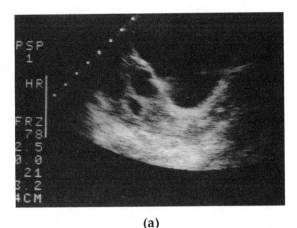

(a)

(b)

ure 1.4). This is called intravaginal culture (IVC) (Ranoux C, Seibel MM, 1989). Two days later, the culture tube is removed from the vagina, and the eggs are examined.

As with eggs fertilized in a petri dish, eggs that are fertilized intravaginally are placed in a thin catheter and transferred into the uterus. The embryo transfer (ET) is usually performed through the cervix (Figure 1.5). If the cervix is narrow or twisted, making embryo transfer difficult, a transuterine transfer (TUT) can be performed by placing a needle through the vagina and anterior wall of the uterus directly into the uterine lining (endometrium) and passing the catheter through the needle directly into the endometrium, bypassing the difficult cervix. If the fertilized egg implants, pregnancy follows as it would normally.

GAMETE INTRAFALLOPIAN TRANSFER (GIFT)

Both sperm and eggs are called gametes. Under natural conditions the ovulated egg is released into the fallopian tube. Following intercourse, the sperm begin reaching the fallopian tube within minutes, and if the egg is present, fertilization occurs. The fertilized egg then migrates to the uterus, where it implants and grows.

The GIFT procedure attempts to mimic this natural event by removing the egg from the ovary just before ovulation and placing it together with sperm into the fallopian tube, where it is hoped that fertilization will occur (Figure 1.6). In contrast to IVF, the GIFT procedure requires that there be at least one patent fallopian tube. In addition, if pregnancy does not occur, it is impossible to determine whether or not the sperm and egg fertilized.

As with IVF, there are several variations of GIFT. Although some centers do perform ultrasound-guided oocyte retrieval for GIFT followed by transcervical tubal canalization and

and placing them together with the egg, usually in a petri dish within an incubator. Alternatively, the sperm and egg (gametes) may be placed into a 3-mL culture tube with a screw cap, covered in a protective plastic sheath, and inserted into the vagina like a suppository (Fig-

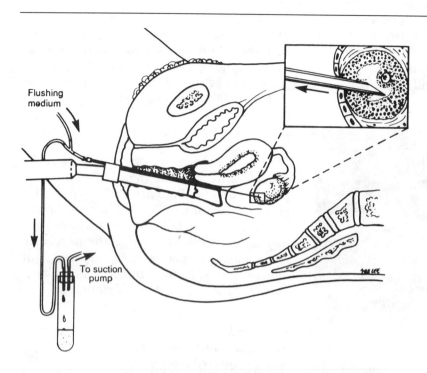

(a)

Flushing medium

To suction pump

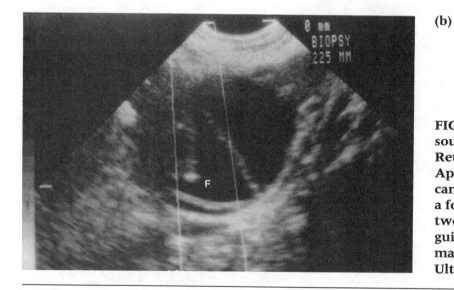

(b)

FIGURE 1.3. Ultrasound-Guided Oocyte Retrieval (Transvaginal Approach). The needle can be seen entering a follicle between the two parallel biopsy guide lines. (a) Schematic drawing; (b) Ultrasound view.

FIGURE 1.4. Culture Tube Used for Intravaginal Culture.

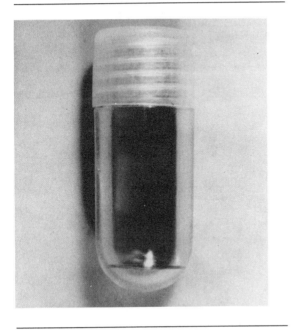

intratubal transfer of gametes (Jansen R, et al., 1988), the majority of centers continue to perform GIFT via laparoscopy because the catheter is difficult to see by ultrasound, making the procedure technically difficult. As a result, GIFT success rates using ultrasound guidance are generally lower.

Pronuclear Stage Tubal Transfer (PROST), Tubal Embryo Transfer (TET), and Zygote Intrafallopian Transfer (ZIFT)

PROST, TET, and ZIFT are all variations of GIFT that differ in one major respect. Instead of transferring sperm and an unfertilized egg into the fallopian tube, the three procedures above describe the transfer of a fertilized egg (Figure 1.7a, b). Therefore PROST, TET, and ZIFT all require IVF to be performed initially to achieve fertilization, followed in one or two days by a laparoscopy to transfer the fertilized eggs into the patient's fallopian tube.

Gamete Uterine Transfer (GUT)

Gamete uterine transfer is a simplified version of GIFT. The major difference between GUT and GIFT is that the unfertilized egg and sperm are placed into the uterus, not the fallopian tube (Figure 1.8). Therefore patent fallopian tubes are not required. Its main advantage is that the entire procedure can be performed by ultrasound, and laparoscopy is unnecessary. Following an ultrasound-guided egg retrieval, the previously collected and washed sperm are placed in a catheter and transferred directly into the uterine cavity. The procedure eliminates the need for incubation and subsequent transfer and therefore also eliminates most of the religious and personal objections to IVF.

Peritoneal Ovum and Sperm Transfer (POST)

Peritoneal ovum and sperm transfer is another variation of GIFT. The major difference between these two procedures is that the unfertilized egg and sperm are transferred via catheter through a needle into the patient's cul de sac using transvaginal ultrasound (Figure 1.9). In contrast to the GUT procedure, the patient must have normal fallopian tubes. As with GUT, the procedure does eliminate the need for laparoscopy, incubation, and subsequent transfer.

ARTIFICIAL INSEMINATION (AI)

Artificial insemination is the mechanical placement of sperm into the woman's repro-

FIGURE 1.5.   Schematic Drawing of Embryo Transfer.

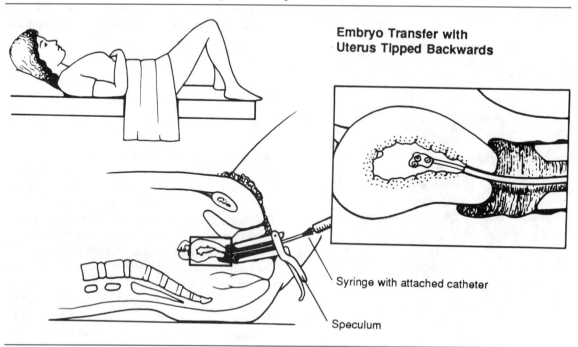

Embryo Transfer with Uterus Tipped Backwards

Syringe with attached catheter

Speculum

ductive tract. If the husband's sperm is used, the procedure is called homologous artificial insemination (AIH). If donor sperm is used, the procedure is called therapeutic donor insemination (TDI) (Loy RA, Seibel MM, 1990). To prevent confusion with the disease AIDS, the abbreviation AID is no longer used for artificial insemination with donor sperm. TDI is used when the man has too few sperm to achieve pregnancy or when he possesses an inherited condition that he does not wish to pass on to his children. In rare cases, TDI is used when the woman is Rh negative, the man is Rh positive, and the woman has become sensitized to a prior Rh positive baby, making the risk to a future Rh positive baby unacceptably high.

Several common insemination methods are performed with a catheter, and their names are usually descriptive of where the sperm are placed (Figure 1.10). Intracervical insemination (ICI) involves placement of the sperm in the upper vagina and lower cervix; intrauterine insemination (IUI) involves washing the sperm and placing it into the uterus; and the least common procedure, transuterine intrafallopian tube insemination (TIFI), involves washing the sperm and placing it through the cervix into the fallopian tube (Figure 1.11).

Additional variations require a needle and include direct intraperitoneal insemination (DIPI), in which the washed sperm are placed into a catheter and threaded through a needle into the cul de sac after transvaginal egg retrieval (Figure 1.12), and direct intrafollicular insemination (DIFI), in which the transvaginal ultrasound is used to place sperm directly into

FIGURE 1.6.   Schematic Drawing of Gamete Intrafallopian Transfer Illustrating (a) the Oocyte Retrieval and (b) the Gamete Transfer.

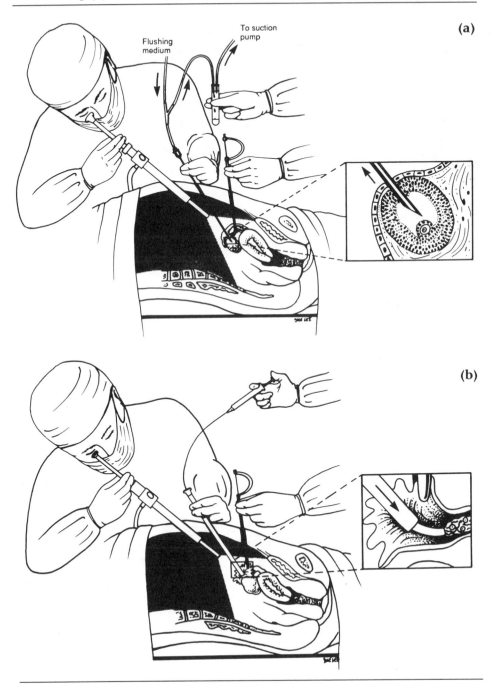

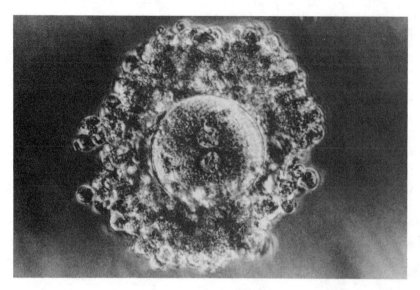

FIGURE 1.7a. A Fertilized Egg at the Pronuclear Stage. The two spheres are the male and female pronuclei.

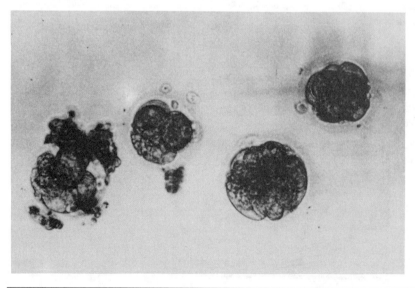

FIGURE 1.7b. Illustration of Four Fertilized Eggs at Various Stages of Division.

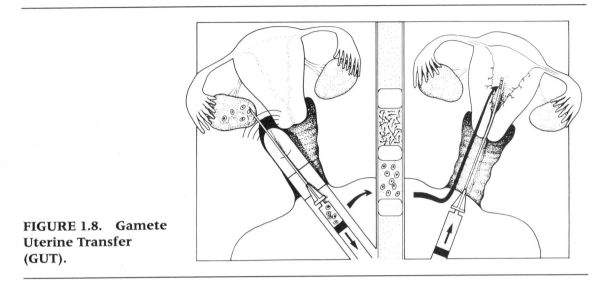

FIGURE 1.8. Gamete Uterine Transfer (GUT).

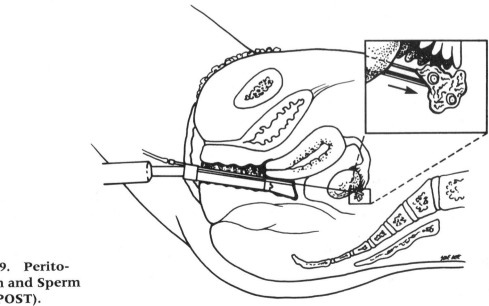

FIGURE 1.9. Peritoneal Ovum and Sperm Transfer (POST).

FIGURE 1.10. Variations of Artificial Insemination.

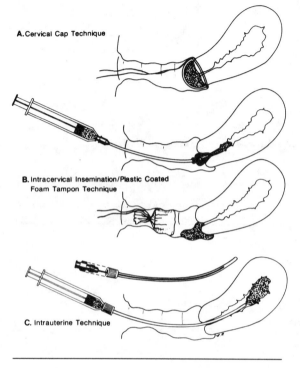

A. Cervical Cap Technique

B. Intracervical Insemination/Plastic Coated Foam Tampon Technique

C. Intrauterine Technique

FIGURE 1.11. Transuterine Intrafallopian Tube Insemination.

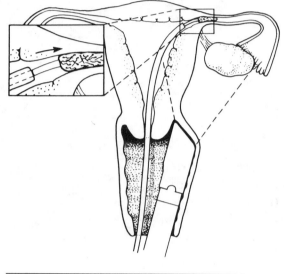

the follicle without ever performing an egg retrieval. All methods of artificial insemination assume that the woman's fallopian tubes are patent and preferably normal.

ASSISTED FERTILIZATION

Assisted fertilization (also called micromanipulation) refers to a group of three procedures designed to aid the sperm in entering the egg (Van Steirtegham AC, et al., 1993). The first is zona drilling, in which a small hole is "drilled" in the zona pellucida or shell of the egg to allow the sperm easier access. This technique allows the sperm to be selected natu-

rally. The second technique is called subzonal insemination (SUZI). In this procedure, approximately five sperm are selected and injected beneath the zona with the hope that one will achieve fertilization. The third procedure is called intracytoplasmic single sperm injection (ICSI) and involves the selection and placement of a single sperm directly into the egg. The ICSI procedure does prevent more than one sperm from entering the egg, but selecting which sperm to use and loading it into a micropipette are technically quite difficult. All of these procedures are performed when fertilization is poor or fails, with the hope that even a low sperm count will result in pregnancy (Figure 1.13). These procedures are no longer considered experimental, but genetic counseling is encouraged for couples choosing these techniques. Micromanipulation offers an alternative treatment to TDI for some couples.

Another micromanipulation technique is called assisted hatching. This procedure as-

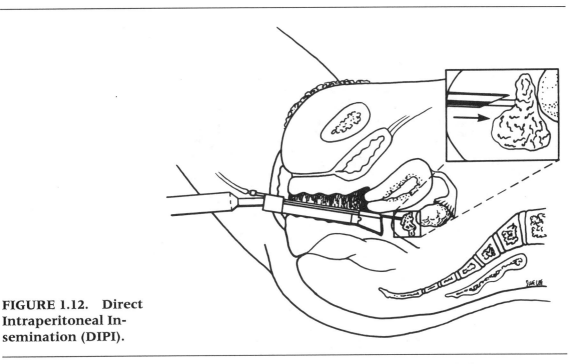

FIGURE 1.12. Direct Intraperitoneal Insemination (DIPI).

sumes that for some couples, pregnancy does not occur because the zona is too thick for the embryo to break through and implantation is prevented. By creating an artificial break in the zona before transferring the fertilized egg into the uterus, some believe that implantation is aided (Zilberstein M, Seibel MM, 1994).

SURROGATE

A surrogate is a woman who is artificially inseminated with the sperm of a man who is not her husband. The surrogate carries the pregnancy, then turns the child over to the man after the delivery; his wife then adopts the child. Surrogates are usually needed only when a woman has had both of her ovaries and her uterus removed. A surrogate could be a friend, a relative, or a stranger identified for

the sole purpose of becoming impregnated and carrying a pregnancy. Because the surrogate bears a child that is genetically half hers, this procedure incorporates many social, legal, and ethical issues. Both clear legal and psychological advice should be obtained in advance.

GESTATIONAL CARRIERS

A gestational carrier is a woman who carries another couple's child. In contrast to a surrogate, the gestational carrier does not use her own egg. In vitro fertilization is performed on the infertile couple, and the embryo is transferred into the gestational carrier. After the child is born, the gestational carrier turns the child over to the couple. The most common reason women need a gestational carrier is

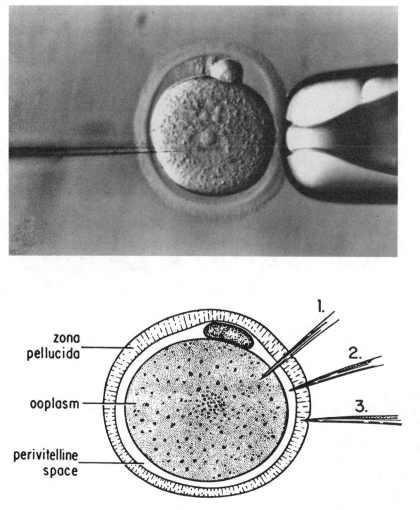

(a)

(b)

zona pellucida

ooplasm

perivitelline space

1.

2.

3.

FIGURE 1.13. Micromanipulation of Egg. (a) The actual procedure. (b) Schematic drawing showing (1) intracytoplasmic single sperm injection (ICSI), (2) subzonal insemination (SUZI), and (3) zona drilling.

that they have had their uterus removed but still have at least one working ovary. Alternatively, a woman may have a uterine condition that prevents her from carrying a pregnancy to term or a medical condition that would make pregnancy an undue risk. As with surrogates, a gestational carrier could be a friend, a relative, or a stranger identified for the sole reason of carrying a pregnancy that is not genetically

her own. Clear legal and psychological advice should be sought in advance.

EGG DONOR

An egg donor is a woman who has an egg retrieval performed and allows her eggs to be used by another woman (a recipient) so that the recipient can become pregnant. The donor's eggs are fertilized with the sperm of the recipient's husband. The recipient's uterine lining is hormonally prepared and synchronized with the donor's cycle, and the resulting embryo is transferred into the recipient, who carries the pregnancy. For egg donation to work, the recipient must have a uterus but does not need ovaries. The usual indications are premature menopause (before age 40) and genetic diseases the woman does not want inherited by her children. More recently, an increasing number of women nearing the end of their reproductive years (perimenopausal) or even in natural menopause are seeking egg donation (see Chapter 12).

Donors are usually divided into two categories: anonymous and known. However, I have listed three types of egg donors to reflect current trends: unknown, known, and well-known. Unknown or anonymous donors are women who never meet the recipient. Well-known donors are close friends or relatives who have known the recipient for a long time. Known donors—or, perhaps more appropriately, identified donors—are strangers who are found by the recipient for the sole purpose of providing eggs. They are not anonymous but have no preexisting relationship with the recipient. As with surrogacy and gestational carriers, legal and psychological support should be sought.

Patients requiring egg donation and who have ovarian failure (are menopausal) may initiate a cycle at any time using the protocol in Table 1.2. Patients receiving oocyte donation for purposes other than ovarian failure, or who have any remaining suggestion of ovarian function (occasional menses, etc.) should apply the protocol as follows. The recipient is asked to maintain a basal body temperature chart (BBT). On day 21 of the recipient's cycle, look for a BBT rise of at least 4 days and obtain a serum progesterone level. If ovulation is deemed to have occurred by either a sustained

TABLE 1.2. Cycle Initiation Protocol

Cycle Medication	Cycle Day	Dose
1. Estradiol	1–5	2 mg/day
	*6–9	2 mg q 12 h
	10–13	2 mg q 8 h
	**14–28	2 mg q 12 h
2. Progesterone in oil	15	50 mg
	16–23	100 mg daily

*Day 6 is the day the donor begins gonadotropin treatment or the day before clomiphene citrate is initiated in partially medicated cycles.

**Day 14 is the day HCG is administered to the donor.

BBT rise or a progesterone value above 4 ng/ml, the recipient is given 3.75 mg of depo-lupron intramuscularly.

Once ovarian down-regulation has been documented by a serum estradiol value of less than 50 pg/ml and by a vaginal ultrasound examination demonstrating no significant ovarian cyst development, the replacement protocol is initiated as outlined for patients without ovarian function (see Table 1.2). The recipient must be down-regulated before the donor starts her ovarian stimulation. Either a fully medicated cycle using lupron and gonadotropins or a partially medicated cycle using clomiphene citrate (Seibel MM, 1995) may be employed.

Serum E_2 levels may be determined on days 11 and 21 and serum progesterone on day 21 of the recipient cycle. No ultrasound is needed in the recipient, although ultrasound verification of endometrial thickness may be helpful in certain circumstances. Blood for serum progesterone should ideally be drawn 6 hours after progesterone injection.

In the event that initiation of the donor's cycle is delayed, the recipient should receive depo-lupron 3.75 mg for a second dose 21 to 28 days after the first dose. It should be possible to get the patient through her monitored cycle and into her replacement cycle by use of two injections of depo-lupron. If the donor is close to beginning her gonadotropins (or clomiphene) and it is nearly time for another depo-lupron injection, the recipient should be switched to daily subcutaneous injections of 0.5 mg lupron which is continued until the donor receives HCG.

If egg donation is carried out in conjunction with a GIFT cycle, the protocol is the same as for an IVF cycle except that a progesterone dosage of 50 mg/day is administered on the day of the GIFT procedure and continued for 3 days. The progesterone dosage is increased to 100 mg/day on the fourth day following the GIFT procedure, and continued until pregnancy is established.

If the recipient becomes pregnant, progesterone in oil 100 mg/day is continued at 9:00 a.m., and one 400 mg progesterone vaginal suppository is administered at 9 p.m. daily, and the Estrace dosage is reduced to 2 mg daily. Treatment is discontinued 14 weeks following embryo transfer.

CONCLUSION

This chapter has defined the major procedures in assisted reproductive technology. I hope it will provide the reader with a better understanding of the chapters that follow. In addition, Appendixes 1-A through 1-J provide several short articles and letters to further clarify some of the major issues surrounding gamete donation.

REFERENCES

1. Glezerman (1981).
2. Jansen R, Anderson JK, Radonic I, Smit J, Sutherland P. (1988) Pregnancies after ultrasound guided fallopian insemination with cryostored donor sperm. Fertil Steril 49:920–923.
3. Loy R, Seibel MM. (1990) Therapeutic insemination. In: Seibel MM, ed. Infertility: A Comprehensive Text. Norwalk, Conn.: Appleton & Lange.
4. Seibel MM. (1988) A new era in reproductive technology: In vitro fertilization, gamete intrafallopian transfer, and donated gametes and embryos. N Engl J Med 318:828–834.
5. Seibel MM. (1995) Toward reducing risks and costs of egg donation: A preliminary report. Fertil Steril 64:199.
6. Seibel MM, Blackwell R. (1994) Advanced Gonadotropin Therapy. New York: Raven Press.
7. Seibel MM, Kiessling AA, Bernstein J, Levin SR., eds. (1993) Technology and Infertility: Clinical, Psychosocial, Legal and Ethical Aspects. New York: Springer-Verlag.
8. Van Steirtegham AC, Liu J, Joris H, Nagy Z, Janssenwillen C, Tournaye H, Derde M-P, Assche EV, Devroey P. (1993) Higher success rate by intracytoplasmic sperm injection than by subzonal insemination: Report of a second series of 300 consecutive treatment cycles. Hum Reprod 8:1055–1060.
9. Zilberstein M, Seibel MM. (1994) Fertilization and implantation. In: Tan SL, ed. Current Opinion In Obstetrics and Gynecology 6:184–189.

Appendix 1-A

Equal Time

To Everything There Is a Season

MACHELLE M. SEIBEL, M.D.

> *To every thing there is a season, and a time to every purpose under the heavens. —Ecclesiastes, Chapter 3, Verse 1*

Assisted reproductive technology has changed forever the way we as a society view childbearing and the options opened to us for building families. With consistent success, in vitro fertilization has allowed women with irreparably damaged fallopian tubes and men with congenitally absent vas deferens to bypass their mechanical obstacles to parenting. Ultrasound-guided oocyte retrieval and refinements in ultrasound-guided gamete and embryo transfer techniques have further reduced the risks and the discomfort of repeating cycles.

For couples fearful of conceiving an abnormal child, the development of preimplantation embryo biopsy, together with diagnostic advances in molecular biology, permits diagnosis of certain inherited disorders prior to embryo transfer. These remarkable advances have offered men and premenopausal women who had previously completed childbearing extended hope for conceiving a healthy baby.[1]

More recently, the boundaries of the reproductive life span have been further blurred by the development of embryo cryopreservation and oocyte and embryo donation.[2] These two conceptual advances have extended the reproductive life span beyond menopause and potentially allow women to continue their efforts at childbearing indefinitely. Perimenopausal women who no longer respond to ovulatory stimulation find it increasingly difficult to feel they have tried sufficiently to allow themselves to stop treatment. Besides the many successes assisted reproductive technology has allowed, it has greatly prolonged the number of years a couple may attempt to carry a pregnancy with their own or donated gametes.

This trend has caused both our patients and our colleagues to struggle with the process of bringing closure to achieving pregnancy.[3] This is compounded by the fact that no absolute data exist to scientifically assess couples' prognosis for conception and limited data are available concerning the psychosocial consequences of prolonging infertility treatment, especially beyond the normal reproductive span.

We have found that more than 90% of in vitro fertilization babies are born within four attempts. Neither age nor diagnosis alter these findings.[4,5]

In a recent epidemiologic study investigating the emotional strain associated with infertility, half of the women and nearly two thirds of men reported they had thought about stopping treatment. The primary reason for want-

Seibel MM. (1992) Equal time: To everything there is a season. Contemp OBGyn 37:153.

ing to stop was emotional drain (72%) followed by lack of success (27%), pain (19%), and life disruption (18%).

However, desire for success increased with length of infertility and acted to prevent patients from stopping. Of patients responding, 30% felt they could not stop and only 4% of patients felt the payback, including pregnancy, would be worth the emotional expense. Nevertheless, half of the patients did not feel the issue of stopping was a matter to be discussed with their doctor.[6]

More than half of the patients were concerned about the effect of infertility on their relationship with their spouse, and 84% were concerned about the emotional drain on themselves. In view of the open-ended nature of current infertility treatment, and the emotional strain of pursuing it, I believe that infertility patients have a strong need for both emotional support and assistance with closure—deciding that it is time to stop. Clinicians should be sensitive to these issues and,

when appropriate, help patients through this process.

References

1. Seibel MM: A new era in reproductive technology: In vitro fertilization, gamete intrafallopian transfer, and donated gametes and embryos. N Engl J. Med 1988; 318:828.
2. Sauer MV, Paulson RJ, Lobo RA: A preliminary report on oocyte donation extending reproductive potential to women over 40. N Engl J Med 1990; 323:1
3. Taylor PJ: When is enough enough? Fertil Steril 1990; 54:772
4. Seibel MM, Ranoux C, Kearnan M: How much is enough? Knowing when to stop in vitro fertilization. N Engl J Med 1989; 321:1052.
5. Seibel MM, Kearnan M, Kiessling A, et al.: Multiple IVF cycles: Diminishing returns. World Congress on in vitro fertilization, Paris, June 30–July 3, 1991. Abstract.
6. Seibel MM, Bernstein J, Levin S, et al.: Epidemiologic insights into the importance of emotional support in infertility treatment. 47th annual meeting of the American Fertility Society, Orlando Florida. October 19–24, 1991. Abstract.

Appendix 1-B

After Office Hours

In Vitro Fertilization Success Rates: A Fraction of the Truth

MACHELLE M. SEIBEL, M.D.

A couple recently came into my office and the wife asked me, "Doctor, we are looking for the best IVF [in vitro fertilization] program. What is your success rate?" I responded, of course, that I would be happy to answer that question. But deep down I knew it would not be a simple response. "I want to tell you the whole truth," I responded. "What do you mean," she replied, "doesn't every IVF program tell the whole truth?" I realized immediately that my answer could be misconstrued. "I am confident," I said, "that doctors and IVF team members do not lie. The problem is mathematical." "Mathematical?" she replied. "Mathematical," I confirmed, and proceeded to explain about a fraction of the truth. "You see, every fraction has a numerator and a denominator. In IVF the numerator is the number of pregnancies." This was so obvious to my patient that she became indignant. "Babies are the numerator," she quipped. "They certainly may be," I agreed. "But the numerator is pregnancies. All

Seibel, MM. (1988) After office hours: In vitro fertilization success rates: a fraction of the truth. Obstet Gynecol 72:2. Copyright © 1988 by The American College of Obstetricians and Gynecologists.

From the Division of Reproductive Endocrinology and Infertility, Department of Obstetrics and Gynecology, Dana Biomedical Research Laboratories, Beth Israel Hospital and Harvard Medical School, Boston, Massachusetts.

pregnancies do not result in babies in a fraction of the truth."

With some hesitation I struggled to explain. "The numerator may represent a positive pregnancy test or a term pregnancy." "I'm beginning to understand," she responded. Her girlfriend had recently conceived by IVF. They had even seen the fetus on ultrasound and called it a clinical pregnancy. It was ongoing for another month. Unfortunately, her friend had a miscarriage a few weeks later. I responded, "I am sorry to hear that, but according to the mathematics of a fraction of the truth, she can still be counted as a pregnancy."

I continued my discussion of a fraction of the truth by talking about the denominator. "The denominator," I said, "is even more confusing to explain. It can represent patients, oocyte retrievals, or embryo transfers." "Can you give me an example to illustrate your point?" she interjected. "I am having trouble understanding the denominator." I never liked math, I mused to myself, but a theoretical model might just do the trick. "Let's pretend a new IVF clinic has one patient who goes through the procedure five times. The first time, they fail to retrieve an egg, and the second time, the retrieved eggs fail to fertilize. The last three cycles result in embryo transfers and the patient conceives on her fifth attempt. What is the success rate?" After some consideration, the patient responded, "The IVF success rate is one pregnancy per five oocyte retrievals or 20%, one pregnancy per three embryo transfers or 33%, or one pregnancy per one patient or 100%, depending on which denominator you choose." "That's right!" I told her, "but don't forget about the numerator in a fraction of the truth."

At this point the husband, who had been largely silent, spoke up for the fist time, close to tears. "My sperm count is low," he confessed. "If IVF success rates are only reported as pregnancy per embryo transfer, then all of the procedures in which fertilization does not occur will not be included. Won't that make the results seem higher?" "That's correct," I agreed. "Omitting the failed fertilizations makes the results seem higher, even though a fraction of the truth is reported correctly."

At this time our interview was drawing to a close. "Are there any other important points about a fraction of the truth?" the wife inquired. "There are two mathematical variables that must also be considered in a fraction of the truth," I responded. "They are time and patient selection. You see, if IVF success rates represent only a particularly successful inter-val of time, the results will seem higher. Results will also seem increased if they exclude older patients or men whose sperm counts are extremely low," I explained. "One of my friends has tried many times unsuccessfully to achieve an IVF pregnancy," the wife admitted. "I guess couples like them make the results seem lower too." "Absolutely," I responded, "but couples with a poor chance of success want a baby so badly that IVF centers differ in opinion about these kinds of issues."

"What is the whole truth?" the couple asked together. For the question they had initially asked had still not been answered. I responded cautiously. The answer they wanted was still not simple. "If one considers all patients, regardless of age or medical problems, the expected term pregnancy rate per oocyte retrieval is approximately ten to fifteen percent at better centers." "And what about centers that claim to have success rates that are so much higher?" the wife blurted out in disbelief. She had expected results that were really much better. "It's possible," I responded, "but be sure you determine whether the results are the whole truth, or a fraction of the truth."

Appendix 1-C

Gender Distribution—Not Sex Selection

MACHELLE M. SEIBEL, M.D., SHARON GLAZIER SEIBEL, MOSHE ZILBERSTEIN, M.D.

Giving birth to a healthy baby is the ultimate goal of most would-be parents. However, for some couples with sex-linked diseases there is a substantial need to undergo prenatal genetic testing to prevent the birth of an affected child through pregnancy termination. While this sequence carries ethical concerns for some individuals, most would accept the decision process as necessary and appropriate. More recently, the availability of preimplantation genetic diagnosis has provided couples with the opportunity to diagnose sex-linked diseases before the mother is pregnant. Only non-affected embryos are transferred into the woman's uterus (Winston and Handyside, 1993).

But what about couples who choose sex selection simply to have a boy or a girl? Each year an increasing number of couples throughout the world are seeking technology to help specifically design their families (Egozcue, 1993). Preconception sex selection using sperm separation and artificial insemination yields unreliable results at best (Johnson *et al.*, 1993). Prenatal diagnosis using amniocentesis or chorionic villus sampling and pregnancy termination on the basis of gender is, in our opinion, morally wrong and could have adverse and potentially unanticipated implications on the composition of societies. Similarly, preimplantation genetic diagnosis for the sake of gender selection only with destruction of the resulting embryos would seem, at best, a tremendously inappropriate use of technology.

However, preimplantation genetic diagnosis may allow gender selection to occur in an extremely ethical way without affecting gender ratio, and help some infertile couples at the same time. Couples desiring sex selection *per se* could be offered preimplantation genetic testing only if they agreed to donate the resulting embryos of the undesired sex to an infertile couple needing embryo donation. If the two couples were synchronized properly, the embryo transfers could be performed on two separate days, thus maintaining anonymity. With this approach there would be no need for pregnancy termination, cryopreservation or destruction of embryos, and no sex selection— only gender distribution.

References

1. Egozcue, J. (1993) Sex selection: why not? *Hum. Reprod.,* **8,** 1777.
2. Johnson, L.A., Welch, G.R., Keyvanfar, K., Dorfmann, A., Fugger, E.P. and Schulman, J.D. (1993) Gender preselection in humans? Flow cytometric separation of X and Y sperm for the prevention of X-linked diseases. *Hum. Reprod.,* **8,** 1733–1739.
3. Winston, M.L. and Handyside, A.H. (1993) New challenges in human in vitro fertilization. *Science,* **260,** 932–936.

Seibel MM, Seibel SG, Zilberstein M. (1994) Gender distribution—not sex selection. Hum Reprod 569–570. By permission of Oxford University Press.

Appendix 1-D

Hysterectomy in Benign Conditions:
A Procedure of the Past?

MACHELLE M. SEIBEL, M.D., CHARLOTTE RICHARDS

Sir,—Advances in reproductive technology offer treatment options which have caused clinicians to rethink the management of certain common gynaecological conditions.[1] Ectopic pregnancy is one example. In the 1970s trainees were often taught that a first ectopic pregnancy should be treated by salpingectomy. A second ectopic pregnancy was managed by removal of the remaining tube and hysterectomy. Today this approach is inappropriate. Linear salpingostomy my conserve one or both fallopian tubes, and in-vitro fertilisation (IVF) provides an excellent chance of pregnancy should bilateral salpingectomy be required.

Let us take this line of thinking one step further. Today, standard teaching is that conditions which require bilateral oophorectomy, such as bilateral ovarian abscess, severe endometriosis, or borderline adnexal neoplasia, should be combined with hysterectomy, even in women who have not completed childbearing. However, this treatment plan may no longer be appropriate, in the absence of uterine disease, thanks to the increasing availability and success of donor embryo programmes.

The first report of establishment of pregnancy from a donated embryo came in 1983.[2] A woman with gonadal failure received exogenous oestrogen and progesterone to prepare her endometrium for implantation. A donated oocyte was fertilised with her husband's sperm and the embryo was transferred into her uterus. A normal healthy baby was delivered nine months later. Since that time, implantation rates above 50% have been reported after the transfer of donor embryos, with a term pregnancy rate approaching 23%.[3,4] This success has been achieved as a direct result of understanding that in women on 28-day steroid replacement regimens the endometrium is most receptive to implantation during a defined window that mimics days 16–19 of the natural menstrual cycle.

An additional breakthrough further supports uterine conservation. Oocytes obtained from unstimulated ovaries removed for benign disease were cultured with follicular fluid from mature follicles; and oocyte maturation, fertilisation, and conception followed in a patient who received these donated embryos.[5] This development paves the way for women postoophorectomy to cryopreserve [their] gametes for "autodonation".

The use of donor gametes is not considered experimental in Massachusetts, where health insurance is required by law to cover assisted reproduction, according to the American Fertility Society bulletin; elsewhere in the US legislation to provide insurance coverage for this procedure is under consideration in seven states, and the matter awaits debate in fifteen state congresses.

Hysterectomy is second to caesarean section among the most common major surgical procedures in the United States, and on current trends 30–50% of women will have had a

Seibel MM, Richards C. (March 10, 1990) Hysterectomy in benign conditions: a procedure of the past? Lancet 335:600–601.

hysterectomy by age 60. The availability of donor embryo programmes and other technological advances should cause clinicians and patients to reassess the management of women of childbearing age who require bilateral oophorectomy for benign ovarian disease. Among this large group of patients, routine hysterectomy may become a procedure of the past.

References

1. Seibel M. A new era in reproductive technology: in vitro fertilization, gamete intrafallopian transfer, and donated gametes and embryos. *N Engl J Med* 1988; **318;** 828–34.

2. Trounson A, Leeton J, Besanka M, Wood C, Conti A. Pregnancy established in an infertile patient after transfer of a donated embryo fertilized in vitro. *Br Med J* 1983; **286:** 835–38.

3. Navot D, Laufer N, Lopolovic J, et al. Artificially induced endometrial cycles and establishment of pregnancies in the absence of ovaries. *N Engl J Med* 1986; **314;** 806–11.

4. Schenker JG. Ovum donation: the state of the art, *Ann NY Acad Sci* 1988: 742–54.

5. Cha KY, Yoon SH, Ko JJ, Choi DH, Han SY, Koo JJ. Pregnancy after in vitro fertilization of human follicular oocytes collected from nonstimulated cycle, their culture in vitro and their transfer according to the donor oocyte program. Presented at 45th annual meeting of American Fertility Society (San Francisco Nov 13–16, 1989): S1.

Appendix 1-E

In Vitro Fertilization: How Much Is Enough?

MACHELLE M. SEIBEL., M.D., CLAUDE RANOUX, MAUREEN KEARNAN

To the Editor: Approximately one in six couples in the United States is experiencing infertility. The aging of the baby-boom generation, delayed childbearing, and a decreased availability of infants for adoption all contribute to the increasing requests for infertility services in the 1980s.[1] In the past, many of these couples remained childless. Now that medical technology offers almost endless hope for infertile couples, however, when to stop has become a difficult question to answer. When the treatment offered is in vitro fertilization (IVF), determined couples may initiate many cycles with the hope that with one more try they will succeed in having a child.[2] Such determination may translate into extreme physical, emotional, and financial costs. The number of office visits for infertility now approaches 2 million per year. In 1987, Americans spent about $1 billion to overcome infertility, of which about 7 percent was spent on IVF. Approximately 14,000 attempts at IVF were performed in 1987.[3]

We analyzed the number of cycles required for the first 50 women we treated who conceived and delivered a baby (Table 1). A cycle was defined by the attempt to induce ovulation, not by the existence of an oocyte or an embryo. Therefore, all cycles in which the procedure was canceled were included. No effort was made to analyze the data by either age or diagnosis.

Of the 95 clinical pregnancies, 50 resulted in births and 12 are ongoing. The remaining 33 resulted in either spontaneous abortions or ectopic pregnancies. Eighty-four percent of the births occurred after two IVF cycles, and births were extremely unlikely after the fourth IVF cycle. At present, only Arkansas, Hawaii, Maryland, Massachusetts, and Texas require that IVF be covered at least in part by insurers. as more states provide coverage, the number of IVF attempts a couple initiates will probably increase.

We conclude that the overwhelming majority of couples who will achieve pregnancy as a result of IVF do so within a relatively short period of time. Couples who do not achieve a viable pregnancy after four to six IVF cycles should be counseled that success with this technique is unlikely and should not be encouraged to pursue IVF further. It may be cost effective for couples to undergo two cycles of treatment before undergoing major abdominal surgery for infertility, which carries a low

Seibel MM, Ranoux C, Kearnan M. (1989) In vitro fertilization: how much is enough? N Engl J Med 321:15.

TABLE 1. Cycles in Which IVF Was Initiated among the First 50 Couples to Achieve Conception and Delivery.

Outcome	No. of Cycles						Total No.
	1	2	3	4	5	6	
	Percent						
Pregnancy	46	31	11	6	2	4	95
Birth	44	40	10	6	0	0	50

success rate. The cost of third-party coverage for up to four IVF cycles is competitive with that for repeated major operations or extended treatment for infertility. Decisions about more than four attempts should be made on an individual basis.

If guidelines similar to these are followed, the physical, psychological, and financial cost of in vitro fertilization may be contained while patients are still given the best chance for success.

References

1. Aral SO, Cates W Jr. The increasing concern with infertility: why now? JAMA 1983; 250:2327–31.
2. Seibel MM. A new era in reproductive technology: in vitro fertilization, gamete intrafallopian transfer, and donated gametes and embryos. N Engl J Med 1988; 318:828–34.
3. Office of Technology Assessment. Infertility: medical and social choices. Washington, D.C.: Office of Technology Assessment, 1988.

Appendix 1-F

Compensating Egg Donors: Equal Pay for Equal Time?

MACHELLE M. SEIBEL, M.D., ANN KIESSLING, PH.D.

To the Editor: The ability to achieve pregnancy after egg donation represents an important recent medical advance, not only because of its scientific merit, but also because of the way in which it benefits society. A woman with ovarian failure or known genetic disease can have a normal child if a healthy egg is available through egg donation.

However, the word "donation" is creating a stumbling block. The American Fertility Society (AFS) clearly stated in its 1990 ethical advisory committee report that "there should be no compensation to the donor for the egg." Yet the next sentence states, "This does not exclude reimbursement for expenses, time, risk and associated inconvenience."

In most states in which insurance coverage for the treatment of infertility is not mandated, egg donors are so compensated. In Massachusetts, where coverage for the treatment of infertility is mandated, one major insurance company's provider contract acknowledges only the first sentence of the AFS report. The insurers will not compensate donors for the time, risk, inconvenience, or mental health screening involved in the process of donation. More important, they do not allow the insured recipient to cover these expenses out of pocket. This entire stance is puzzling, since the same insurance company does compensate for sperm

donation. Sperm donors are generally paid a minimum of $25 as compensation for approximately one hour of time and any inconvenience and travel involved. Using this scale, we calculated the time involved in egg donation (Table 1). According to our calculations, an egg donor could expect to receive $1,400 for her time alone, exclusive of any compensation for travel, risk, or inconvenience.

Although some women are fortunate enough to have a sister or friend who will go through mental health screening, days of injections, blood tests, ultrasonography, and a minor surgical procedure to provide them with an egg, many women are less fortunate. Luckily, some young women are willing to brave the risks and inconvenience to help

TABLE 1. An Analysis of the Time Involved in Egg Donation

	Hours Spent
Initial interview	1
Minnesota Multiphasic Personality Inventory	2
Mental health evaluation	3
History and physical examination	1
Cycle initiation	1
Daily blood sampling, ultrasonography (1 hr/day × 10)	10
Egg retrieval	12
Postoperative recovery	24
Follow-up visit (1 to 4)	2
Total	56

Seibel MM, Kiessling A. (1993) Compensating egg donors: equal pay for equal time? N Engl J Med 328:737.

someone they do not know. Most donor programs across the United States compensate anonymous egg donors in amounts ranging from $1,000 to $2,000. By neither providing nor allowing compensation for the donors' time, risk, inconvenience, or mental health screening, insurance companies negatively influence egg-donor selection and standards of care. In February 1993 the AFS guidelines for oocyte donation were changed to the following: "Donors should be compensated for direct and indirect expenses associated with their participation, inconvenience, time, risk and discomfort." Since it is standard to compensate men for sperm donation, shouldn't the policy be equal pay for equal time?

Appendix 1-G

More on Compensating Egg Donors

To the Editor: Seibel and Kiessling (March 11 issue)* invoked equal worth of the sexes and the nationwide practice of paying sperm donors to justify their proposal to pay oocyte donors. The risks and benefits associated with paying donors are not mentioned. Although oocyte donation has not been demonstrated to transmit infectious disease, hepatitis and human immunodeficiency virus (HIV) are transmissible through sexual intercourse, artificial insemination, and organ and tissue transplantation. Transfusion from paid blood donors is associated with a higher risk of transmitting infectious disease from donors to recipients than transfusion from donors who do not receive monetary reimbursement or incentives.

This increased risk is not balanced by a demonstrated need to pay egg donors to ensure their availability. Nationwide programs involving voluntary donors of bone marrow who are unrelated to the recipients have succeeded without paying the donors. Many were skeptical that people would volunteer to donate marrow to nonrelatives; yet, over 700,000 have registered with the national program as potential donors. In the St. Paul, Minnesota, program, the time spent on the donation of bone marrow to an anonymous recipient is comparable to the time spent on oocyte donation.

Perhaps it is time to develop community programs of anonymous oocyte donation by volunteers to meet the needs of patients with infertility, as has been done for bone marrow and blood donations.

D. Ted Eastlund, M.D.
David E. Stroncek, M.D.

The authors reply:

To the Editor: Drs. Eastlund and Stroncek raise an important point in suggesting that a registry of unpaid volunteers for anonymous oocyte donation be compiled as has been done for bone marrow and blood donations. Perhaps this concept should be considered at the national level. The prospect of a national registry, however, has been made difficult by a moratorium by the National Institutes of Health on sponsoring research in assisted reproduction.

Oocyte donation differs from blood donation in many respects. Blood and marrow donors are identified in the open forum of a drive for donations, and their identity is known. Oocyte donation does not solve a problem of life and death. The donation does not remain in the recipient; it becomes a child. When the donor allows another woman to have a baby, complex issues of parenthood arise for the donor, the recipient, and the child. The identities of some oocyte donors are known, but as in sperm donation, the opportunity for confidentiality remains essential for optimal protection of all parties.

The number of recipients of donated eggs is increasing rapidly, as women wait longer to have children and the number of babies available for adoption dwindles. In addition, 3.5 million women a year are reaching menopause, and some will want to continue childbearing. Egg donation could become as

---

*Seibel MM, Kiessling A. Compensating egg donors: equal pay for equal time? N Engl J Med 1993; 328:737.

Eastlund DT, Stroncek DE. (July 22, 1993) More on compensating egg donors. N Engl J Med 329:278.

common as adoption or sperm donation. At present, the number of acceptable oocyte donors is marginally sufficient.

Not all oocyte donors are paid. Historically, anonymous sperm donors were paid. The same approach was applied to anonymous oocyte donors. In our program, about 50 percent of oocyte donors remain anonymous. Altruism is an important criterion for acceptance. Potential donors motivated by financial reasons alone are refused. Applicants undergo intensive psychological screening as well as testing for HIV infection, hepatitis, and other infectious diseases. Not all applicants are emotionally well suited to donate oocytes.

In our original letter, we took issue with the contractual agreements with insurance companies that currently limit patient access, affect standards of care, and determine treatment policy. Perhaps adequate numbers of acceptable, unpaid volunteers for oocyte donation do exist. This letter could serve as a call for a national meeting on the topic of a registry, the contrast between oocyte donation and other organ donations, and the opportunity to standardize care. But today there is no registry. Compensating oocyte donors is the norm, in accordance with the ethical guidelines of the American Fertility Society. The medical community, not the insurance industry, should make these decisions.

MACHELLE M. SEIBEL, M.D.
ANN A. KIESSLING, PH.D.

Appendix 1-H

Cadaveric Ovary Donation

MACHELLE M. SEIBEL, M.D.

To the Editor: Egg donation to help an infertile woman achieve pregnancy is now an accepted procedure worldwide. Yet there is a shortage of available eggs, even if compensation is provided to donors for time, risk, and inconvenience.[1] This has been most clearly shown in Britain, where scientists have proposed taking ovaries from aborted fetuses, maturing the eggs in a laboratory, fertilizing them with sperm, and implanting a resulting embryo in the womb of a infertile woman. This proposal has met with "unease, distaste and surprise."[2] Perhaps most unsettling is the notion that a child could have as a biologic mother an aborted fetus. Such a donor could never give consent to the ovary donation. In addition, critics express concern about the potential for abuse, misuse, or coercion—for instance, a pregnancy could be conceived solely for the purpose of obtaining fetal ovaries after an abortion.

Cadaveric organ donation after death is a common and accepted procedure. Many people have living wills or organ-donor cards that stipulate the donation of such organs as the kidneys, liver, or heart. The possibility of including the donation of ovaries in a living will should be considered. Both immature murine eggs[3] and immature human eggs[4] have now been cultured to maturity in vitro without prior hormonal manipulation. Immature eggs from murine cadavers have matured and been fertilized after hours of refrigeration.[5] Harvesting immature eggs shortly after death for egg donation could become a reality.

Biologically, the eggs of a female fetus begin to enter the prophase of the first meiotic division at approximately 11 to 12 weeks of gestation. This stage is exceedingly long, because egg maturation is arrested until after puberty, when each month a few of these immature eggs resume meiosis and one is selected to ovulate. Although atresia reduces the number of eggs available for donation, the immature eggs obtained from a premenopausal adult are biologically comparable to those obtained from a fetus. The recipient would have the added advantages of knowing the health of the donor (before death) and the presence of any genetic mutations, which would be unrecognized in a fetus.

In my opinion, using ovaries from a person who has given her consent to egg donation before her death would accomplish the objective of making additional eggs available without stretching existing boundaries of acceptable and standard medical practice.

References

1. Seibel MM, Kiessling A. Compensating egg donors: equal pay for equal time? N Engl J Med 1993; 328:737.
2. Miller W. British debate: does fertility science break "natural law"? Boston Globe. January 9, 1994:2.
3. Carroll J, Gosden RG. Transplantation of frozen-thawed mouse primordial follicles. Hum Reprod 1993; 8:1163–7.
4. Cha KY, Koo JJ, Ko JJ, Choi DH, Han SY, Yoon TK. Pregnancy after in vitro fertilization of human follicular oocytes collected from nonstimulated cycles, their culture in vitro and their transfer in a donor oocyte program. Fertil Steril 1993; 55:109-13.
5. Schroeder AC, Champlin AK, Mobraaten LE, Eppig JJ. Developmental capacity of mouse oocytes cryopreserved before and after maturation in vitro. J Reprod Fertil 1990; 89:43–50.

Seibel MM. (March 17, 1994) Cadaveric ovary donation. N Engl J Med 330:796.

Appendix 1-I

Becoming Parents after 100?

MACHELLE M. SEIBEL, M.D., MOSHE ZILBERSTEIN, M.D., SHARON GLAZIER SEIBEL

Sir—A few months ago, when a 63-year-old celebrity was interviewed about his baby, people hardly batted an eye. But a 62-year-old woman expecting a child through egg donation sparked international concern,[1,2] reflecting an entrenched bias that women above a certain age should not become pregnant.[3] The unease probably stems from the former evolutionary absolute that menopausal women could not conceive[4] while men can father children into old age. In addition, before 1940 or so, the life expectancy of women was 20 years less than it is today so that women in their 60s were nearing the end of their lives.

The man and the woman referred to have something else very important in common—namely, a younger spouse. With myopic focus on the age of the individual, too little attention has been paid to the couple who will become the child's family. Men are becoming much more involved in child rearing and in some families the father is the primary care-giver. Single parent adoption by both men and women is commonplace, as is artificial insemi-

nation of single women. Should a mother die early in her child's life, her younger husband can provide good and sustained parental care.[5]

We propose that instead of focusing on the upper age limit for a woman to become a parent[5] the debate should be redirected at the combined ages of the couple, with case-by-case consideration of the health and vigour of the older partner. If one parent is old, the other should be young. If both are old, limits should be set. We suggest that gamete donation be considered in the context of the family unit it will establish. An appropriate guideline could be that couples refrain from initiating parenthood when their combined ages exceed 100.

References

1. Dean M. New controversies over assisted conception. *Lancet* 1994; **343**:165.
2. Anon. Too old at 59? *Nature* 1994; **367**:2.
3. Benagiano G. Pregnancy after the menopause: a challenge to nature? *Hum Reprod* 1993; **8**:1344–45.
4. Sauer MV, Paulson RJ, Lobo RA. Pregnancy after age 50: application of oocyte donation to women after the natural menopause. *Lancet* 1993; **341**:321–23.
5. Flamigni C. Egg donation to women over 40 years of age. *Hum Reprod* 1993; **8**:1343–44.

Seibel MM, Zilberstein M, Seibel S. (1994) Becoming parents after 100? Lancet 43:603.

Appendix 1-J

In-Vitro Fertilization and Health Care Coverage

MACHELLE M. SEIBEL, M.D., MOSHE ZILBERSTEIN, M.D., MAUREEN KEARNAN

Sir—The recent emphasis on in-vitro fertilization and its associated costs has raised questions about the reasonableness of providing this procedure as part of any overall health care plan.[1] One of the most important arguments raised against its use is the presumption that were it to be a covered procedure, individuals would abuse the privilege of having it provided and go on to repeat six or more cycles if necessary. This has not been our experience.

In Massachusetts, in-vitro fertilization is a mandated procedure covered by insurance policies and most of its citizens have an opportunity to be treated without restriction. Of our last 823 consecutive cycles, 73% were in patients having the procedure only three times and 84% of cycles were in patients having the procedure no more than four times. Only a few of our patients were willing to have invitro fertilization for more than four cycles. This information indicates the tremendous physical and emotional strain in-vitro fertilization places on patients.[2]

We have previously shown that more than 95% of babies resulting from in-vitro fertilization are conceived within four treatment cycles, irrespective of the patient's age or diagnosis.[3] Because most patients seem ready to undergo no more than four treatment cycles, and because the majority of successes occur within that window of treatment, it seems that providing in-vitro fertilization coverage in the USA would not unduly add to the cost of health care. The USA and Canada define infertility as a health problem whose treatment is regarded as a health act.[4] In Massachusetts, the average increment to a family policy is about $2.40 per family contract per month to cover all infertility services. Surely, the right to build a family is worth that?

References

1. Neumann PJ, Soheyla D, Gharib MD, Weinstein MC. The cost of a successful delivery with in vitro fertilization. *N Engl J Med* 1994; **331**:239–43.
2. Seibel MM, Levin S. A new era in reproductive technology: the emotional stages of in vitro fertilization. *J In Vitro Fert* 1987; **4**:135–40.
3. Seibel MM, Ranoux C, Kearnan M. How much is enough? Knowing when to stop in vitro fertilization. *N Engl J Med* 1989; **321**:1052–53.
4. Knoppers BM, LeBris S. Ethical and legal concerns: reproductive technologies 1990. *Curr Opin* 1993; **5**:630–35.

Seibel MM, Zilberstein M, Kearnan M. (January 7, 1995) In-vitro fertilization and health care coverage. Lancet 345:66.

2

Therapeutic Donor Insemination

MACHELLE M. SEIBEL, M.D.

Evaluation for Therapeutic Donor Insemination (TDI)

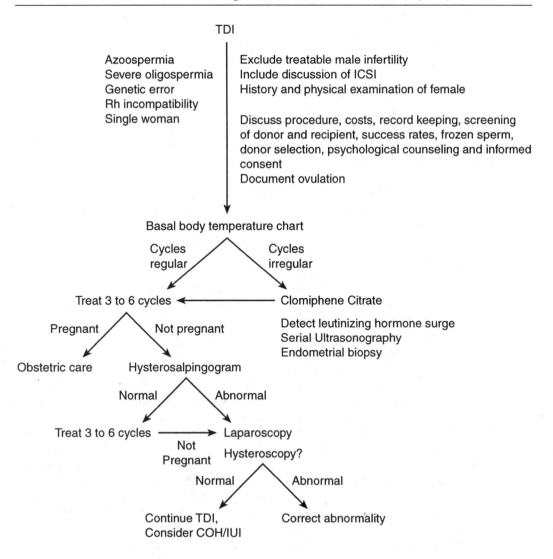

TDI

Azoospermia
Severe oligospermia
Genetic error
Rh incompatibility
Single woman

Exclude treatable male infertility
Include discussion of ICSI
History and physical examination of female

Discuss procedure, costs, record keeping, screening
of donor and recipient, success rates, frozen sperm,
donor selection, psychological counseling and informed
consent
Document ovulation

Basal body temperature chart

Cycles
regular

Cycles
irregular

Treat 3 to 6 cycles ← Clomiphene Citrate

Pregnant   Not pregnant

Obstetric care   Hysterosalpingogram

Detect leutinizing hormone surge
Serial Ultrasonography
Endometrial biopsy

Normal   Abnormal

Treat 3 to 6 cycles → Laparoscopy

Not
Pregnant   Hysteroscopy?

Normal   Abnormal

Continue TDI,
Consider COH/IUI

Correct abnormality

Artificial insemination is noncoital reproduction. It involves the mechanical placement of semen into the female reproductive tract. When semen from a woman's partner is used, the procedure is called homologous artificial insemination (AIH). When semen from another male is used, the procedure is called donor artificial insemination (AID). Because of the similarity in sound between AID and AIDS (acquired immune deficiency syndrome), most practitioners in reproductive medicine prefer the term therapeutic donor insemination (TDI) (Loy R, Seibel MM, 1990).

Although TDI is frequently grouped with the new assisted reproductive technologies, it is far from a new procedure. Documentation of its use can be found as early as the third century A.D. in a collection of Jewish law called the Talmud (Bernstein J, 1993). The first record of donor insemination in the United States was performed in 1884 by William Pancoast of Jefferson Medical College (Reuben B, 1965). Almost without question, the procedure continued to be practiced beyond that point, but little was written about it for more than half a century, until Sophie Kleegman (Kleegman S, 1954) in America and Margaret Jackson in the United Kingdom (Jackson MCN, Richardson DW, 1977) actively promoted the procedure through aggressive clinical use and widespread public awareness. The first reported pregnancies using stored frozen semen occurred in 1953 (Bunge RG, Sherman JK, 1953) and initiated what could appropriately be called the modern era of donor insemination. Along with the potential for widespread utilization, TDI at that time, like egg donation today, brought with it a number of medical, legal, ethical, and social concerns.

Today, TDI is used extensively (Shapiro S, et al., 1990). In the United States, more couples build their families through donor insemination than through adoption of newborns (Office of Technology Assessment, 1988). This translates into nearly 30,000 newborn children annually, a number that is probably greatly underrepresentative of the true number of donor births, owing to underreporting. Nevertheless, a review of the worldwide medical literature reveals follow-up reports on fewer than 1,500 TDI pregnancies and fewer than 800 offspring (Bernstein J, 1993), most of whom were followed for less than five years.

There are many reasons for the widespread use of donor insemination. The largest reason for using TDI is male factor infertility and the poor success rates ascribed to its treatment. Few male factor patients respond to hormonal treatment, and even micromanipulation procedures such as intracytoplasmic single sperm injection overcome only a portion of male factor problems (Van Steirtegham AC, Liu J, et al., 1993). Some men prefer donor insemination to adoption because it allows them to keep their sterility a secret. The second most prevalent indication for using donor insemination is to prevent the transmission of genetic diseases to one's offspring (Jalbert P, et al., 1989). Examples of inherited diseases that could be prevented include Rh-factor incompatibility in the face of severe Rh isoimmunization, cystic fibrosis, glycogen storage diseases, hemophilia, Huntington's disease, muscular dystrophy, Tay-Sachs disease, and chromosomal abnormalities transmitted by the male. With the emerging availability of preimplantation genetic diagnosis, genetic diseases can be detected before implantation, and only the unaffected embryos can be replaced. As the procedure becomes more widespread, using donor insemination to prevent genetic diseases may diminish over time. The third most prevalent indication for donor insemination is single women who desire pregnancy. This latter indication appears to be increasing; a growing number of lesbian couples seek conception, and an increasing number of unmarried or divorced women want to have children despite currently not being in a traditional relationship.

PSYCHOLOGIC ASPECTS OF TDI

For most men the realization that they will require TDI to have a child represents a major crisis and a blow to their self-esteem (Czyba JC, Chevret M, 1979). Many couples leave the consultation that initially explains the need for donor insemination and do not return to begin treatment for long periods of time, occasionally as long as years later. Whether this is due to feelings experienced by the man or his partner's protection and concern for him is unknown, but it is clear that donor insemination is an evolution and not a revolution in thinking.

David and Avidan (David A, Avidan D, 1976) observed that 80% of men who were questioned after their recent completion of TDI expressed guilt that they were unable to meet their marital expectations by producing a biologic child. The majority of their wives experienced guilt because they did not share the failure and felt that it introduced an inequality into their relationship. Unfortunately, the conflict between these two feelings created discomfort, and nearly one third of couples reported frank clinical depression. Others have also reported major symptoms such as insomnia, depression, weight loss, and reduced libido in the months following the diagnosis of severe male factor infertility (Berger DM, et al., 1986). Delaying treatment for at least six months after the diagnosis is made seems to increase marital satisfaction and improve self-concept. Patients who do not do so are more likely to experience marital strain, anxiety, and depression.

Understanding the need for emotional preparation is an important part of the discussion. In our program, all donor patients, both egg and sperm recipients, married and single, heterosexual and homosexual, are required to meet with a member of our mental health team before initiating treatment. We purposely have both a male and a female therapist to prevent any discomfort surrounding gender issues. Asking all patients to be evaluated eliminates any suggestion that a particular individual or couple is being asked to see a therapist because they have a particular problem or lifestyle and allows the focus to be appropriately placed on the need for support.

Once the inseminations are begun, many women experience a temporary irregularity in their menstrual pattern. This usually resolves over the next few months. Anticipating this occurrence and warning the patient that this could occur are helpful for most patients and prevent the stress from being compounded.

EVALUATING THE PATIENTS

Patients presenting for TDI are initially required to be interviewed together with their partner. Obtaining a careful social history at this visit is essential. If the man was married before and had children followed by a vasectomy, no evaluation of the male is warranted, assuming that he is aware that vasovasostomy or intracytoplasmic single sperm injection combined with either testicular biopsy or epididymal aspiration can be performed and understands their potential for success. Similarly, no evaluation is needed if the man is azoospermic due to gonadal failure as evidenced by an elevated serum level of follicle-stimulating hormone (FSH) and the presence of fructose in his semen. If fructose is absent in the semen and serum FSH levels are normal, the diagnosis of obstruction must be excluded. Azoospermic men who have low levels of FSH and luteinizing hormone (LH) are likely to have hypogonadotropic hypogonadism and may respond well to gonadotropin therapy.

Men with abnormal semen parameters (oligozoospermia-reduced number of sperm, asthenospermia-decreased sperm motility, or teratozoospermia-increased number of abnormally shaped sperm) who choose to pursue TDI require more consideration. The potential benefits of reviewing treatment such as homologous artificial insemination, in vitro fertilization, or micromanipulation must be weighed against the emotional pain created by continuing to discuss the use of the man's sperm. If the man is informed of alternative options and desires TDI, in most instances it is usually preferable to proceed along that course of action.

Evaluation of the woman also depends on her history. If there is no suggestion of possible tubal disease and her cycles are regular, it is reasonable to initiate TDI with no infertility evaluation. A hysterosalpingogram is recommended if pregnancy does not occur in three months, and a laparoscopy is recommended if pregnancy does not occur in six months. A positive history for possible tubal disease requires that the hysterosalpingogram be performed before initiating TDI. Ovulatory inducing agents are recommended if the woman's cycles are irregular. We use a basal body temperature chart (BBT) for all of our TDI patients to determine whether the inseminations were performed at the correct time. The best time to perform an insemination is one to three days before the midcycle temperature rise. While ovulation prediction kits have attained wide popularity and are supplemental, in my opinion they are no better than, and do not replace, the BBT for donor insemination.

In addition to the above-mentioned evaluation, all patients in our program initiating TDI are required to be screened for HIV, hepatitis, and other infectious diseases as recommended by the American Society for Reproductive Medicine. Patients are also screened for rubella and are immunized if they do not possess antibodies. Although the risk is small, treatment should be delayed three months following immunization to ensure that immunization does not cause inadvertent infection of an early pregnancy. We also advise patients to begin taking supplemental folic acid as soon as they initiate treatment, to decrease the possibility of having a child with a neural tube defect (Centers for Disease Control, 1992).

SCREENING AND SELECTING THE DONOR

It is difficult to believe how much things have changed in less than a decade. Until approximately the mid l980s, the task of identifying and screening semen donors was a private and individual one. Physicians would identify medical students, residents, or other graduate-level males; test them for gonorrhea and syphilis; and match them by phenotype with patients accordingly. Cryopreservation techniques were good but had not reached the level of excellence they have attained today. Few commercial sperm banks were available, and post-thaw semen quality was variable. As a result, pregnancy results were much greater with fresh than with frozen semen—a circumstance that is no longer accurate. However, because of the desire to attain pregnancy as rapidly as possible, virtually all donor insemination treatments were performed with fresh semen until the 1980s. In the mid to late l980s, testing for HIV and hepatitis was added to donor screening, but fresh semen continued to be used. It is believed that the use of frozen donor sperm increased from 31% of practices in 1978 to 79% of practices in 1988 (Shapiro S, et al., 1990).

The current screening of potential semen donors and the use of semen cryopreservation is much more standardized (see Appendixes 2-A and 2-B). Donor semen must now be quarantined for six months and the donor must be retested as negative before frozen semen can be released. There has been a proliferation of sperm banks with standardized basic quality assurances, allowing TDI to be available even where there are inadequate numbers of sperm donors. The donors themselves are often white, unmarried, middle-class students in the health sciences between 20 and 27 years of age with excellent semen parameters (Currie-Cohen M, et al., 1979). They are typically of above-average intelligence.

MATCHING DONORS AND RECIPIENTS

In the past, donors and recipients were matched by the physician who performed the procedure. Race, eye color, hair color, and height were the most important priorities. Issues such as Rh factor were seldom considered unless the recipient insisted or Rh incompatibility was the indication. A patient was typically asked for a photograph, to be placed in his medical record, which assisted in selecting a donor. Great care and effort were made to match donors and recipients

Today, most semen is obtained from sperm banks that provide a catalogue of the available samples and a brief description of the donor. The physician performing the procedure has no more information about the donor than the patient does. Some sperm banks will provide semen samples directly to the patient; others require that semen samples be delivered only to physicians. This may be due to the fact that the laws of some states require that TDI be performed under the supervision of a licensed physician, certified medical doctor, or person duly authorized to practice medicine. Although most sperm banks provide semen only from anonymous donors, a few will provide access to the donor's identity.

In our center, patients are given a short list of appropriately matched donors to choose from. This is done to relieve the patient of the daunting task of selecting one donor from a catalogue containing many pages of donor descriptions. The center then orders the semen sample for the donor. It is the responsibility of the sperm bank to reliably provide excellent donor screening, excellent-quality donor samples, and on-time delivery. However, the clinical facility must do its best to ensure that the sperm bank is capable of providing those services.

ORDERING SEMEN SAMPLES

Because the overwhelming majority of TDI cycles use frozen semen, each center must determine how it will obtain the samples. Some TDI programs prefer that patients order their own samples; others prefer to order the samples themselves. At our center, both ways are options, but our policy is that the sample must be shipped to the center to ensure that the sample that is received and inseminated is indeed the sample that was ordered. Unused semen specimens are returned to the sperm bank to prevent future treatment errors. In the unusual circumstance requiring a sample to be stored at the center, the specimen is kept in a separate cryopreservation tank.

Patients are given a choice of two sperm banks. We have found that using a larger number of sperm banks creates stress for the TDI team by increasing the potential both for errors to occur and for the cycle not to run smoothly. If more than one person is involved in ordering the semen sample, it is useful to have a stamp that clearly states who ordered the sample, when it is due, and when it is received (Figure 2.1). This system is particularly useful on weekends and vacations, when the person who ordered the sperm may not be available. Because shipping costs can be considerable, it is important that the patient be made aware of them before initiating a cycle.

FIGURE 2.1. Suggested Stamp for Ordering Frozen Sperm.

	DATE	INITIALS
Ordered	_____	_____
Due	_____	_____
Received	_____	_____

LEGAL CONSIDERATIONS OF TDI

Because TDI involves a third party in the reproductive process, a discussion of the legal considerations is warranted. The first consideration is to be certain that the couple (or the individual if the patient has no partner) is comfortable with the decision to proceed with donor insemination. As obvious as this concept seems, some individuals begin TDI without being ready to do so. In such instances, smoldering feelings ignite after the child is born, when it may be too late to intervene.

The treating physician must be absolutely certain whether or not the recipient wishes to have information concerning the TDI forwarded to her obstetrician and must clearly mark the chart accordingly. All members of the team should understand how to find this notation, including clerical workers who might inadvertently photocopy confidential records. If recipients anticipate that they may want to use the same donor for a future pregnancy, they should be advised to purchase samples ahead of time and store them, to be certain that they will be available and that recipients were aware of the possibility.

While every effort will undoubtedly be made to maintain donor anonymity, one cannot guarantee that future offspring will be unable to trace the identity of the donor. Similarly, as one is usually depending on a sperm bank to screen for infectious diseases, the physician must be as certain as possible of the quality of screening being done. An example is that of a donor insemination pregnancy becoming infected with cytomegalovirus as a result of the donor sample being infected. In such instances the treating physician could be held accountable for the adverse outcome.

The recipient couple must also be informed that while donor insemination does not increase the risk of chromosomal anomalies, a small percentage of children will be born with birth defects (Appendix 2-B). If the patient's concern is great, the recipients can be offered genetic counseling. In addition, the donor can be screened for genetic diseases by having a chromosomal analysis if the recipient is uncomfortable having only a negative history for significant genetic diseases (see Chapter 6).

INFORMED CONSENT

Informed consent represents a particularly important consideration in TDI. Not only are there potential medical risks to the patient; there are also potential risks to the child. In addition, consideration must be given to issues related to paternity, infection, confidentiality, and genetics, among others.

Both the woman and her partner must provide their consent for donor insemination in order to receive the rights and responsibilities of parenthood. There are additional considerations if the donor sperm is being used for a single woman or for in vitro fertilization (Appendixes 2-C, 2-D, and 2-E). The donor consent form can contain the medical, genetic, and sexual history as well as help to maintain confidentiality. However, no consent form is as protective to the program as the time spent explaining things to the couple. Table 2.1 lists the states that have statutes regarding TDI. Some

TABLE 2.1.   Therapeutic Donor Insemination Statutes

State	Has TDI Statute	MD Involvement	Refers to Married Woman or Wife	Husband Consent	Legitimates Child	Record Keeping Requirement	Requires Screening of Donor	Limits Number of Offspring per Donor	Miscellaneous
Alabama	yes	yes	yes	yes	yes	yes	no	no	
Alaska	yes	yes	yes	yes	yes	no	no	no	
Arizona	yes	no	yes	yes	yes	no	no	no	
Arkansas	yes	yes	yes	yes	yes	no	no	no	
California	yes	yes	yes	yes	yes	yes	no	no	
Colorado	yes	yes	yes	yes	yes	yes	no	no	
Connecticut	yes	yes	yes	yes	yes	yes	no	no	
Delaware	no						yes		HIV screening and confidentiality requirements
District of Columbia	yes	no	no	no	no	no	no	no	
Florida	yes	no	yes	yes	yes	no	no	no	
Georgia	yes	yes	yes	yes	yes	no	no, but allows recovery for negligence	no	
Hawaii	no								
Idaho	yes	yes	yes	yes	yes	yes	yes	no	
Illinois	yes	yes	yes	yes	yes	yes	no	no	
Indiana	no						yes	yes	HIV screening law; exempts AIH
Iowa	no								
Kansas	yes	no	yes	yes	yes	yes	no	no	
Kentucky	no								
Louisiana	yes	yes	no	yes	yes	yes	yes	no	
Maine	no								
Maryland	yes	no	yes	yes (pre-sumed)	yes	no	no	no	

Continued

39

TABLE 2.1. *Continued*

State	Has TDI Statute	MD Involvement	Refers to Married Woman or Wife	Husband Consent	Legitimates Child	Record Keeping Requirement	Requires Screening of Donor	Limits Number of Offspring per Donor	Miscellaneous
Massachusetts	yes	no	yes	yes	yes	no	no	no	
Michigan	yes	no	yes	yes	yes	no	no	no	
Minnesota	yes	yes	yes	yes	yes	yes	no	no	
Mississippi	no								
Missouri	no								
Montana	yes	yes	yes	yes	yes	yes	no	no	
Nebraska	no								
Nevada	yes	yes	yes	yes	yes	yes	no	no	
New Hampshire	yes	no	no	yes	yes	yes	no	no	
New Jersey	yes	yes	no	yes	yes	yes	no	no	
New Mexico	yes	yes	yes	yes	yes	yes	no	yes	
New York	yes	yes	no	yes	yes	no	no	no	
North Carolina	yes	no	no	yes	yes	no	no	no	
North Dakota	yes	no	no	yes	yes	no	no	no	Exempts AIH
Ohio	yes	yes	no	yes	yes	yes	yes	no	
Oklahoma	yes	yes	no	yes	yes	yes	no	no	
Oregon	yes	yes	no	yes	yes	yes	yes	no	
Pennsylvania	no								
Rhode Island	no								
South Carolina	no								
South Dakota	no								
Tennessee	yes	no	yes	yes	yes	no	no	no	
Texas	yes	no	yes	yes	yes	no	no	no	
Utah	no								Only applies to surrogacy
Vermont	no								
Virginia	yes	no	yes	yes	yes	no	yes	no	
Washington	yes	yes	yes	yes	yes	yes	no	no	Exempts AIH
West Virginia	no								
Wisconsin	yes	yes	yes	yes	yes	yes	no	no	
Wyoming	yes	yes	yes	yes	yes	yes	no	no	

Prepared by Ami S. Jaeger, J. D., November 5, 1995

states mandate that a record-keeping body receive a copy of the executed consent. The treating physician must clearly explain his or her philosophy and policy on record keeping.

In the past, when fresh semen was used and the only records kept were in the office of the treating physician, the information was destroyed after one to two years, once it was fairly certain that the resulting child had no medical problems. This was done to ensure anonymity. This approach was common in the past and may or may not be commonplace today. The guidelines on donor insemination issued by the American Fertility Society (1988) suggest that permanent and confidential records be kept, maintained, and available anonymously for the infertile couple, the offspring, or both. However, whatever one's views on record keeping and confidentiality, it is much harder to guarantee anonymity today using frozen sperm, owing to the need for long-term record keeping by sperm banks and the number of individuals that are now involved. The impact this will have on future generations of TDI offspring and their potential need and desire to search for their biologic parents remains to be seen.

RATES OF SUCCESS

Patients requiring TDI are both women who have normal fecundity but whose partners are azoospermic and women who have subnormal fecundity and whose partners are oligospermic. Women in the former group can anticipate pregnancy rates of 70%, compared with 48.8% in the latter group (Loy R, Seibel MM, 1990). The difference in success rates is probably due to the fact that the latter group has a lower fecundity and those with a higher fecundity will have already conceived (Emperaire JC, et al., 1982). Evidence for this belief is found in the British experience, in which waiting lists required years of waiting for couples to receive TDI (Table 2.2).

TABLE 2.2. Correlation Between Oligospermia and Pregnancy

Motile Sperm Count (millions/cc)	Pregnancy, 5 years	Rate (%), 12 years
0.1–1	3.9	8.7
1–5	11.9	26.6
5–10	22.1	34.3
10–15	45.0	58.5
15–20	68.6	82.0

With sufficient time, even individuals who had severely reduced semen counts were capable of impregnating their partners. These types of data strongly suggest that in instances of longstanding infertility in which the semen parameters are poor, it is imperative that the female be evaluated to be certain that she does not have reduced fecundity that can be corrected.

Overall, patients who receive donor insemination can anticipate results between 40% and 85% and a mean of 70–75%. Part of the differences in success rates are due to study design. Another important variable is the age of the recipient (Figures 2.2, 2.3). Women beyond age 35 should be counseled to anticipate a lower rate of success, a longer time to conceive, and a higher percentage of spontaneous abortion. However, in general, most women who achieve pregnancy using donor insemination do so within six treatment cycles (Figure 2.4).

Several papers have suggested using the term fecundability, which is the ratio of the number of pregnancies to the number of treatment cycles, to reflect the influence of dropout and to facilitate the application of life-table analysis (Guzick D, et al., 1982). The overall fecundability for TDI has ranged between 7% and 12% (Shapiro S, 1991). Results are generally reported as being higher for fresh semen than for frozen semen. However, because freezing methods have been developed to improve

FIGURE 2.2. Success Rates for Donor Insemination Depend on the Number of Treatment Cycles and Maternal Age.

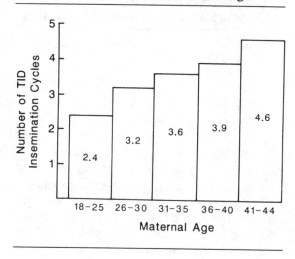

FIGURE 2.4. Donor Insemination Pregnancy Rates.

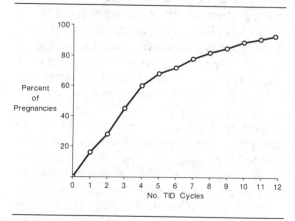

sperm survival rates and because the use of frozen-quarantined sperm is now considered standard of care, discussions surrounding fresh sperm are moot. Freezing affects outcome by reducing semen motility upon thawing, short-

ening the life span of the thawed sperm, and reducing the thawed sperm's ability to penetrate cervical mucus (Keel B, et al., 1987). In addition, frozen semen samples usually contain 0.5 cc or less of semen combined with an equal volume of cryoprotectant. Therefore the amount of sperm that is actually available for insemination after thawing is actually much less, with lower motility and survival, than is the case with fresh semen and probably accounts for the slightly lower success rates.

To compensate for these reduced semen parameters, many centers perform inseminations on two consecutive days around the time of ovulation. Other centers prefer to skip one day between insemination treatments. The majority of physicians do perform two inseminations per cycle, while approximately 20% perform either one or three inseminations per cycle. Ovulation is timed by using either BBTs, ovulation monitoring with urinary LH surge predictor kits, or ovulation-inducing medications combined with human chorionic gonadotropin (Shapiro S, 1991). Inseminations can be performed as either intracervical or intrauterine procedures (Figure 2.5). A stamp can help greatly in record keeping (Figure 2.6).

FIGURE 2.3. Success Rates of Donor Insemination Based on Maternal Age.

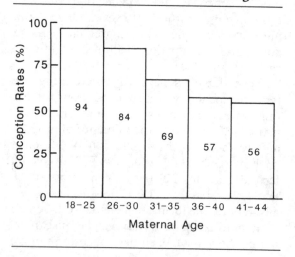

FIGURE 2.5.   Methods of Artificial Insemination.

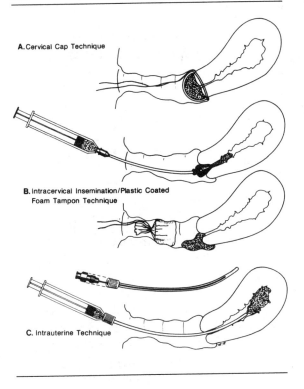

A. Cervical Cap Technique

B. Intracervical Insemination/Plastic Coated Foam Tampon Technique

C. Intrauterine Technique

FIGURE 2.6.   Stamp Used for Record Keeping of Insemination Cycles.

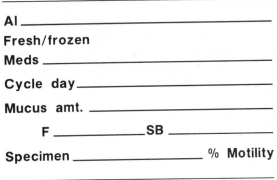

AI _____
Fresh/frozen
Meds _____
Cycle day_____
Mucus amt. _____
    F _____SB _____
Specimen _____ % Motility

TECHNIQUES OF TDI

For intracervical insemination (ICI) a syringe and small cannula are used to place approximately 0.3 cc of semen just within the external cervical os. The remainder of the semen may be placed into the back of the vagina. The speculum is then loosened, and the patient is asked to lie in the examination room for another ten minutes so that the additional sperm can mix with the cervical mucus. A plastic-covered sponge with a string attached is inserted into the vagina to prevent leakage, and the speculum is removed. The patient is then released and asked to remove the sponge two to three hours later.

Intrauterine insemination (IUI) is performed by washing the semen sample in culture medium to remove the seminal plasma from around the sperm. The washed sperm are then separated from the culture medium by one of several techniques, and the concentrated pellet of sperm is injected into the uterus by using a syringe attached to a thin plastic tube. No anesthesia is used, and the procedure is usually painless. Some individuals who have a narrow cervical canal may require instrumentation of the cervix for the catheter to press through it.

Each of these variations has its proponents. It does appear that women who have had a prior pregnancy—whether it ended in abortion, ectopic pregnancy, or viability—have a higher success rate with TDI than do those who have never been pregnant (Yeh J, Seibel MM, 1987).

DISCONTINUATION OF TREATMENT

Women who have experienced longstanding infertility, who are from low socioeconomic groups, and whose husbands convey reluctance to undergo TDI are more likely to discontinue treatment (Glezerman M, 1981). Most studies report decreased participation after six months of unsuccessful treatment, a trend that continues with more extended periods of time. Reasons contributing to discontinuing treatment include discouragement, relocation, adoption, marital problems, and the realization of additional fertility problems. Discontinuation is probably the single most common cause of failure with TDI (Corson SL, 1980).

FOLLOW-UP OF TDI

Despite its widespread acceptance and use, there remains limited follow-up of TDI families or their offspring. Clearly, TDI is not for every couple. However, the risk of divorce is low for couples who have conceived through TDI (Amuzu B, et al., 1990). Many couples have returned for second and even third children. Occasionally, the male has more of an adjustment to having a male child than a female child, perhaps because this is the child who will carry on his name. In addition, couples who choose not to tell about TDI and who achieve multiple births due to the use of fertility drugs may face awkward situations when they are praised for their "stud" capabilities.

Children resulting from TDI tend to score higher than the norm on intelligence tests (Iizuka R, et al., 1977) (Figure 2.7). The number of birth defects following donor insemination are within the normal range. Similarly, birth weight and developmental milestones were normal, and more than 10% were found to be gifted. There is a tendency toward a higher number of male offspring resulting from TDI. However, the total number of studied cases for all parameters remains small.

CONCLUSION

Therapeutic donor insemination has become a widespread and widely accepted form of treat-

FIGURE 2.7. Intelligence Quotients of Children Conceived Through Donor Insemination.

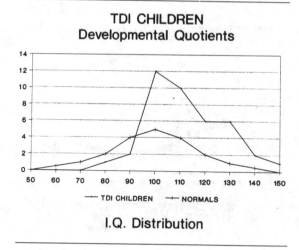

ment for male factor infertility. However, it is not for everyone. Couples who cannot accept TDI should be given every opportunity to conceive with aggressive treatment of the male, including homologous artificial insemination and in vitro fertilization combined with micromanipulation. At the same time, couples who are unable to accept TDI should be helped with closure and encouraged to pursue adoption or child-free living. Mental health support should be strongly encouraged at this time as well.

For couples who choose to pursue TDI, a psychological consultation is extremely important. Open discussion concerning fears and issues that could arise is helpful in averting future problems. Often, both partners are not at the same level of readiness simultaneously. In such instances, time must be allowed for processing to occur. Both the physician and the patient must come to realize that TDI is a second choice, not second best. Once that occurs, TDI becomes an extremely gratifying method of family building.

REFERENCES

1. Amuzu B, Laxova R, Shapiro S. (1990) Pregnancy outcome, health of children, and family adjustment after donor insemination. Obstet Gynecol 75:899.
2. Berger DM, Eisen A, Shuber J, Doody KF. (1986) Psychological patterns in donor insemination couples. Can J Psychiatry 31:818.
3. Bernstein J. (1993) The long-term psychologic and social effects of gamete donation. In: Seibel MM, Kiessling AA, Bernstein J, Levin SR, eds. Technology and Infertility: Clinical, Psychosocial, Legal and Ethical Aspects. New York: Springer-Verlag. pp 337–346.
4. Bunge RG, Sherman JK. (1953) Fertilizing capacity of frozen human spermatozoa. Nature 172:767.
5. Centers for Disease Control. (1992) Recommendations for the use of folic acid to reduce the number of cases of spina bifida and other neural tube defects. MMWR 41:1–7.
6. Corson SL. (1980) Factors affecting donor artificial insemination success rates. Fertil Steril 33:415.
7. Currie-Cohen M, Luttrell L, Shapiro S. (1979) Current practice of artificial insemination by donor in the United States. N Engl J Med 300:585.
8. Czyba JC, Chevret M. 1979. Psychological reactions of couples to artificial insemination with donor sperm. Int J Fertil 24:240.
9. David A, Avidan D. (1976) Artificial insemination donor: Clinical and psychological aspects. Fertil Steril 27:528.
10. Emperaire JC, Gauzere-Saimireu E, Audebert AJM. (1982) Female fertility and donor insemination. Fertil Steril 37:90.
11. Guzick D, Bross D, Rock J. (1982) A parametric method for comparing cumulative pregnancy curves following infertility treatment. Fertil Steril 37:503.
12. Iizuka R, Sawada Y, Nishina N, Ohi M. (1977) The physical and mental development of children born following artificial insemination. Int J Fertil 13:24.
13. Jackson MCN, Richardson DW. (1977) The use of fresh and frozen semen in human artificial insemination. J Biosoc Sci 9:251.
14. Jalbert P, Leonard C, Selva J, David G. (1989) Genetic aspects of artificial insemination with donor semen: The French CECOS Federation Guidelines; Am J Med Genet 33:269.
15. Keel B, Webster B, Roberts D. (1987) Effects of cryopreservation on motility characteristics of human spermatozoa. J Reprod Fertil 81:213.
16. Kleegman SJ. (1954) Therapeutic donor insemination. Fertil Steril 5:7.
17. Loy RA, Seibel MM. (1990) Therapeutic insemination. In Infertility: A Comprehensive Text. Edited by MM Seibel. Norwalk, Conn.: Appleton & Lange, pp. 199–215.
18. Office of Technology Assessment. (1988) Artificial Insemination Practice in the U.S. Washington, D.C.: U.S. Government Printing Office.
19. Reuben B. (1965) The psychological aspects of human artificial insemination. Arch Gen Psychiatry 13:121.
20. Shapiro S. (1991) Can timing improve therapeutic donor insemination fecundability? Fertil Steril 55:869.
21. Shapiro S, Saphire D, Stone W. (1990) Changes in American AID practice during the past decade. Int J Fertil 35:284.
22. The American Fertility Society. (1994) Guidelines for therapeutic donor insemination: Sperm Fertil Steril 62:995.
23. Van Steirteghem AC, Liu J, Joris H, Nagy Z, Janssenwillen C, Tournaye H, Derde M-P, Assche EV, Devroey P. (1993) Higher success rate by intracytoplasmic sperm injection than by subzonal insemination: Report of a second series of 300 consecutive treatment cycles. Hum Reprod 8:1055–1060.
24. Yeh J, Seibel MM. (1987) Artificial insemination with donor sperm: A review of 108 patients. Obstet Gynecol 70:313.

Appendix 2-A

Guidelines for Therapeutic Donor Insemination: Sperm

FAULKNER CENTRE FOR REPRODUCTIVE MEDICINE

I. Indications

    A. Irreversible azoospermia of the male partner.

    B. Obstruction of the male partner's reproductive tract, either acquired or congenital, that cannot be repaired or the male partner wishes not to have surgically corrected.

    C. The male partner has severe oligospermia or severely impaired semen parameters and does not desire or has failed conception using intracytoplasmic single sperm injection (ICSI) or other assisted reproductive technologies.

    D. The male partner possesses a known inherited or genetic disorder such as Huntington's disease, hemophilia or chromosomal abnormality that places a biologic offspring at significant risk.

    E. Non correctable ejaculatory dysfunction in the male partner.

    F. Severe Rh-isoimmunization in an Rh-negative female partner who has an Rh-positive male partner.

    G. A human immunodeficiency virus (HIV) positive male partner.

    H. A single female.

II. Preparation

    A. Couples or individuals interested in pursuing TDI should receive detailed explanation of the procedure, its benefits and risks including the potential risk of acquiring an infection, the need for them to be screened, and out-of-pocket expenses.

    B. Couples or individuals should understand how and from where donors are selected, how they are screened and how they are matched, and any days, if any, that TDI is not performed (i.e., weekends, holidays, etc.).

    C. Informed consent forms should be signed by the couple or the individual if she is single.

    D. Discussion of the need to obtain and store additional semen samples if the couple/individual anticipates desiring subsequent pregnancies.

    E. Psychological counseling of the couple/individual by a trained mental health professional to minimize the emotional risk, and to explore such issues as when and if to tell.

    F. Both partners should be tested for HIV I-II antibody, hepatitis B surface antigen, hepatitis C antibody, and serologic test for syphilis.

    G. The female recipient should also be tested for her blood type, Rh factor, cervical cultures for gonorrhea and chlamydia, and rubella titers with vaccination offered to patients without immunity.

    H. The female recipient should be examined and evaluated for potential infertility factors prior to initiating treatment if there is a suspicious female factor history or within three months of initiating TDI if there is a negative female factor history and pregnancy has not occurred.

Modified by Machelle M. Seibel, M.D., from American Society for Reproductive Medicine. Guidelines for gamete donation. (1994) Fertil Steril 62: 1045.

III. Donor Selection

    A. Donors for TDI should be of good general health, should not possess a genetic abnormality or a strong family history for a major abnormality, and should be between legal age and 40 years of age.

    B. Established fertility is desirable but not an absolute requirement.

    C. Anonymous donors are recommended but not required.

    D. If known donors are used they should have the same evaluation and treatment as anonymous donors including specimens being quarantined for six months.

    E. Owners, operators, physicians, or employees of a facility performing TDI should not be a donor for that program or for patients treated by that program.

IV. Donor Screening

    A. Donors should be found to have normal semen samples on several occasions, and the samples should have a cryosurvival of $\geq$ 50% of initial motility.

    B. Genetic screening is important including a pedigree to exclude hereditary and familial diseases, but chromosome analysis is not mandatory.

    C. Donors should be of good general health and not be at high risk for HIV (intravenous drug use or a sexual partner who uses intravenous drugs) or have multiple sexual partners.

    D. Donors should have a complete medical examination with special attention given to exclude urethral discharges, genital warts or ulcers.

    E. Laboratory testing including Rh factor testing and blood type initially, and serum hepatitis B antigen (HBsAg) and hepatitis C antibody, serologic tests for syphilis, semen or urethral cultures for gonorrhea and chlamydia, and cytomegalovirus antibody testing initially and at 6 month intervals. Cytomegalovirus antibody positive donors are recommended to be used only with cytomegalovirus antibody positive recipients.

    F. Donors should be tested initially for HIV antibodies, and if negative, their specimens should be cryopreserved, quarantined for 6 months and released only if a repeat HIV antibody test is negative.

    G. Donors should sign a form denying any known risk factor for HIV.

    H. Donors should be willing to provide nonidentifying information about themselves that can be made available to the recipient and/or resulting offspring.

Appendix 2-B

Genetic Screening for Gamete Donors

FAULKNER CENTRE FOR REPRODUCTIVE MEDICINE

I. Donor History:

   A. Minimal genetic screening requires a three generation genetic history and establishing that the donor is of general good health. Information beyond minimal screening is defined by B to G below.
   B. Should not have or had a major mendelian disorder (e.g. hemophilia) or major malformation. Although major is a matter of judgment, the term implies serious handicap of a functional or cosmetic nature.
   C. Should not be a carrier for a detectable autosomal recessive gene that is prevalent in the recipient's ethnic background (e.g., α-thalassemia in Southeastern Asians and Philippinos, β-thalassemia among Mediterranean populations, sickle cell disease in African-Americans, and Tay-Sachs disease in Jews of Eastern European descent and other defined populations) unless the recipients approve and are ready to be tested themselves.
   D. Should never have possessed a major malformation of complex cause (e.g., spina bifida or heart malformation). The term major must be viewed as a matter of judgement.
   E. Should not possess a familial disease known to have a major genetic component.
   F. Known carriers of chromosomal rearrangement that could result in an unbalanced gamete should not be used as donors.
   G. Should ideally be below 35 years for egg donation and below 40 years for sperm donation to reduce the potential transmission of chromosomal aneuploidy (women) and new mendelian mutations (men).

II. Donor Family History: First degree relatives (parents or offspring)

   Should be free of:

   A. Major malformations
   B. Major mendelian disorders within the following categories:
      1. Autosomal dominant or X-linked disorders where age of onset typically occurs beyond the time of donation (e.g., Huntington's disease).
      2. Autosomal dominant inheritance with variable penetrance.
   C. If a chromosome abnormality exists in a donor's family history, chromosome analysis of the donor may be required.
   D. Donors found to be unacceptable based on genetic or family history may need appropriate genetic counseling.

III. A nonidentifying permanent record of the donor including genetic work-up, should be maintained and should be made available to the recipient and/or any resulting offspring upon request. Programs may wish to provide such information to potential recipients prior to using a given donor for them.

Modified from Minimal genetic screening for gamete donors. Ethical considerations of assisted reproductive technologies. Fertility and Sterility 62:995, 1994.

Appendix 2-C

Consent Form: Therapeutic Insemination— Donor (Single Recipient)

FAULKNER CENTRE FOR REPRODUCTIVE MEDICINE

I, _____ an unmarried woman 18 years of age or older, authorize Dr. _____ and his/her designated assistants to perform one or more artificial inseminations on me with the sperm obtained from an anonymous donor(s) for the purpose of making me pregnant.

I agree to rely on the judgment and discretion of the FCRM Clinical team to select an appropriate donor(s) whose characteristics are compatible with mine. If applicable, I accept responsibility for selecting my own donor(s). I will never seek to identify the donor(s), nor shall the donor be advised of my identity. I understand and agree that it cannot be guaranteed that the same donor will be utilized for each insemination. I also agree that donor sperm that has been frozen (for storage purposes) may be used.

I understand that there is no guarantee that these inseminations will result in pregnancy. I further understand that within the normal human population a certain percentage (approximately 4%) of children are born with physical or mental defects, and that the occurrence of such defects is beyond the control of physicians. I therefore understand and agree that Faulkner Centre for Reproductive Medicine and its physicians do not assume responsibility for the physical and mental characteristics of any child or children born as a result of artificial insemination. I also understand that within the normal population approximately 20% of pregnancies result in miscarriages and that this may occur after donor insemination as well. Similarly, obstetrical complications may occur in any pregnancy. I also understand and accept that the artificial insemination procedure carries with it the risk of sexually transmitted diseases including but not limited to gonorrhea, syphilis, herpes, hepatitis, and acquired immune deficiency syndrome (AIDS). This agreement therefore is not a contract to cure, a warranty of treatment, nor a guaranty of conception. By these presence I do hereby absolve, release, indemnify, protect and hold harmless from any and all liability for the mental or physical nature of character of any child or children so conceived or born, and for affirmative acts or acts of omission which may arise during the performance of this agreement, the Faulkner Centre for Reproductive Medicine.

I further agree that I am assuming entire responsibility for any child or children conceived or born. I agree that I will not seek support for the child or children, or any other payment from the donor, physicians or nurses associated with the Faulkner Centre for Reproductive Medicine. I further agree that if the child or children should seek support or any other payment from the donor, physicians or nurses I will indemnify and hold harmless the donor, physicians, nurses, and Faulkner Centre for Reproductive Medicine.

It is further agreed that the nature of this agreement is such that it must remain confidential; therefore, I agree that a sole copy of this agreement may be retained in the above-named doctor's files and shall not be disclosed except with my express written permission.

Faulkner Centre for Reproductive Medicine may use the agreement as necessary in connection with any legal proceeding to which it is relevant.

Date_____ , 19_____   Signature _____

_____ o'clock _____   Witness_____

Rev. 3/94

Appendix 2-D

Consent Form: Therapeutic Insemination— Donor (Married Recipient)

FAULKNER CENTRE FOR REPRODUCTIVE MEDICINE

We _____ and _____ being partners authorize Dr. _____ and his/her designated assistants to perform one or more artificial inseminations on the wife with the sperm obtained from an anonymous donor(s) for the purpose of making her pregnant.

We agree to rely on the judgment and discretion of the FCRM Clinical team to select an appropriate donor(s) whose characteristics are compatible with ours. If applicable we accept responsibility for selecting our own donor(s). We will never seek to identify the donor(s), nor shall the donor be advised of the identity of either husband or wife. We understand that it cannot be guaranteed that the same donor will be utilized for each insemination. We also agree that the donor sperm that has been frozen (for storage purposes) may be used.

We understand that there is no guarantee that these inseminations will result in a pregnancy. We further understand that within the normal human population a certain percentage (approximately 4%) of children are born with physical or mental defects and that the occurrence of such defects is beyond the control of physicians. We therefore understand and agree that Boston Center for Reproductive Health, D.B.A. Faulkner Centre for Reproductive Medicine, and its physicians do not assume responsibility for the physical and mental characteristics of any child or children born as a result of artificial inseminations. We also understand that within the normal population approximately 20% of pregnancies result in miscarriages and that this may occur after artificial insemination as well. Similarly, obstetrical complications may occur in any pregnancy. We also understand and accept that despite careful screening, the insemination procedure carries with it the risk of sexually transmitted diseases including but not limited to gonorrhea, syphilis, herpes, hepatitis, cytomegalovirus and acquired immune deficiency syndrome (HIV).

This agreement therefore is not a contract to cure, a warranty of treatment nor a guaranty of conception. By these presence we do hereby absolve, release, indemnify, protect and hold harmless from any and all liability for the mental or physical nature of character of any child or children so conceived or born, and for affirmative acts or acts of omission which may arise during the performance of this agreement the Boston Center for Reproductive Health D.B.A. Faulkner Centre for Reproductive Medicine and its staff.

We understand that, if a woman is artificially inseminated with the consent of her husband, the husband is treated in law as if he were the natural father of a child thereby conceived.

It is further agreed that from conception, I _____, as husband accept the act of insemination as my own and agree:

a. That such child or children conceived or born shall be my legitimate children and heirs of my body, and
b. That I hereby waive forever any right which I have to disclaim or omit the child or children as my legitimate heir or heirs, and
c. That such child or children conceived or born shall be considered to be in all respects, including descent and distribution of my property, a child or children of my body.

Husband _____   Wife _____

Date _____   Witness/Physician _____

Date _____

Appendix 2-E

Consent Form: Request for Donor Insemination of Oocytes for IVF

FAULKNER CENTRE FOR REPRODUCTIVE MEDICINE

We, _____ and _____ both being of legal age, authorize Dr. _____ and any such physician, scientist or technician as he or she may designate to inseminate oocytes of the above named female patient with donor sperm in an attempt to produce a pregnancy. We are extremely anxious to have a child and believe that this donor insemination will promote our mutual happiness and well-being.

We understand that even though the insemination by donor may be repeated in several cycles there can be no guarantee of pregnancy resulting. Should pregnancy occur, we understand that it is susceptible to all of the common complications of pregnancy occurring in the usual manner, including but not limited to a 3–5% incidence of serious congenital defects, and all of the potential complications inherent in In Vitro Fertilization. We also understand that there is no increased probability of complications from donor insemination once a pregnancy is established, during childbirth or delivery, but that offspring could possibly have undesirable hereditary tendencies and other health problems that cannot be foreseen. We release the above named physician and associates from any and all liability or responsibility of any delivery or for hereditary tendencies of any such issue, or for any other adverse consequences which may arise in connection with, or as a result of donor insemination of oocytes during In Vitro Fertilization.

We have been fully informed by the above named physician of the hazards and risks of this procedure which may include the transmission of venereal disease or other diseases, and nevertheless, individually and collectively, agree to hold the physician and such assistants as he may utilize and the donor or donors free and harmless from any claims, demands or suits for damages, or for injury or complications which may result pursuant to this agreement. We shall refrain from bringing legal action of any kind, refrain from aiding and abetting anyone else in bringing legal action for or on account of any matter or thing which might arise out of the insemination herein contemplated. Under no circumstances shall we require that the name of the donor of the semen be divulged to us or anyone else, and accordingly forever waive all rights, if any, that we have to name, identity or any information of any kind concerning the donor. We shall rely on the discretion of the FCRM clinical team in the selection of qualified donor(s). If applicable, we accept responsibility for selecting our own donor(s). Should any action of any kind evolve surrounding donor insemination, we shall indemnify the above named physicians and assistants, the donor or donors, for attorney's fees, court costs, damages, judgments or expenses incurred.

Finally, we individually and collectively acknowledge our obligation to care for, support and otherwise treat any child which results from donor insemination in a fertilization cycle as if it were a naturally conceived child.

_____   _____
Signed   Date

_____   _____
Signed   Date

_____   _____
Physician/Witness   Date

Rev. 3/94

3

Psychologic Issues Associated with Donor Insemination

R. TRACY MacNAB

Before the 1970s, psychologic attention to infertility focused on psychopathology as an etiology. Since that time, investigators have begun to recognize infertility as a life crisis. This chapter continues the current emphasis on studying the traumatic impact of frustrated wishes for parenthood, the responses to the treatment process itself, and the psychosocial impact of living with involuntary childlessness on couples who do not have a preexisting psychiatric diagnosis.

When the already complex issues of infertility are mingled with the additional complexities of therapeutic donor insemination (TDI), it becomes even more important to find a consistent perspective from which we can view the couple's situation as an adaptational challenge rather than as evidence of psychological dysfunction. Normal disruptions are normal and expectable aspects of such circumstances. These disruptions can be grouped into four categories: (1) the impact on narcissistic development and an intact sense of self; (2) issues of sickness, loss, and mortality; (3) jealousy, oedipal concerns, and the "other man"; and (4) sexual dysfunction.

SENSE OF SELF

Kohut's psychology of self (Kohut H, 1977) has established the centrality of a stable and sustainable sense of self to human happiness. The self, the organizing force of the personality that guides how we live our lives, can be disrupted by a disappointment or frustration of a person's innermost hopes and expectations. When the disappointment is severe enough, there can be a perceived deficit of the self, with a concomitant loss of hopefulness about life and a depression of other psychosocial functions. The primary affect of a deficient or faulty self is shame. A couple facing decisions about TDI must face one such potentially shame-producing disappointment.

Many investigators have noted that patients work through the traumatic impact of infertility on the self system in a series of steps (Wieche V, 1976; Menning BE, 1980; MacNab RT, 1985). Further, it has been noted that women and men experience their infertility differently. Women are more likely than men to report infertility-related changes in their lives (Klock SC, Maier D, 1991). There has been considerable attention to the fact that women perceive their inability to conceive as a self deficiency, and there have even been references to women as having more shame (Lewis HB, 1971). However, it is probably more accurate to state that women do not experience shame more than men, but they do tend to talk about it sooner and more readily (Wright F, et al., 1989). The pattern observed in counseling with couples during and after the process of TDI often bears out this assumption. During the early stages of decision making about TDI, there is often a predominant focus on the feelings of the woman. The man typically focuses on her disappointment and on the trouble he is forcing her to go through. There is also concern as to what she will now think of him as a man and a partner. It is frequently necessary in counseling to draw attention to the man's affective experience. Regrettably, it is often difficult for either partner to allow the man the necessary time and space he needs to express his emotions about these events. After a period of delay, however, men's reactions do eventually become a more significant part of the picture. This often occurs about the fourth year of the infertility struggle (MacNab RT, 1993; Osherson S, 1986; Wieche V, 1976).

Another testimony to the importance of shame in the TDI experience is the controversy surrounding the issue of secrecy. There are strong voices arguing for disclosure, especially to the child (Brown MR, 1994; Rowland R, 1985; Daniels K, 1988). There is also concern about the impact of family secrets on the functioning of the family system (Bernstein J, 1993; Penochet JC, et al., 1979). Others, however, counsel the advisability of confidentiality (Curie-Cohen M, et al., 1979; Mahlstedt P, Probasco K, 1991). Despite available professional opinions, most couples continue choosing not to reveal that they have been through TDI (Klock S, 1993). Perceptions that the child's self-esteem or the bond with the parents will be threatened are common. Other concerns include possible social ostracism of either the couple or the child, prejudices against TDI within the larger family system, potential legal complications, and the fear that the child may some day want to search for his or her genetic father.

Case Example.   The Whites are a couple who sought TDI early in their marriage. They knew from the start of their marriage that some form of assisted reproductive technology would be necessary if they were to have children because Mr. White had previously been evaluated and found to have a congenital absence of a vas deferens. This diagnosis had been a considerable shock to him, and he had suffered what he described as a "real bad time" for several months thereafter. His first marriage ended in divorce, and Mr. White had been open about his diagnosis with his current wife from the start of their courtship. They mutually agreed that they wanted to have children, using TDI if necessary. Upon evaluation, Mrs. White was diagnosed with sufficient tubal blockage to require IVF.

In initial counseling sessions the Whites presented themselves as having no concerns about TDI. Most of the emotional issues had to do with Mr. White's concerns for his wife's feelings about the medical procedures. Mrs. White denied any misgivings about the IVF procedures but seemed very concerned about the issue of confidentiality. They had agreed early in their discussions together that the TDI would be a secret they would never reveal. They couched their desire for privacy in concerns about the child feeling alienated from Mr. White and perhaps wishing to search for the biological father. The only conflict that this decision presented for them was that they had no one with whom they could discuss issues of infertility, IVF, and so on. This was particularly hard on Mrs. White because she could not rely on her usual sources of support (her mother and a close friend). The desire for secrecy was contributing to a sense of isolation and shame about the entire process.

With further discussion the Whites were able to loosen the denial about the impact of TDI on their lives. They could admit that their wish for secrecy had at least as much to do with their own emotional conflicts as it did with concern for the prospective child. Mrs. White discussed her worries about the emotional impact of Mr. White's diagnosis on him, her anxiety about how hurt he was by this blow to his manhood, and even her fantasy that Mr. White's first marriage had ended over the issue of infertility. Only then was Mr. White able to talk about how distressing that period of time had been for him and to allow himself (outside the session) some tears about the loss this represented for him.

Without the counseling sessions, Mr. and Mrs. White might well have continued to present a united front of denial about their own emotional struggles. Mrs. White might not have explored her misgivings about her husband's emotional vulnerability, and Mr. White would have had to find another channel for the expression of his grief. One can speculate about the impact of such unresolved conflicts on a future child, but there were immediately observable adaptive changes in the couple. First, each was able to speak and be heard by the other. Second, they reaffirmed their belief in the importance of open communication between them. Finally, though their resolve to keep TDI a secret did not change, they were talking about the possibility that Mrs. White might discuss some of her experience with a trusted friend.

It is apparent that couples collaborate and collude in the creation and maintenance of a self system that they believe will weather the emotional trials of infertility. In the case of TDI, attention is drawn to the male factor. The feared damage to the man's narcissism leads to a defensive refocusing of attention to the woman's emotional responses. There is an unconscious assumption in such cases that the man's self-esteem is too frail and vulnerable to bear the emotional impact of what is perceived to be a failure of his masculinity. Couples' counseling can be quite useful in such cases because it can use existing defensive structures (e.g., the highlighting of the wife's emotional responses) to redirect attention to the source of the distress (e.g., the perception of narcissistic vulnerability in the husband). Through these means, the salient issues can be brought to light and given the opportunity for healing.

SICKNESS, LOSS, AND MORTALITY

Becker (1973), in his dramatic revisioning of Freud, puts mortality at the psychological core of human identity. He writes (of menopause) that changes in a woman's reproductive cycle impose

---

a definite physical milestone on the person, putting up a wall and saying, "You are not going any further into life now, you are going toward the end, to the absolute determinism of death." As men don't have such . . . specific markers of a physical kind, they don't usually experience a . . . stark discrediting of the body . . . . But the woman . . . is put in the position of having to catch up psychologically with the physical facts of life (p. 215).

Male factor infertility places men in the unaccustomed role of measuring the scope and span of their lives with physiological milestones. This circumstance jars the more typical sociocultural notion that manhood is distinct from anatomical maleness (Gilmore DD, 1990) because in contrast to women, who define their reproductive maturity from menstruation through menopause, the ascension to manhood seems less a physiologic event and more a culturally and socially created condition. The process of TDI serves as a reminder to men that they also cannot transcend aging and the cycle of life and death. The introduction of another man's genetic line into the family harshly confronts fantasies of a connection to immortality. These realizations can be profoundly unsettling to a man and thereby also to the marriage. If the male factor diagnosis is related to a prior illness or medical condition, the confrontation can be particularly harsh.

Case Example. Mr. Greene was referred for psychotherapy because of a depression that began after he and his wife undertook the initial stages of TDI. He did not believe that his depression could be related to the TDI process, because he felt that he had dealt with the issue years before. He had been told in early adolescence, following chemotherapy and radiation treatment for testicular cancer, that he could never have children. He related that this had always been a fact of his life and that he had undergone a semen analysis before his marriage that had confirmed his diagnosis. He and his future wife had discussed the matter and agreed that they would pursue TDI. They both considered the subject closed. After some exploratory probing, Mr. Greene revealed that he was having some frightening nightmares about being a child alone in a hospital room. This led to a vivid recounting of his experiences with cancer and a realization that he had suppressed his overwhelming terror and fear of dying because it would not be manly and it would alarm his parents if he cried or complained. He came to see that his depression was the result of the conflict between his and his wife's desire to have a child and his rejection of TDI (and, consequently, the child it might produce) as reminders of his repressed emotional trauma. Over the following year, Mr. Greene reworked his memories of the painful cancer experience and was able to finally grieve for the real and symbolic losses he was suffering. His depression resolved, the couple successfully went through TDI, and he wholeheartedly accepted the child as his own.

TDI can be a reminder of one's mortality because it represents the ending of the man's blood line. This impression gathers extra strength from the medicalization of the process of conception. Even for people without a prior history of major illnesses, childbearing can seem to be more a matter of sickness, loss, and disappointment than of assisted reproduction.

OEDIPAL RIVALRY AND THE OTHER MAN

In a culture that largely lacks consensually validated rites of passage, (Raphael R, 1988), parenthood is often seen as the entry into adulthood. As noted above, males do not have some of the biological markers of this development, and therefore the identification of the self as masculine and mature is a more vulnerable arrangement (Krugman S, 1994). Paternity provides some ameliorative opportunities for restructuring the unsatisfactory experiences of childhood as well as for identification with the positive aspects of one's father (Osherson S, 1992; Colarusso CA, Nemiroff RA, 1982). TDI can place obstacles in the path of this generational reckoning with the legacy of the father and development of an adult, masculine identification. The extreme reluctance of couples to tell the husband's father about TDI (Bernstein J, 1993) seems to be testimony that this aspect of the process is highly conflictual.

Case Example. Six months after the birth of his son, Mr. Black sought psychotherapy for a series of anxiety attacks. The child was his first, conceived through TDI, and Mr. Black had been very happy with the success of the intervention. His wife, who had initially been very distressed at their failure to get pregnant, was now glowing with happiness. During the pregnancy, Mr. Black felt a reprieve from his guilty feeling that his azoospermia was depriving his wife of the thing she most wanted, to be a mother. He loved his son very much and found fatherhood more fulfilling than he had imagined. However, he would find himself closely examining his son's face for signs of another man's features. He and his wife had decided to keep the TDI a secret, and each time a friend or family member commented on how much his son looked like him, he had the uncomfortable feeling that he was a fraud. When his son developed colic, depriving the entire family of needed sleep, he was alarmed at the intensity of his anger. He feared that the absence of a biologic bond would make it likely that he would grow to hate this child. He feared the extremes of his anger and condemned himself for his failures as a father.

Psychotherapy focused on an examination of his reasons for keeping TDI a secret. Both he and his wife had been concerned about his father's reaction to this news, and so they had decided that they would not tell members of the family about the situation. Mr. Black saw his father as a perfectionist whom he had always striven to please. He anticipated that the news of his infertility would lose forever the chance to be approved as a whole man by his father. As these feelings were articulated, Mr. Black learned a more forgiving self-regard. It was possible to reassure him that hateful feelings were a normal part of being a parent of a colicky child, rather than the aberrant responses of an unloving outsider. The Blacks continued to keep the TDI a secret between them but developed a much improved communication between themselves about the trials and conflicts of the process.

TDI can activate intrafamilial struggles that might otherwise be resolved by the arrival of a grandchild. These conflicts need not be severe to become part of the TDI picture, but instead are emphasized by the presence of male factor infertility and the perceived intrusion of the donor into the couple's family planning.

SEXUAL DYSFUNCTION

Several investigators point out the relatively high frequency of sexual dysphoria or frank dysfunction in couples seeking TDI (deVries K, et al., 1984; Glezerman M, 1981; Cooper S, 1993). Changes in sexual drive, ovulatory function, and potency (Berger DM, 1980; Penochet JC, et al., 1979; Vere MF, Joyce DN, 1979) have been observed in a large percentage of this population. Because infertility workups and treatment focus sexuality almost exclusively on the goal of producing children, there is less room for sexual expression of pleasure, mutual sharing, and communication. Depending on the couple's intimate history and habits and on the ease with which they can talk about their own sexuality, this interruption of the usual pathway for negotiating physical and affiliative needs is usually destructive. No couple escapes at least a temporary alteration in their relational pattern. The medical intrusions into the couple's private life also heavily emphasize the man's responsibility for the problem. This emphasis can feel like blame or rubbing salt in a wound. Since sexuality is a performance issue for many men, the increase in shame and anxiety can impair their pleasure as well as their sexual capacity. Such impairments may draw out a protective response from many wives (Cooper S, 1993).

Case Example. Mr. and Mrs. Gray sought marital therapy because of tension over their sexual incompatibility. This was the second marriage for Mr. Gray, who had fathered a daughter (now an adolescent living part-time with them) before having a vasectomy. The Grays had known that TDI would be necessary because their health insurance did not cover vasectomy repair and they could not afford to pay for a vasovasostomy. However, from the onset of their decision to begin the process, their sex life virtually halted. They made several efforts at lovemaking, but Mrs. Gray had no interest. Mr. Gray, feeling that his advances were unwelcome, withdrew into a quietly resentful silence. Until this time the Grays had maintained a regular and mutually satisfactory sexual life. On the fourth cycle of TDI,

Mrs. Gray conceived and bore a son, after which all pretenses at sexual involvement ceased. Mr. Gray became absorbed in his work, and Mrs. Gray devoted herself to being a mother and continuing her job on a part-time basis. When the child was six months old, Mr. Gray insisted that the couple seek marital therapy to improve their sexual relationship.

In sessions, Mr. Gray complained of feeling unloved and rejected by his wife. She had been aware of Mr. Gray's displeasure but was surprised to learn how angry he was. She stated that rather than deal with an irritated partner, she had instead concentrated on the more pleasurable activity of caring for her son. Her long-deferred dream of being a mother had come true, and she wanted to enjoy it while she could. She found Mr. Gray's anger unsupportive and perceived it as a personal attack on her. Mr. Gray took her defensiveness as further evidence that she was no longer interested in him and that she had, in effect, found a better man.

Considerable time and hard work were necessary to resolve the difference between the Grays. Mrs. Gray eventually admitted that she had experienced a loss of libido after the birth of the child, and during that time she was not as interested in her husband as a sexual partner. Mr. Gray shared his own insecurities about his role in the family, since he had no biologic link to his son. The couple also reworked issues about the combined family that they had created. Mrs. Gray had seen Mr. Gray's irritability as selfish because he already had a child. Mr. Gray had seen his son as another man who had won his wife's affection. Eventually, they were able to come to terms with the changes in their family and to see that all of the relationships within their family system needed to be reexamined. They agreed that their marriage needed a renewed courtship, although a very different courtship from their original one. A three-year follow-up revealed that though their sex life had not re-turned to the pre-TDI frequency, both Mr. and Mrs. Gray were satisfied with their marital adjustment. Both of them also felt that they had learned about the value of communication from the experience.

TDI can leave a couple in a double-bind style of communication. The man feels that his status in the marriage is reduced by both physiologic limitation and his wife's preoccupation with becoming pregnant. He feels that he can't complain about this change in the marriage because he views himself as responsible for causing the problem. She senses his emotional vulnerability and tries to make things better by avoiding the topic. Although communication may be more necessary than ever, both partners feel constrained by their circumstances not to discuss the problem. Unaddressed binds of this sort can produce long-term sexual dysfunctions in a marriage. Seeing the couple together in such cases is often highly useful. In this manner, the man does not have to begin as the focus of attention and thereby feel that his deficits are the cause for concern. Attention can be initially directed to the emotional responses of the partner who is most able to communicate about the trouble and can gradually be redirected to the hidden and shameful aspects of the difficulty.

CONCLUSION

The case examples cited above are not intended to exhaustively cover all of the psychological issues associated with TDI, nor are they intended to suggest that all couples react in these specific fashions. They are offered as an insight into the growing body of knowledge and speculation about the short- and longer-term impact of this widely employed procedure. We still have much to learn, particularly longitudinally, about the consequences of our efforts to help couples conceive.

It is increasingly clear that infertility, and the assisted-reproductive technology we use to treat it, can have a significant traumatic impact on the couple and on each of the individuals in the marriage. This impact appears to be mediated but not eliminated by foreknowledge of the need for TDI (such as prior vasectomy or medical condition). Even when the couple know well in advance about the male factor infertility and there will be no shock or surprise when the diagnosis is discovered, there can still be significant impact on self-concept, sense of well-being and hopefulness, and sexual communication and satisfaction. There is reason to suspect that this impact is still quite great even in cases of secondary infertility or when there is a child from a prior marriage.

There is also a series of questions that remain to be explored. What role does age play in the impact of TDI on the couple? Are younger couples less troubled by this intrusion into their conceptualizations about mortality and the intactness of the self system? What about the psychodynamic structure of this technology as it is applied to single mothers or lesbian couples? How are our biases and preconceptions influencing our decision making about suitable candidates for the process? What is the meaning of the reluctance to use known sperm donors when the known egg donor process is so frequently practiced? How are cultural and social perceptions about TDI changing, and how are we contributing to this change in assumptions about conception, family building, and the rearing of children? Finally, and most important, what is the impact on the children whom we are helping into this world? Data and hypotheses are being assembled, but we are far from having a clear picture (Bernstein J, 1993).

What is apparent from an anecdotal clinical perspective is that the couples and individuals who seek counseling or psychotherapy are frequently better able to accept the experience of TDI, and couples are better able to re-establish the bond between them and to grieve for their losses. Whether or not their future includes parenting, processing the traumatic interruption of their adult development helps them to get on with their lives.

REFERENCES

1. Becker E. (1973) The Denial of Death. New York: Free Press.
2. Berger DM. (1980) Impotence following the discovery of azoospermia. Fertil Steril 34:154–156.
3. Bernstein J. (1993) The long-term psychologic and social effects of gamete donation. In: Seibel MM, Kiessling AA, Bernstein J, Levin SR, eds. Technology and Infertility: Clinical, Psychological, Legal, and Ethical Aspects. New York: Springer-Verlag.
4. Brown MR. (1994) Whose eyes are these, whose nose? Newsweek March 7:12.
5. Colarusso CA, Nemiroff RA. (1982) The father in midlife: Crisis and the growth of paternal identity. In: Cath SH, Gurwitt AR, Ross JM, eds. Father and Child: Developmental and Clinical Perspectives. Boston: Little, Brown.
6. Cooper S. (1993) Paradise lost: Sexual function and infertility. In: Seibel MM, Kiessling AA, Bernstein J, Levin SR, eds. Technology and Infertility: Clinical, Psychological, Legal, and Ethical Aspects. New York: Springer-Verlag.
7. Curie-Cohen M, Luttrell L, Shapiro S. (1979) Current practice of artificial insemination by donor in the United States. N Eng J Med 300:585–590.
8. Daniels K. (1988) Artificial insemination using donor sperm and the issue of secrecy: The views of donors and recipient couples. Soc Sci Med 27:377–383.
9. deVries K, et al. (1984) The influence of the post coital test on the sexual function of infertile women. Psychosom Obstet Gynaecol 3.
10. Gilmore DD. (1990) Manhood in the Making: Cultural Concepts of Masculinity. New Haven, Conn.: Yale University Press.
11. Glezerman M. (1981) Two hundred and seventy cases of artificial donor insemination: Management and results. Fertil Steril 35:180.
12. Klock S. (1993) The psychological aspects of donor insemination. Infertil Reprod Clin N Amer 4:455–469.

13. Klock SC, Maier D. (1991) Psychological factors related to donor insemination. Fertil Steril 56:489–495.

14. Kohut H. (1977) The Restoration of the Self. New York: International Universities Press.

15. Krugman S. (1994) Male development and the transformation of shame. In: Levant R, Pollack W, eds. A New Psychology of Men. New York: Basic Books.

16. Lewis HB. (1971) Shame and Guilt in Neurosis. Hillsdale, N.J.: Lawrence Erlbaum Associates.

17. MacNab RT. (1985) Infertility and men: A study of change and adaptive choices in the lives of involuntarily childless men. Dissertation Abstracts International 774–778.

18. MacNab RT. (1993) Male infertility: The psychologic issues. In: Seibel MM, Kiessling AA, Bernstein J, Levin SR, eds. Technology and Infertility: Clinical, Psychological, Legal and Ethical Aspects. New York: Springer-Verlag.

19. Mahlstedt P, Probasco K. (1991) Their attitudes providing medical and psychosocial aspects of donor insemination. Infertil Reprod Clin N Amer 4:455–469.

20. Menning BE. (1980) The emotional needs of infertile couples. Fertil Steril 34:313–317.

21. Osherson S. (1992) Wrestling with Love: How Men Struggle with Intimacy, Women, Children, Parents and Each Other. New York: Ballantine.

22. Osherson S. (1986) Finding our Fathers. New York: Free Press.

23. Penochet JC, Moran P, Jarrige A. (1979) Psychiatric complications linked to AID. Ann Med Psychol 137:635.

24. Raphael R. (1988) The Men from the Boys: Rites of Passage in Male America. Lincoln: University of Nebraska Press.

25. Rowland R. (1985) The social and psychological consequences of secrecy in artificial insemination by donor (AID) programmes. Soc Sci Med 21:391–396.

26. Vere MF, Joyce DN. (1979) Luteal function in patients seeking AID. Br Med J 6182:100.

27. Wieche V. (1976) Psychological reactions to infertility. Psych Rpts 38:863–866.

28. Wright F, O'Leary J, Balkin J. (1989) Shame, guilt, narcissism and depression: Correlates and sex differences. Psychoanal Psych 6:217–230.

4

Program Design for Successful Egg Donation

JUDITH BERNSTEIN, R.N.

Over the last hundred years, therapeutic donor insemination (TDI) has come of age, maturing dramatically from its first known use, in which a physician reportedly inseminated an anesthetized woman without the knowledge of the patient or her husband. Donor insemination today is understood to have significant psychological and social ramifications (Bernstein J, 1993; Mahlsted PP, Greenfield DA, 1989). To that end, the American Society for Reproductive Medicine (ASRM) developed guidelines for counseling, consent, screening, and matching to describe responsible TDI practice (Ethics Committee of the American Fertility Society, November, 1994). Because the ASRM already had an ethics committee in place that had pondered current practices in sperm donation, it was well positioned to respond to the rapid evolution of egg donation and to develop standards designed to protect all parties involved: recipient couple, donor, and potential offspring.

The guidelines that resulted are significant in that they address a number of important issues and recommend minimum standards. However, they are not sufficiently comprehensive to totally standardize care among the hundreds of egg donation programs that are springing up all over the United States in response to the demand for this successful new technology. This is at least in part due to unanticipated issues that continually occur in association with egg donation. Consequently,

programs have frequently "reinvented the wheel," causing standards to differ widely between clinics (Braverman et al., 1993). A modification of the ASRM guideline is provided in Appendix 4-A.

Although the medical aspects of egg donation have become simplified (Rosenwaks Z, 1987), the social and ethical issues raised by egg donation are complex and difficult (Robertson JA, 1989; Schenker JG, 1992; Grodin MA, 1993). Egg donation challenges traditional views of women, reproduction, and family by permitting a woman of almost any age to gestate a child that is not genetically her own. As a result, family relationships become blurred (an aunt may be a genetic mother, or a woman might gestate her mother's or daughter's genetic child), and chronologic relationships become distorted (a child's mother could be the same age as his friend's grandmother). Social relationships also become blurred and awkward as children who are raised in the same social circle with the donor and her children could find themselves biologically related but totally unaware of their genetic connection.

Another set of concerns arises from the relationship between donor and recipient(s). As in sperm donation, the egg donor is a third party involved in creating another family through gamete donation. In contrast to the sperm donor, however, the egg donor must commit to an extensive and intensive time involvement with considerably more risk. Thus there is increased potential for miscommunication, manipulation, and victimization of either party. Both donors and recipients may enter the arrangement psychologically vulnerable and become devastated by an adverse outcome. Contracts may be broken or, over time, regretted. In addition, social support for the process, both culturally and intellectually, is inadequate, causing considerable disagreement about family policy without benefit of tested legal or ethical principles. Consequently, all participants, including medical professionals, potential donors, and egg recipient candidates must understand that they are operating in a relative vacuum, traversing a country without roads for the foreseeable future. For all these reasons the medical team that decides to establish a program must be prepared to engage in lengthy ethical discussion and extensive and ongoing review of detailed policies and procedures for recruitment, counseling, selection, matching, and follow-up. Similarly, potential donors and recipients should be encouraged to carefully examine the policies and guidelines of programs with which they affiliate.

Each egg donation site will have special issues to consider that are related to the nature of its specific community, its cultural and religious values, and its institutional relationships and organization. The purpose of this chapter is to provide general principles for use in developing and reviewing an egg donation program and to help potential donors and patients formulate questions and make informed decisions.

SETTING UP AN EGG DONATION PROGRAM: THE ETHICAL DEBATE

Ethical debate is a guaranteed part of any egg donation program, whether it is planned for or not. Each patient who walks through the door potentially brings issues that were never anticipated or raised in program planning. On the new frontier of advanced reproductive technologies, the unlikely is probable, and the unusual often becomes the norm. In situations in which immediate precedent is not available, three general principles of medical ethics, applied through the centuries, can provide a focus for discussion: beneficence (the commitment of healers to relieve suffering), nonmaleficence (the injunction to do no harm), and autonomy (the goal of respect for the individual person).

Beneficence

For the donor the concept of relieving suffering takes on an altogether new slant because the donor is neither a patient, with all the commitment that status implies, nor suffering. Yet care must be taken because medical professionals are indeed performing "patient care" in the form of invasive procedures. Although the donor does not present in the usual format with a complaint, egg donation can provide beneficence, or benefit, in the form of gratification through altruism, increased self-esteem, or fulfillment of a desire to rework a negative past experience with a better outcome, such as a donor who has had an earlier abortion helping a couple have a child through egg donation. As in most medical decisions, the key feature is the risk-benefit analysis. Since the potential benefit to the donor is both abstract and nonessential for continued well-being, the ratio must be weighed individually and with extreme care (Frydman R, et al., 1990; Lessor R, et al., 1993; Sauer M, et al., 1989; Bolton V, et al., 1991).

Benefit may also imply financial terms. The ASRM guidelines appropriately define financial benefit, with reimbursement permitted for time, trouble, and risk but not for sale of body parts. There is concern that monetary exchange may contribute to depersonalization of the donor and provide undue pressure for donation. Programs that opt for direct remuneration of donors are advised to develop financial policies that explicitly preclude sale of eggs and establish a reimbursement schedule that is directly tied to amount of time and risk involved at each stage of the process (Seibel MM, Kiessling A, 1993). The various steps involved in egg donation, such as screening, ovulation induction and retrieval, for example, create convenient places for prorating donor compensation in the case of cancellations. Programs that leave financial arrangements to private negotiation between donor and recipient should suggest that each party have separate legal counsel to protect individual rights and indirectly to provide some safeguard for the program. Such an agreement should not contain compensation clauses or other stipulations that are ethically inappropriate.

Issues of beneficence for the recipient are related to the vulnerability experienced by an individual who desires something desperately (Kirkland A, et al., 1991). However, suffering is not always relieved by the relentless pursuit of a biologic child. For a particular couple, permission to stop and either adopt or pursue a life without parenting may be of far greater benefit than repeated cycles of egg donation that exhaust both finances and spirit (Seibel MM, 1992). For this reason, many programs require counseling to assess the emotional reserves of potential recipients and assist them with values clarification and decision making.

The principle of beneficence must also be considered for the offspring of egg donation. A child born to older parents who do not live to see him or her through adolescence (Seibel MM, et al., 1994) or who experiences a family that is distressed by the burden of blurred relationships may not as an adult accept the premise that egg donation has been beneficial. "It's a terrible burden," says a leader of a national TDI peer support group, "to be created as a solution to my parents' problems."

Some programs choose to refer recipients for counseling when there are questions about parenting potential or emotional stability. Others set limits for age, exclude mother-daughter donation, or reject prospective recipients on psychologic grounds. Programs may limit recipients to married heterosexual couples in the belief that children have a right to a traditional family, although the majority of children in the United States are no longer raised within a nuclear family and the definition of "traditional" is changing (see Prologue). As long as the same services are available elsewhere in the community, differing policies based on reasonable criteria do not limit candidates' access to egg donation. The only characteristic that programs must share is adherence to a medical standard of thorough consideration of medical, ethical, and legal rights.

Nonmaleficence

For the donor the principle of "do no harm" means frank discussion of both emotional and physical risks (Vernale C, Packard SA, 1990; Lancet Editorial Board, 1993). The prospective donor who has been the victim of sexual abuse, lost parents at an early age, grown up in a disturbed household, or experienced any other traumatic event may be placed at risk by egg donation. Evaluation should consider prospective donors beyond their ability to reliably provide eggs (focus on the vulnerability of the recipient) and attempt to anticipate the possibility of an adverse psychological outcome (focus on the vulnerability of the donor). In an initial consultation with a prospective donor, potential physical risks and pain during procedures should be described in detail, including possible complications of retrieval, hyperstimulation, or compromise of future fertility. Research that tentatively suggests an increase in ovarian cancer after ovulation induction should be discussed, for example, along with a description of the flaws in the study. A prospective donor who is concerned about possible drug effects might prefer a natural cycle (Seibel MM, et al., 1995) or a partially medicated one (Seibel MM, 1995) to a fully stimulated one.

To do no harm, the medical team must get to know the donor as well as the recipient, who is often already a familiar patient. It is not uncommon in known donor situations for tremendous pressure to be brought to bear on the prospective donor. As one recipient with premature menopause phrased it, "My sister got all the luck and all the good eggs—she owes me a baby." Similarly, a mother may threaten to break off communications if one sister does not help the other. Screening protocols should detect this type of manipulation and protect the donor's right to refuse donation in the face of family pressure.

Another major concern is avoiding pregnancy for the donor, since donors must discontinue hormonal contraception in order to donate. Donors may already have small children of their own and fear conception in an egg donation cycle if one egg is left behind. All donors should be provided with adequate barrier contraception and should be impressed with the need to use it scrupulously.

For the recipient, "do no harm" requires strict adherence to standard screening procedures for genetic risk and infectious diseases. In addition, a recipient who is concerned about sequelae for offspring from ovulation induction medications might be offered a natural cycle donation of a donor who receives limited medication. Clear and precise policies and guidelines related to information about the donor must be discussed initially so that issues of genetic contribution will not surface after a pregnancy has already been established. Recipients should be told at the time of their initial consultation how much information they will receive about their anonymous donor so that there is still time to act on concerns about protecting future offspring. Care

must be taken not to set up unrealistic expectations for success or to offer guarantees. Medical professionals, in their eagerness to help, could be misinterpreted by patients who are looking for promises.

For offspring, "do no harm" means careful evaluation of donor history to reduce potential risks from transmitting genetic disease. Similarly, every reasonable precaution should be taken to prevent multiple pregnancy. Many programs initially underestimate the fertilization and implantation rates of eggs from young, healthy donors and transfer the same numbers of embryos they are accustomed to returning in their IVF patients. The result is often multiple gestation, and the risk of those infants being born prematurely and having a poor prognosis creates a potential nightmare for infertility patients. Protocols for transfer should be developed that take into account the differences in egg donation implantation rates.

Autonomy

Autonomy issues are similar for both donor and recipient. Respect for person implies equal standing between patient and medical professional and shared decision making based on mutual understanding. For the patient to be an equal partner in medical planning, both counseling and extensive education are necessary to provide to the participants self-knowledge as well as knowledge of their medical alternatives.

The last decade has seen a major transition away from the medical model of "doctor knows best," which places responsibility for the patient's well-being squarely on the physician and limits patients' ability to make their own decisions. This type of relationship does not fit the construct of modern reproductive technology and does not best meet the needs of patients or physicians. Current infertility treatments, especially those involving third parties, are both financially and emotionally expensive and have long-range ramifications. Today's decisions will require justification to offspring decades from now, long after all connection has ceased between physician and patient. Physicians may also be called to account many years in the future, as society's mores and ethical precepts change (Koval R, 1990; Raymond JG, 1994). Such a burden is best shared.

There are also autonomy issues to be taken into account for the yet-unborn offspring. What rights will the child have to information about his or her genetic parent? Will lack of information compromise the child's sense of identity and/or self-esteem, or will too much information cause confusion and anxiety? Will the child's right to identifying information about the donor at a future date supersede the donor's right to privacy? If so, what ethical decisions will the program make about availability of facts for future release? The egg donation program is obligated to provide to the recipients nonidentifying information about the donor that could later be released to children, even if parents state that they will opt for secrecy and do not plan to use it. However, at present there is no consensus on the amount of information that is appropriate for release. As research data becomes available, medical professionals may be in a better position to answer these questions. For the present, the team must rely on ethical debate to achieve consensus on which to base policy.

A model for sharing ethical decision-making responsibility that works quite well is affiliation of an egg donation team with a separately constituted ethics advisory board. A general institutional ethics board can serve the purpose if a good working relationship exists and the board members are familiar with reproductive issues. Otherwise, a special advisory group can be constituted containing clergymen, scientists, attorneys, and laypeople who are interested in the ethics of reproductive policies (see Chapter 11).

A board of this type serves three purposes. First, it can examine in depth the general ethical issues related to egg donation. From this analysis comes guidance for developing program policies and procedures. Second, it can focus on particular patient problems, discuss troubling incidents and events, and give guidance for specific patient care. Third, by serving as both check-and-balance and validation of program efforts, an ethics advisory board reassures patients, reduces team anxiety, and decreases the likelihood of future adverse legal action.

DEVELOPING A TEAM

The egg donation team may be organized in a variety of ways and may be composed of several subgroups. The individuals who are commonly involved are the medical director, physician responsible for day-to-day operation of the egg donation program, nurse-coordinator, embryologist, ultrasonographer, laboratory personnel, counselor, office manager, insurance biller, financial manager, liaison with outside services (operating room, radiology, recovery room, etc.), liaison with hospital administration, and liaison with the ethics committee. One individual may wear several hats, but all roles should be identified in advance, and their responsibilities should be clearly defined. Teams often function best if divided into small working groups, three or four key people being involved at different stages in the process. Matching of donor and recipient, for example, might be done by a nurse, counselor, and physician, while budget planning might involve the medical director, insurance biller, and financial manager. Clinical members might gather each week with the embryologist to review upcoming cycles and evaluate the results of completed cycles. Agendas and minutes are especially helpful if the entire team meets infrequently.

THE COUNSELING COMPONENT

Three types of decisions must be made about a counseling component in setting up an egg donation program: (1) Who will be involved? (2) What mandate will the mental health person receive from the program? (3) What will the relationship be between the counseling staff and the egg donation team?

Mental health professionals have different levels and types of training as well as different approaches, and no one individual can provide all the necessary resources. Most teams use a psychologist for administering psychometric tests, although clinical evaluations can be done by a social worker, psychologist, clinical nurse specialist in psychiatry, or psychiatrist. If a psychiatrist is not directly involved in the program, it will be necessary to have a referral relationship for patients who are taking psychotropic medications or may need to do so. A critical factor in the success of a mental health division is the previous experience of the mental health professionals with infertility patients. Issues related to infertility are rarely covered in counseling training and are neglected in the psychiatric literature. As a result, mental health professionals may either overdiagnose or underdiagnose the stresses and miseries of infertility patients.

The issue of mandate also requires decision making. Will all donors and recipients be expected to be interviewed before acceptance into the program, or will the mental health professional be used only occasionally as a resource when obvious problems emerge? Will evaluation consist of written testing, clinical interview, or both? What procedures will be established for either donors or recipients who are described by the counselor as being at risk? If patients can be rejected, what will they be told, and who will disclose the information? Is any psychological follow-up planned for either donor or recipient for research or clinical purposes? Although patients may initially balk at the expense of mental health sessions or feel reluctant to disclose private information to a stranger, resistance usually disappears if policies are clearly described from the very beginning and the goal of protection of patients is explained. Persistent resistance to participate in mental health sessions usually heralds a problem patient. Whatever answers your team arrives at, the next step is distillation into written material for patient handouts.

Finally, there is the matter of the relationship of the mental health professional to the team. Some programs simply refer and get written reports, but both patient and team benefit if it is possible to include the counselor or psychiatrist in weekly team meetings. In such a case the mental health person can play a triple role: evaluation of the patient, problem solving for the patient, and problem solving for the team.

THE PATIENT EDUCATION MODULE

Both egg donors and recipients are different from typical IVF patients, and established educational practices may need to be adapted for them. Because donors are presumed to be fertile, they may have knowledge deficits about infertility and its therapy and may have formed unrealistic expectations about the intensity of the process or the likelihood of success. The infertility patient approaches IVF forewarned, knowing that treatment is emotionally invasive, often uncomfortable, and generally disruptive to personal and work life. The egg donor does not have that background experience to rely on in deciding to go ahead. Nor is the donor as motivated; there is no direct benefit to her as great as the promise of a child, against which infertility patients balance distress and pain. So the natural optimism and desire to please that are inherent in the altruistic act of egg donation must be tempered with repeated information about the details of the commitment and potential for complications.

The recipient may also be in a compromised situation. If ovarian failure is the result of cancer, early menopause, or traumatic surgery, the recipient, like the donor, may lack adequate information. If she has been through repeated infertility procedures, including many failed IVF cycles, she may be emotionally exhausted and have difficulty retaining or accepting information.

In both of these situations the answer is information, repeated and presented in several ways. The goals of education are to obtain a truly informed consent, to establish reasonable expectations, to prepare patients for medication and procedure routines and possible emotional sequelae, to assist in decision making, and to reduce anxiety.

Educational materials can begin with a detailed program description packet sent out at first telephone contact. After the first consultation, patients can be given an acceptance packet explaining required tests, insurance validation, counseling process, and information about whom to call with which questions. Before beginning medications, patients also need information about the instructions necessary for receiving medication, testing, and pre-op requirements. In addition, one-on-one teaching is a valuable reinforcement that can take place at several points: after the first consultation, during the preparation phase, at the time of cycle start, and during daily callbacks for test results and medication instructions. A phone call is helpful to both donor and recipient in the post-retrieval and post-transfer period, before the outcome is known. Support groups and seminars are also useful, particularly if they permit networking of recipient couples.

Education is usually the responsibility of the nurse-coordinator. Because of the enormity of detail involved, egg donation is labor-intensive. A nurse who is assigned to egg donation will be able to handle about half the number of patients she or he previously coordinated for IVF, and additional time must be allocated for accurate record keeping, emotional support of patients, and the volume of educational activity.

RECRUITMENT, SCREENING, AND MATCHING PROCEDURES

Recruitment policies and methods will influence the character of the donor pool. Hospital employees represent an easily available source of young, healthy women, but they may also have relatively easy access to recipients' records. College students are also young and healthy women, but many have unproven fertility, and they themselves may develop infertility at a later date and regret being a donor. If a patient population is affluent and middle-class, does advertising in working-class communities risk the appearance of marketing body parts and charges of discrimination and victimization? If a potential donor has survived a chaotic family of origin and is doing well herself but has siblings in jail or on drugs, does that mean she is too vulnerable to donate, or is she a good candidate because she is a demonstrated survivor? What medical conditions will be listed as causes for exclusion, and which will be accepted? If a donor has no insurance coverage herself, who is financially responsible for complications that might occur?

Decisions must be made about these and other possible parameters of donor acceptability including age, marital status, family and personal medical history, genetic history, reproductive record, occupation, educational level, income level, emotional stability, drug and alcohol history, sexual orientation, history of trauma and loss, relationship with recipient (if known donation). Exclusions may also be established for recipients based on age, relationship, medical factors such as recent cancer history, concerns about emotional stability, and other criteria. Some decisions must be made on a case-by-case basis, as circumstances will inevitably arise that no one anticipated. Nevertheless, it is helpful to list as many scenarios as possible before beginning and to continuously attempt to set consistent limits.

Protocols must also be established for screening. The order of the process will vary depending on the circumstances of each program, but the common elements are a nurse interview to provide and obtain information; a physician interview to examine, assess, and counsel; a mental health visit to assess, educate, and provide a context for donor and patient self-examination; and laboratory testing for infection and systemic illness. In a team approach, once information is collected, a subgroup of the team meets to review and discuss. Topics that are commonly considered in accepting a donor or a patient are medical status; genetic and emotional history; psychometric test results; apparent motivation; medical, nursing, and mental health assessment of reliability and stability; results of physical exam and infection-screening panel; and physical and psychologic risk factors.

If a donor is rejected, she may either be informed of the specific reason or simply be told that there is no match at present. If the reason for rejection is related to an identified emotional vulnerability, it may not be necessary to communicate this information unless she is thought to be experiencing a treatable disorder, in which case a referral should be made. If the donor is rejected for a medical cause, she should be informed and either treated or referred. At Faulkner Center for Reproductive Medicine, potential donors are informed at their initial visit that the screening process might uncover information about themselves that they were unaware of. They are asked whether or not they would like to have that information revealed to them.

Donor and patient matching may also occur as a team effort. This is especially helpful when no individual knows both parties well. Matching criteria may be as broad as eye, hair, and skin color and phenotype or may be much more specific and include occupation, educational level, hobbies and interests, or specific patient requests such as athletic ability. Minimal criteria for matching should be described in a policy statement that is made available at the start of both donor and recipient involvement. It is often helpful for a blank disclosure form to be included in the initial information packet.

The disclosure statement should also contain clinic policy concerning refusal of a donor. For instance, if a recipient does not want a particular donor for reasons that appear trivial to the program but have great import for a couple, what is the clinic policy how refusal affects a couple's chances for a future donor? Will the couple stay at the top of the list or go to the bottom? If the reason is clearly nontrivial, such as a history of alcoholism in the donor's immediate family, will it still count as a rejection?

Information about a prospective donor should be provided, in writing, to recipients in advance of the need for a decision, to allow time for serious consideration. Any appearance of rush or pressure may contribute to doubts and anxieties during pregnancy and early parenthood.

THE ROLE OF THE COORDINATOR: PRACTICAL CONSIDERATIONS

The cornerstone of successful egg donation is a well-functioning IVF program, but special procedures and guidelines will need to be developed and the role of the IVF coordinator will need to be expanded to address complex emotional needs and privacy issues of egg donation patients.

Issues of confidentiality must be ironed out before the first procedure is begun. All staff members, both program and hospital, who interact with donors and recipients will need special in-service training sessions that should cover goals and procedures. Otherwise, staff members will be attempting to figure out who is whom or will ask inappropriate questions through natural curiosity and good intentions. Similarly, if staff members do not understand the principles behind special requirements, such as the use of codes for anonymous donors, they may not comply with the extra work that is involved.

For known donors, privacy should be protected. The following scenario illustrates the point: Suppose that a recipient's husband (John) and his mother-in-law (Mrs. Brooks) are sitting together in the waiting room on the day of retrieval, waiting to hear how many eggs have been obtained from John's wife's sister Mary (Mrs. Brooks's other daughter). The nurse knows that Mrs. Brooks has been involved all along in the decision to use egg donation. She approaches John and tells him in front of Mrs. Brooks that she needs a sperm specimen now. John becomes horribly embarrassed. He was uncomfortable about masturbation in the first place but is overwhelmed at having it discussed in front of his mother-in-law. He wants to know how many eggs they got but doesn't ask because he doesn't want Mrs. Brooks to think he's just after her daughter Mary's eggs. Mrs. Brooks want to ask how Mary is doing but doesn't want John to think she's a worrywart or that she blames him for subjecting Mary to risk. They both want to be able to call John's wife Joan (Mrs. Brooks's older daughter), who is at work, to tell her the news, but neither wants to appear to vie for who is more important to Joan. Through not understanding the difference between privacy and confidentiality, the nurse can step into the hornet's nest of family relationships. Even among known donors and recipients, it is important to evaluate at each step the privacy needs of each individual involved and provide for individual time for information giving and receiving.

Provisions for confidentiality can be even more difficult in anonymous donation. It may be necessary for a donor to assume an alias for the operating room record sheet if it is widely distributed on the day of retrieval. In the medical record, however, all information must go under the donor's own name for her future access and for legal accountability. Special coding procedures may also have to be worked out for hospital registration and billing, since the donor should not generate a bill in her own name. It is also preferable not to release the donor's name to insurance companies, which may be less than circumspect about protecting the information.

In many cases, procedures for confidentiality will require hand posting of charges and special billing mechanisms worked out in advance with other departments such as radiology, anesthesiology, and outside laboratories that provide services for the donor. Unique arrangements may have to be made with pharmacies that provide medications paid for by the recipient but designated for the donor.

Billing procedures for egg donation must also be worked out in advance. Cycle charges vary greatly with the type of practice and region of the country. A detailed fee structure and written billing policies should be made available initially to all potential recipients. Inquiry should be made before program start-up to each insurance carrier that is likely to be involved, since coverage can be either minimal, partial, or complete, and restrictions may apply to type of diagnosis and selection criteria. Some companies will cover egg donation directly. Others will compensate under organ donation. Still others will refuse all related claims. State insurance commission regulations may affect billing formats. Although the final responsibility for payment rests with the patient, the financial office should assemble as much information as possible to smooth the process along. Finally, the party who is responsible for bills in case of complications to the donor should be clearly identified before egg retrieval.

Record keeping should be meticulous, because information may be requested many years later. The name of the donor should never appear in the recipient's record, nor should the recipient's name appear in the donor's record. Numerical coding procedures should be described in detail, and the record of assigned codes should be protected by the medical director under lock and key with a back-up copy available. From a practical point of view, flow charts (see Appendix 4-B) provide useful organization for administrative issues, genetic screening, medical history, matching characteristics, physical examination, and laboratory results and cycle information (Seibel SG, 1995). Practice records should provide the donor long-term access to her health information, matching criteria, genetic screening, and consent forms. The program will also have to make decisions in advance about disclosure to the donor of information about egg quality or cycle outcome. Any photographs taken for purposes of matching and recall should be kept in a locked location with numerical codes.

A decision should be made before program start-up about future handling of requests for information from either the donor or the recipient. Provision should be made for requests of medical necessity, and the possibility of future laws requiring disclosure of identifying offspring should be considered, discussed, and documented with both donor and recipient. All programs should seriously consider acquiring and maintaining extensive nonidentifying information for potential release to adult offspring.

The days of actual procedures (retrieval and transfer) require considerable organization to keep all parties separate. In known donation the multiplicity of individuals involved makes such organization complicated. On the day of retrieval a known donor's mother may be sitting in the waiting room waiting for a report. Her husband might be at work and need telephone notice that his wife is doing well. The donor's sister who is the designated recipient may also be at work and want to know how the donor is doing and how many eggs were obtained. The recipient's husband must also be called at work to arrange for a sperm specimen. In the midst of all this, another sister may call and say she is worried because it has taken so long, and by the way, could the nurse go find her mother in the waiting room and pass on a message. The coordinator functions as juggler for many, but on the books this is one patient and one procedure.

For anonymous donation the juggling act is even more complex because it involves keeping geographical separation between parties as well. The donor must have ultrasound at a different time and place than the recipient, and care must be taken to make sure both parties are never in the waiting room or the laboratory at the same time. On the day of retrieval, anxiety levels are flying, fantasies abound, and husbands who have been called in to provide a semen sample have been known to stake out the operating room waiting area to try to catch a glimpse of someone who might be the donor as she exits the hospital. If a GIFT procedure is requested, ZIFT, which involves tubal transfer one day later than GIFT, might be substituted instead to avoid having both donor and recipient in the operating room at the same time.

On the day of transfer, there is opportunity for similar complications. If a donor's eggs have been split between two recipients, transfers should not be scheduled for the same day to avoid the possibility that the husbands of both recipients will meet over the coffee pot in the recovery area. Because there is an acceptable window for implantation between days 17 and 19, embryo transfers can be timed to protect confidentiality without compromising the outcome. One can't control for everything, but one has to try. Clearly, procedures for geographical separation of parties must be carefully thought through, written down, and discussed among team members. One individual may have primary responsibility for an egg donation program, but several people on the medical staff should be cross-trained to provide back-up in the event of illness or other absences.

Although coordination is a major part of the coordinator's role, it is only half the story. In most programs, coordinators provide the day-to-day emotional support that has to be integrated into all phases of egg donation to ensure a positive experience.

Emotional support provided by the coordinator as part of all interactions is as important to program success as good fertilization results and pregnancy rates are. This is especially true if one approaches egg donation with the goal of assisting patients to carry out a well-considered plan with their self-respect and dignity intact, whether or not a pregnancy results.

FOLLOW-UP PROTOCOLS

Follow-up policies should be developed for both donors and recipients. Donors who have received medication for ovulation induction should be discharged after retrieval with written warnings about symptoms of hyperstimulation and should be seen immediately if problems develop. There should be documentation of any complications and medical follow-up until normal. If there have been no complications, donors are usually seen two weeks after retrieval, after a menses, and then are medically cleared. Some programs also re-

quire a follow-up visit with the mental health professional to assess emotional risks and post-donation attitudes. This is of value clinically to the individual donor and of immense value to the program in obtaining information for refining guidelines and policies.

Recipients are usually followed medically, if pregnant, through the end of the first trimester and then referred to their obstetrician of choice. Information about egg donation should be provided to the obstetrician, who may not have much information about the technology and may have questions about appropriate screening and counseling. It is also useful to provide data to the nurse in the obstetrician's office about any special needs this patient may have for emotional support or reassurance. The patient will have been previously advised of this sharing of information in the event of pregnancy.

The patient who is not pregnant is usually seen after menses for a follow-up evaluation and discussion of the cycle. A decision is often made at that time about trying again. If a follow-up counseling session is available, however, decisions about future plans are often best postponed until after that visit.

CONCLUSION

Although ASRM guidelines for egg donation are helpful, they do not provide practical guidance for setting up or evaluating programs. This chapter has explored some of the basic principles involved in egg donation: ethical constructs; the team concept; establishment of a counseling component; development of educational materials, delineating policies and standards for selection, screening, and matching; the nursing role in coordination, protection of privacy and confidentiality, and emotional support; and follow-up requirements.

At present, programs achieve quality on the basis of clinical experience, ethical debate, and good judgment. Research studies must be developed to follow donors, recipients, and offspring longitudinally to establish a data base for developing and refining guidelines for ovum donation.

REFERENCES

1. American Fertility Society. (1994) Guidelines for gamete donation. Fertil Steril 62:105s–107s.

2. American Fertility Society. (1994) Donor oocytes in in vitro fertilization. 62:47s–49s.

3. Bernstein J. (1993) The long-term psychologic and social effects of gamete donation. In: Seibel MM, Kiessling A, Bernstein J, Levin S, eds. Technology and Infertility: Clinical, Psychosocial, Legal and Ethical Aspects. New York: Springer-Verlag.

4. Bolton V, Golombok S, Cook R, Bish A, Rust J. (1991) A comparative study of attitudes toward donor insemination and egg donation in recipients, potential donors and the public. J Psychosom Obstet Gynaecol 12:217.

5. Braverman et al. (1993) PSIG Survey Results on the current practice of egg donation. Fertil Steril 59: 1216, 1220.

6. Ethics Committee of the American Fertility Society. (1990) Ethical considerations of the new reproductive technologies. Fertil Steril 53:1s.

7. Frydman R, et al. (1990) A protocol for satisfying the ethical issues raised by oocyte donation: The free, anonymous and fertile donors. Fertil Steril 53:666.

8. Grodin MA. (1993) The new reproductive technologies: Ethical, social and public policy concerns. In: Ormiston GL and Sassower R, eds. The Dissemination of Medical Authority. New York: Greenwood Press.

9. Kirkland A, et al. (1991) An analysis of the psychological aspects of women who have delivered babies after ovum donation. Human Reprod 6:224.

10. Koval R. (1990) The commercialization of reproductive technology. In J Scutt, ed. The Baby Machine. London: Merlin Press.

11. Lancet Editorial Board. (1993) Too old to have a baby? Lancet 341:344.

12. Lessor R, et al. (1993) An analysis of social and psychological characteristics of women volunteering to become oocyte donors. Fertil Steril 53:65.

13. Mahlsted PP, Greenfield DA. (1989) Assisted reproductive technology with donor gametes: The need for patient preparation. Fertil Steril 52:908.

14. Raymond JG. (1994) Women as Wombs. San Francisco: Harper.

15. Robertson JA. (1989) Ethical and legal issues in human egg donation. Fertil Steril 52:353.

16. Rosenwaks Z. (1987) Donor eggs: Their application in modern reproductive technologies. Fertil Steril 47:895.

17. Sauer M, et al. (1989) Establishment of a non-anonymous donor oocyte program: Preliminary experience at the University of Southern California. Fertil Steril 52:433.

18. Schenker JG. (1992) Ovum donation: Ethical and legal aspects. J. Asst Reprod Gen 9:411.

19. Seibel MM. (1992) To everything there is a season. Contemp OB GYN 37:153.

20. Seibel MM. (1995) Toward reducing risks and costs of egg donation: a preliminary report. Fertil Steril 64:199.

21. Seibel MM, Kearnan M, Kiessling A. (1995) Parameters that predict success for natural cycle in vitro fertilization—embryo transfer. Fertil Steril 63:1251.

22. Seibel MM, Kiessling A. (1993) Compensating egg donors: equal pay for equal time? N Engl J Med 328:737.

23. Seibel MM, Zilberstein M, Seibel SG. (1994) Becoming parents after 100? Lancet 343:603.

24. Vernale C, Packard SA. (1990) Organ donation as gift exchange. Image 22:239.

Appendix 4-A

Guidelines for Oocyte Donation

FAULKNER CENTRE FOR REPRODUCTIVE MEDICINE

I. Indications

    A. Ovarian failure (either premature, medically induced or natural) or gonadal dysgenesis.

    B. Avoidance of transmitting a genetic defect.

    C. Perimenopause or declining ovarian function.

    D. Persistently poor oocyte and embryo quality.

II. Preparation

    A. Couples or individuals interested in pursuing oocyte donation should receive detailed explanation of the procedure, its benefits and risks including the potential risk of acquiring an infection, the need for them to be screened, and out-of-pocket expenses. The donor should receive similar information appropriate for her with particular emphasis on ovulatory inducing medications and oocyte retrieval.

    B. Recipient couples should understand how and from where donors are selected, how they are screened and how they are matched.

    C. Recipient couples should understand that they are responsible for expenses resulting from any complications sustained by the donor that are not covered by the donor's own insurance.

    D. Recipient couples should agree in writing to accept their donor after reviewing their potential donor's history.

    E. Informed consent forms should be signed by the recipient couple and the donor. Legal consultation should be offered for further clarification.

    F. Discussion of cryopreservation of "extra" embryos should be discussed.

    G. Psychological counseling of the couple by a trained mental health professional to minimize the potential emotional risk. The donor should receive similar psychological counseling with the recipient if a known donor is used and separately if the donor is anonymous.

    H. Both partners should be tested for HIV I-II antibody, hepatitis B surface antigen, hepatitis C antibody, and a serologic test for syphilis.

    I. The female recipient should also be tested for her blood type, Rh factor, cervical cultures for gonorrhea and chlamydia, and rubella titers with vaccination offered to patients without immunity.

    J. Recipients 45 years of age or older should obtain medical evaluation to exclude potential cardiovascular or metabolic conditions that would be adversely affected by pregnancy. A high-risk obstetrical consultation is advisable.

    K. The female recipient should be examined and evaluated to exclude potential uterine factors that could lead to miscarriage and cervical factors that could impede embryo transfer.

    L. Donors should be instructed to use barrier contraception to avoid inadvertent pregnancy during the egg donation cycle.

Modified by Machelle M. Seibel, M.D. from The American Fertility Society, Guidelines for oocyte donation. (1994) Fertil Steril 62:105s–107s.

III. Donor Selection

    A. Both known and anonymous donors are acceptable. Known donors whose relationship is limited to egg donation represent a less desirable situation.

    B. Egg donors should be of good general health, should not possess a genetic abnormality or a strong family history for a major abnormality.

    C. Potential donors should be between legal age and 34 years of age. Known donors 35 years of age or older may be used if the recipient couple is aware and understands there is an increased risk of chromosomal abnormality in resulting offspring and a decreased chance of optimal ovarian stimulation.

    D. Established fertility is desirable but not an absolute requirement.

    E. Known donors should have the same evaluation and treatment as anonymous donors.

IV. Donor Screening

    A. Genetic screening is important including a pedigree to exclude hereditary and familial diseases, but chromosome analysis is not mandatory.

    B. Donors should not be at high risk for HIV (intravenous drug use or a sexual partner who uses intravenous drugs) or have multiple sexual partners.

    C. Donors should have a complete medical examination with special attention given to exclude urethral discharges, genital warts or ulcers.

    D. Laboratory testing including Rh factor testing and blood type initially, and serum hepatitis B antigen and hepatitis C antibody, serologic tests for syphilis, toxoplasmosis and cytomegalovirus antibody.

V. Donor Compensation

    A. Donors should be compensated for their time, risk, inconvenience, and discomfort.

    B. Compensation should not be sufficiently excessive to constitute a significant financial incentive.

    C. Unanticipated complications experienced by the donor should be the responsibility of the recipient.

    D. Payment should be prorated based on the number of steps completed by the donor.

Appendix 4-B

Donor Egg Paradigm—Donor

FAULKNER CENTRE FOR REPRODUCTIVE MEDICINE

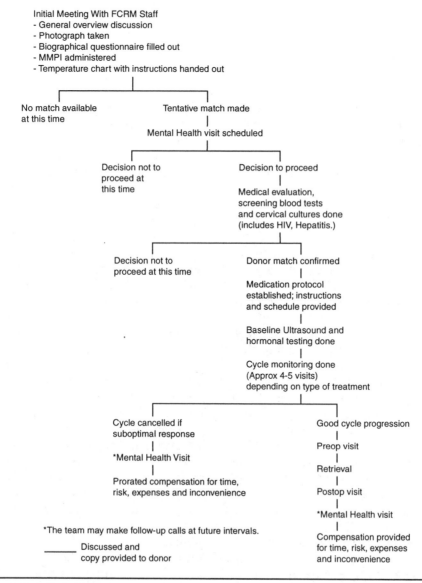

Initial Meeting With FCRM Staff
- General overview discussion
- Photograph taken
- Biographical questionnaire filled out
- MMPI administered
- Temperature chart with instructions handed out

No match available at this time

Tentative match made

Mental Health visit scheduled

Decision not to proceed at this time

Decision to proceed

Medical evaluation, screening blood tests and cervical cultures done (includes HIV, Hepatitis.)

Decision not to proceed at this time

Donor match confirmed

Medication protocol established; instructions and schedule provided

Baseline Ultrasound and hormonal testing done

Cycle monitoring done (Approx 4-5 visits) depending on type of treatment

Cycle cancelled if suboptimal response

*Mental Health Visit

Prorated compensation for time, risk, expenses and inconvenience

Good cycle progression

Preop visit

Retrieval

Postop visit

*Mental Health visit

Compensation provided for time, risk, expenses and inconvenience

*The team may make follow-up calls at future intervals.

_____ Discussed and copy provided to donor

Developed by S.G. Seibel, 1995.

5

Psychologic Counseling and Screening for Egg Donation

MARA BRILL, M.D.
SUSAN LEVIN, LICSW

Infertility is a chronic state of grief and loss. Even if an infertile couple eventually conceive a genetic child of their own, the psychological scars they sustain may stay with them forever. Egg donation overcomes some types of infertility and allows a couple to conceive a child that is in part genetically linked to them. Nevertheless, for most couples it is a very difficult decision.

Some women (and their husbands) have known for a long time that egg donation is their only means of achieving pregnancy (e.g., patients who had radiation/chemotherapy early in life for a tumor or who have had both ovaries removed). Usually, these women have mourned the lost possibility of having their own genetic offspring in the more remote past. Other women, such as those who have recently been diagnosed with a genetic defect, may have learned only a short while ago of their need to consider egg donation. Patients who experience premature ovarian failure have the double burden of coming to terms with egg donation and also being thrust suddenly and unexpectedly into the physical and emotional world of menopause. Finally, there are also women who either have been involved in lengthy infertility treatments or started trying to conceive later in life (e.g., early to middle forties). For all of these patients, egg donation is the last possible means of having a child who is still genetically linked to the husband and can be carried by the wife. Although it is not the same as having their own biologic child, it is very different from adoption. Egg donation allows a couple to share in the experience of pregnancy and childbirth and to retain control over pregnancy and prenatal care, which would not be possible in an adoption situation.

The American Fertility Society's guidelines for gamete donation (Fertil Steril Nov 1994) include only very general specifications. They acknowledge that because of "pragmatic considerations," such as difficulty in recruiting suitable (anonymous) donors, programs should accept known oocyte donors. The guidelines go on to say, "It is suggested that psychological counseling be offered to all parties involved in oocyte donation." No parameters or further recommendations are offered.

There are so many psychological factors associated with oocyte donation that virtually all egg donor programs require couples to have a consultation with a mental health professional, usually to help couples decide whether they are ready to proceed. Couples tend to use these consultations to continue processing their emotional readiness to start the procedure. It introduces them to mental health professionals who are providing supportive, as well as educational, counseling. It is also an opportunity for couples to learn how to talk constructively about the complicated issues that are associated with using donated eggs. Although the couple may not be aware of it, this mental health consultation will initiate a lifelong process.

Many couples initially feel enormous pressure to begin treatment and want to bypass this consultation because they have gone through so many infertility procedures or have been involved with many programs. They are usually unaware that these sessions facilitate discussions concerning normal ambivalence about the procedure, the use of a donor, and dealing with their loss.

Oocyte donation programs vary considerably in their approach to recruiting, accepting, and screening donors as well as their attitudes toward counseling and support of the donor and the recipient couple (Braverman, et al., 1993). The screening and counseling that are provided at the Faulkner Centre for Reproductive Medicine ("Faulkner Centre") represent an evolution that has spanned several years. The refinement of our framework of care emerged from specific questions and individual needs and scenarios that the patients themselves provided. We could not have anticipated many of the dilemmas that arose.

The result of our evolution is a firm belief that the best way to achieve a modicum of comfort—medically, psychologically, ethically, and socially—with egg donation is through mandatory and careful screening and counseling of both the donors and the recipients. Through providing an environment for these patients to process and analyze their motivations, hopes, plans, fantasies, worries, and personal, marital, and eventual parental relationships, the counselor must strive to ensure that this will be a decision the couple can be comfortable with now and remain comfortable with in the future. Obviously, individual programs will need to tailor their approach to suit their particular concerns, patient requests, donor availability, medical standards, and ethical dilemmas. A

TABLE 5.1. Evaluation of Egg Donors and Recipients

Donor Evaluation
1. Donor egg coordinator information session and interview
2. Psychological testing (MMPI and others)
3. The team evaluation
4. Mental health consultation
5. Medical screening

Recipient Evaluation
1. Initial contact with the physician
2. Donor egg coordinator information session and interview
3. Mental health consultation
4. Medical screening

summary of our approach is provided as an example (see Table 5.1).

DONOR EVALUATION

Information Session and Interview

After the physician has verified the patient's indication and need for egg donation and has provided an explanation of the procedure and its associated benefits and risks, a suitable donor must be identified and screened. At Faulkner Centre the potential egg donor is initially interviewed by the donor egg program coordinator. The interview includes an overview of the egg donation procedure, including information about any medication that must be taken, the egg retrieval, and other necessary information. The donor is asked to fill out a questionnaire that provides demographic information; personal medical, psychiatric, and surgical information; her gynecologic and obstetric history; and her family medical and psychiatric history (Table 5.2). Also included are questions about alcohol and drug abuse and any current use of prescription or nonpre-

TABLE 5.2. The Mental Health Evaluation of the Known and Anonymous Egg Donor

1. Demographic information
2. Motivation for egg donation
3. Current level of functioning
4. Mental status including competence and intellectual ability to understand procedures and possible risks
5. Past adaptation to developmental stages, including scholastic, work, and sexual history
6. History of alcohol or drug abuse
7. Psychiatric history
8. Previous trauma (e.g., sexual abuse, rape, early parental losses and adaptation to them)
9. Previous pregnancies and outcomes, as well as adaptation to pregnancy loss(es), pregnancy interruptions, and/or giving up a child for adoption
10. Family history, including alcohol or drug abuse, medical and psychiatric history
11. History of how she has dealt with previous major decisions in the past and their outcomes
12. Time availability for the cycle
13. Ability to follow through on major life decisions
14. Attitude toward medications, medical procedures, and recuperative phase
15. Support systems and who knows of the decision to use egg donation
16. Ability to think about the impact of the donation on herself, her spouse, and her children for now and for the future

scription medication. The intake interview provides the basis for considering whether or not to allow a potential donor to participate. Information thus obtained will subsequently be presented to the egg donation team.

Psychological Testing

If the team believes the candidate is likely to be a suitable donor, she will be asked to complete the Minnesota Multiphasic Personality Inventory (MMPI) (Dahlstrom WG and Welsh GS, 1960). Although the MMPI was not originally intended for screening potential anonymous egg donors, its use is becoming the standard of care in the United States. This evolution is not without its detractors, who argue that it may not be appropriate to screen potential donors with a test that was originally designed as a standardized measure of potential psychopathology in psychiatric patients. However, the growing consensus among mental health professionals is that the MMPI does provide a degree of standardization of potential psychopathology. As such, its use could be beneficial in the event of future litigation surrounding the choice of a particular egg donor or in helping the team to eliminate biases or blind spots that an interviewer may have. At our program, would-be donors are told that the test is designed to pick up when they are trying to "look good," and therefore they should answer all the questions as truthfully as possible. If the test results show an area of concern, such as potential for impulsivity, violence, thought disorder, or sociopathy, that potential donor may not tolerate the cycle and the procedure well and should not be used.

A potential dilemma occurs when known oocyte donors are required to take the test. Unlike anonymous donors, recipients usually know their known donor very well, have a relationship with them, and believe that they do not need a test to tell them whether their potential donor is problematic. On the other hand, if there is a question of psychopathology, it is unfair to the donor, the recipient, and the potential child not to screen or pick up potential problem areas. Therefore the MMPI can cause as well as prevent problems. How does one convey information to a recipient couple about using their potentially problematic known donor while at the same time maintaining the donor's confidentiality? Is the donor seen as a patient who has a right to confidentiality, or is she an "employee"—a person who is providing a service and who does not have a right to keep information private from the potential recipient couple? Despite these complexities, we have elected to administer the MMPI to potential known oocyte donors in the interest of protecting the recipient and the future child.

The results from the MMPI, which is computer-scored and psychologist-reviewed, fall into one of three categories: (1) no evidence of psychopathology—accept; (2) some questionable area of pathology that should be further investigated and correlated with the clinical interview; or (3) evidence of psychopathology—reject. We use the areas of concern delineated by the second category of the MMPI as a starting point to question the potential donor in depth at her mental health interview (see below). Examples of questions that are touched on in the mental health evaluation that may stem from the MMPI results include: What is the extent of this woman's mood swings and how extreme are they? How much is she really drinking? How often is she so depressed that she has thought of suicide or that life is not worth living?

After reviewing the results of the MMPI, the egg donation team decides whether or not to send the potential donor on to mental health counseling. If the MMPI suggests rejection of a potential anonymous donor, we generally inform her of the results and make the appropriate referral if indicated. Occasionally, the potential donors want to have feedback about this extensive psychological test they have taken. Most of the time, there is no problem letting a donor know the results. In more ambiguous results, the counselor can use the MMPI to address any areas of concern with the donor applicant.

The Team Evaluation

After the evaluations are completed, the couple and potential donor are discussed among the members of the egg donation team, who decide whether the people involved should proceed through the egg donation cycle. We find the team approach to be very helpful in egg donation so that no one person feels the burden of making the crucial decision of whether to accept or reject a donor. What makes these decisions occasionally very difficult are particular circumstances that stir up biases or moral or ethical dilemmas within the treatment team. By using a team approach, we are able to arrive at a common decision through a very interesting and helpful group process.

Mental Health Evaluation and Consultation

The complexity of egg donation appears to be best handled with a multifaceted counseling and evaluation process. Ideally, one mental health professional should perform the initial evaluation and counseling of the known donor, and another member of the mental health team should meet with the recipient couple. Separating the initial evaluation helps to eliminate bias that a single counselor might experience as a result of his or her desire for the couple to have a child. As such, a counselor can serve as an advocate for the donor. When evaluating an anonymous donor, it is helpful for the counselor to not know the couple who is tentatively matched to her so as to avoid possible conflict of interest.

KNOWN EGG DONORS AND THEIR RECIPIENTS

During the course of the counseling sessions, certain special issues are brought up by both known and anonymous egg donation. Most couples request known ovum donation for an obvious reason: control of the genetic background. Many view the eggs of the wife's sister or close friend as the next best thing to the wife's own eggs. Many couples like the idea of "keeping it in the family." They know what the children in that family look like and the donor's ethnic and religious background (which is occasionally an important factor for couples), and they believe that it would be beneficial for their child to be an actual grandchild/niece/nephew not unlike the other biologic children and grandchildren in a particular family. Without the unknowns of an anonymous egg donor, they feel that the child would more likely be accepted as part of the family. Also, a prolonged waiting period to identify an anonymous donor and many associated costs are often eliminated. For couples who have postponed childbearing, reducing the waiting time can be an important issue.

Known donors often state that they want to donate their eggs because of their close relationship with their sister or good friend. They want to help them obtain a child by experiencing the biologic connection of pregnancy and childbirth. In addition, if the known donor is a sister, the resulting child will be genetically linked to both the mother and the father. Some donors have had children of their own, others have not completed their family, and some have never had children. Some plan to have children in the future; others don't plan ever to be parents. They, too, speak of the wish to help create a child who would be "part of the family" and who would be a "special niece or nephew."

The desires and hopes of the recipient couple and the altruistic motivation of the donor are apparent in these situations. The mental health professional must evaluate and counsel the parties involved to ensure that egg donation is in the best psychological interests of both the recipient and the donor.

In evaluating people's motivation for becoming an oocyte donor, we find that there may also be nonaltruistic factors. Examples include family coercion, guilt about having children when a sister is childless, a wish to undo

a past abortion or giving up of a child for adoption, or simply a masochistic, victimized stance in which the sister cannot say no. One example of the usefulness of the split evaluation occurred in a sister pair in which the donor sister lived far away and had financial difficulties yet felt unable to ask her sister for travel compensation. She was about to become engaged but experienced difficulty putting her own needs first by delaying the donation cycle to attend to her marriage plans. The counseling sessions allowed the donor sister to prioritize her own life plans and communicate those wishes to her sister. She subsequently did go through the cycle at a more appropriate time for her and was able to ask for travel expenses.

In another sister donor situation the mother was coming to all the medical appointments with her two daughters. The team became concerned that the mother's constant presence might be felt as coercion by the donor sister. In this situation the counselor used the information provided by the team to inquire into the mother's involvement. Work with the sisters clarified the mother's subtle and not so subtle pressure and uncovered that the recipient sister had been the favorite, the "baby" in the family. The donor sister resented the burden of taking care of her younger sister, especially when it proved not to be in her own best interests (e.g., when she wanted to go out on dates). She cared deeply for her younger sister but was fearful of the danger to her own health posed by the hormones involved. She needed help in verbalizing these concerns, even though they contradicted her mother's expectations that she do anything possible to help. The recipient sister understood, and the two were able to come to a comfortable decision to do a natural, unmedicated cycle.

These examples reflect situations in which the donor sister required an advocate to support her need to set limits. In other situations, the recipient couple needs help in deciding not to use a willing sister. The donor sister may be in her late thirties and have reduced or unproven fertility. The recipient couple should be made aware that an anonymous younger donor would provide them with a better chance at pregnancy and not let the pressure of time coerce them.

In a more complicated situation, Jennifer and her husband experienced multiple pregnancy losses (including a second-trimester loss). Her sister, Julie, made an independent decision to become an egg donor for Jennifer and informed the couple that she was going to "give them a baby and that they should fly out to participate in doing their part of the cycle." More history from Jennifer revealed that Julie had an impulsive lifestyle and that she planned never to have a family of her own. In this situation the counselor advised the couple to consider an anonymous donor or to approach another donor.

In evaluating the known donor (Table 5.2), several questions need to be answered, keeping in mind the welfare of the recipient couple, the potential child, and the donor herself. Every care should be taken to assess the donor's current level of functioning and the constellation of her family (husband, partner, children) and to have a thorough understanding of her life until this time. Particular attention should be paid to the question of substance abuse, past history of psychiatric illness (asking specific questions about psychiatric symptoms such as anhedonia, insomnia, decreased libido, and impaired ability to concentrate and work or frankly suicidal ideation, rather than simply asking "Have you ever been clinically depressed?") and to inquire about past pregnancies and their outcomes. Also very important is the prior and current adaptation to previous pregnancy interruptions or losses as well as a more general history of any physical or sexual abuse she has suffered. Schover et al. (Schover LR, et al., 1990) have shown that oocyte donors were more likely to have suffered from either childhood

trauma, sexual trauma, or reproductive losses than were matched controls. However, this has not been studied in known egg donors and thus cannot be generalized to that particular population.

In the closing five minutes of one interview, a donor sister made reference to the invasiveness of the retrieval procedure and associated it with having been raped on a date. Additional discussion was necessary to more carefully assess whether going through the vaginal ultrasound and the pelvic examinations with a male doctor, as well as the retrieval procedure, would stir up previous feelings of trauma that would destabilize her. At times, such situations may require consultation with the donor's therapist (if there is one) to more carefully assess whether past trauma has been adequately dealt with. Referrals to outside therapists are also sometimes indicated.

The issue of exclusion criteria is a complex one, especially in known donor situations. For our program, frank psychosis or evidence of a thought disorder, an incapacitating mood disorder that requires psychotropic medications, and active substance abuse that interferes with everyday functioning are indications to exclude a donor, regardless of the recipient couple's wishes. More subtly complicated situations require work with the donor and her recipient over the course of several sessions to work out a mutually agreeable plan. Occasionally, this may involve additional meetings or referral to an outside therapist or another member of the mental health team if he or she was not the original mental health professional involved. One extra complicating factor is the potential for a genetic predisposition to schizophrenia and bipolar illness (which have been more worked out) and to alcoholism (which is less clearly hereditary). These issues will become even more complicated as new genetic diseases become diagnosable as a result of the Human Genome Project. The recipients of known and anonymous egg donors must be made aware of the genetic risk to their future offspring and must provide informed consent to use donors who pose a risk.

It is also necessary to thoroughly assess the donor's support systems and look for evidence that she has processed and weighed the pros and cons of the egg donation. Has she talked it over with friends, family, a minister, priest, or rabbi? What possible problems does she see with egg donation? How will she feel seeing her genetic offspring if she is a known donor? How does she view that child? Is it hers or the sister's and brother-in-law's, or is that child symbolic of someone else in her life? Has she had any striking dreams as she approaches the donation cycle? Is she concerned about the risks of the medications and of the surgical procedure on her health? Has she considered the possible effects of the donation cycle on her own children? Will she tell them as the cycle is going on? If not, how will she respond if they see her getting injections or feeling more moody or anxious about the retrieval or the recuperative phase after the retrieval? How will she explain to the children that their cousin is actually their half-sister or half-brother?

Our advice to donors who have children is the same as it is for our in vitro fertilization couples who have children, and that is to avoid involving the children in the actual exposure to injections and invasive medical procedures such as repeated blood drawing and vaginal ultrasounds. Otherwise, children might mistakenly believe that their mother is getting shots and going repeatedly to the doctor to get blood drawn because she is seriously ill.

At least part of the screening visit with a donor should be spent talking to her husband or partner. The intent is to ascertain that the decision to donate eggs is a mutual one, since it will affect both of them for the duration of the cycle and could affect their current or future relationships and children. In one situation, Kathy, a woman in her thirties, came to our center to be an identified donor for a close friend. She painted an idyllic picture of her seventeen-year marriage, her three wonderful children, and her successful career alongside a fervent wish to help her close friend. She balked strongly at the insistence that she bring in her husband for the screening appointment, stating that she was a feminist and did not see the point of involving a man in something that affected only her body and what she wished to do with it. She canceled the next appointment for her and her husband and called back a few weeks later to say that she was separated from her husband but still wished to do the egg donation. A decision was made that despite her resolve, her life was currently in too much upheaval and she should wait six months. Although the recipient couple was understandably upset about the need to wait, the need for the donor to be in a stable life situation while undergoing egg donation was explained. The fact that she would not divulge the truth about her marital problems either to the counselor or to her friend suggested that she might also be unable to deal with other complicated feelings and life circumstances that might arise if a child were conceived.

Screening and Counseling the Recipient Couple

The counterpart of screening and counseling the donor involves the recipient couple. The objective is to assemble a picture of the recipient couple through most of the same questions that are asked of the donor. Motivation to be an egg recipient; medical, psychiatric, and gynecologic history; substance abuse; adaptation to life events; and ability to live successfully with major decisions undertaken summarize the main areas covered. Questions must be addressed as to how each member of the couple has dealt with adversity and conflict as well as successes in his and her own life, in the marriage between each other, and in the relationship with the donor. Essential information includes understanding the qualities the donor possesses that the couple are attracted to and sources of possible conflict they anticipate in using a particular donor. One must probe the degree of involvement they desire from the donor in the pregnancy, birth, and future rearing of this offspring. The recipient couple must consider how they see the rest of the donor family's role in the child's life. The recipient needs an avenue to talk about her own guilt in having to subject her donor to possible danger from the medications or the retrieval procedure. Often, recipients must be encouraged to bring up these concerns in the meeting between the donor and the recipient or in the session in which the men are also present. This is especially true when the genetic mother is someone who will be well known to the child, such as a relative or friend of the family who will be in constant contact with the child.

The other major focus of the initial evaluation is the relationship between the donor and the recipient. This could begin with their current relationship but must also probe more deeply into any childhood relationship and how it has evolved over the years.

Usually, the known egg donor pairs are sisters. Areas to discuss with sisters include their degree of closeness, their level of involvement with each other and with their partners, whether or not they are envious of each other's situations, and how they have handled difficult situations in the past such as sibling rivalry, loss, or gain by one of the sisters. Some insights might be gained by asking what reactions they anticipate from friends and family members if they decide to tell. How do they feel about the fact that the genetic mother will also be the maternal aunt? Does the recipient feel comfortable with the notion that the child will genetically be her sister's and her sister's husband's? Can the donor relinquish control of how the sister will handle the pregnancy,

including such issues as whether or not the sister and her husband will decide to have a fetal reduction? Will she accept an amniocentesis, and if it is abnormal, would she feel comfortable if they choose to abort? Will the recipient want the donor present at the birth? Other questions to discuss in the counseling session have to do with whether the sister donor could accept not being the child's guardian and how she would handle situations in which she might not be in agreement with the recipient's child-rearing practices. This latter issue was particularly pertinent to a sister donor who knew that both her sister and her brother-in-law were previously addicted to drugs and had been abstinent for several years. The donor worried about what she would do if they resumed their prior habits and how she would secure the welfare of the child. She was able to tell them honestly in their counseling session that she would wish to step in and take care of her niece or nephew in the event of their resuming their drug abuse, whether or not the child were conceived through her egg donation.

Sibling rivalry can also be stirred up by the oocyte donation. In one sister pair the recipient said, "My sister always borrowed my pearls. Why shouldn't I be able to use her eggs?" In this situation the recipient sister felt that "my sister owes me" some of her "good eggs." The goal of counseling is to make sure that a recipient's feeling of entitlement does not lead to coercion of the potential donor.

Obviously, not all possible problems can be anticipated. It is therefore necessary to identify an atmosphere in which sisters (or close friends) are comfortable with each other separately and together and in which they have a forum and a history in place for discussing conflicts that may arise or sharing both positive and negative experiences that they are having.

Although every precaution is used to maintain confidentiality for both the donor and the recipient, there is a risk that the donor may be asked to divulge important personal history that she has kept secret from her sister and the rest of the family until now, such as prior pregnancies and abortions or a test that comes back positive for a sexually transmitted disease. Donors must be made aware of the possible loss of privacy, and they must agree to it.

For sister donors who have not been pregnant in the past, one important aspect of the counseling session involves sharing with them the ramifications of their finding out something new about their own fertility potential or even about their medical status. This can become problematic. Some donor sisters may have the same difficulties with ovulation induction and the ability to produce good-quality eggs as their infertile sister. This is a devastating piece of information to find out during an egg donation cycle. Not only does the donor sister have to deal with the disappointment of not being able to help her sister conceive, but she must now fact the prospect of possibly being infertile herself. The interview must assess whether these potential donor sisters would be able to tolerate such unfortunate news and the narcissistic injury inherent in that potential diagnosis.

For some, this situation leads to resorting to another sister, who is de facto the one who was initially less preferred by the couple for the egg donation. This may stir up feelings of resentment in the sister who was not initially asked, as well as in the sister who has "failed." Furthermore, the recipient couple must again mourn not being able to get pregnant even with her sister's egg.

Another major area of discussion during the counseling sessions is the issue of secrecy with the child and/or everyone else. In known ovum donation the pairs most commonly have chosen (at least at this point) to reveal the truth to the potential child. Only rarely do these sister pairs decide to keep the information secret from the rest of the family. It is essential to explain to these patients that if more than two people

know, it is no longer a secret, and they may no longer have the option of secrecy.

Most mental health professionals have a bias that family secrets lead to family problems, especially in the children who grow up not knowing the truth but sense that something is being talked about. With the exception of adoption studies (Baran and Paron, 1989) (Nickman S, 1994) (and egg donation has some differences from adoption), there is no concrete research that has proven or dealt with the issue of whether there is a long-term psychological benefit to the child who grows up knowing the truth of his or her genetic roots (Klock S, Maier D, 1991). Further research is crucial to study the short- and long-term psychological effects of egg donation on the donor and her children, the recipient couple, and the child with comparisons between parents who choose to tell and those who do not. Specific questions that must be addressed include when to tell the child, under what circumstances, and the relationship between the donor and the recipient related to the egg donation (see Chapters 16 and 17).

Sister pairs who are not particularly close either emotionally, chronologically, or sometimes geographically don't appear to envision the donor's having a close relationship with the offspring. Only prospective research will establish what actually happens in these families over the course of time. Egg donation between very good friends is also done when it is apparent they have a longstanding relationship built on a solid base of knowledge and understanding of each other accompanied by altruism as the major motive for the egg donation. We have not accepted known donors who are recruited for purely financial remuneration, since we feel that the fabric of the relationship is not in place and thus is too precarious to sustain what may be conflicts in the future.

Unlike the anonymous donor evaluation, in which in our program the counselor routinely has an exit interview with the donor after her egg donation cycle, such interviews are seldom performed with known donor pairs. Most of the feedback is obtained from the nursing and allied office team who report at team meetings how the patients in the cycle are doing, how they appear to relate with each other, and so on. Occasionally, interactions are noticed that cause the staff concern, and these patients are referred back to the counselor.

Some of the psychologic issues for known and anonymous donors overlap, and some are unique for each procedure. The issues around known donors have been described above. The psychological dilemmas that are present for the use of the unknown donor are discussed next.

ANONYMOUS EGG DONORS AND THEIR RECIPIENTS

Women who choose an unknown donor must deal with additional loss. They must give up any genetic connection to their child. They must also forfeit direct access to the donor and information about her. This requires giving up enormous control by entrusting the medical team to provide an appropriate donor.

Why choose an anonymous donor? Some women would prefer to use a relative but do not have an appropriate one to choose. Such women and couples may feel that a genetic link is important and must work through this loss before they can proceed in an anonymous donor program. This could mean dealing with other losses as well; for example, one woman's sister would have been a wonderful donor, had she not died in a car crash. Using an anonymous donor resurfaced the woman's grief about the earlier loss of her sister at the same time she was dealing with the loss of her capacity to have a genetic child.

Another patient who was considering

anonymous donor versus adoption spoke often of her sadness and apparent reexperience of her loneliness growing up as an only child. She was simultaneously reflecting that if she was lucky enough to succeed with the ovum donor, her child would probably be an only child too.

Some women and couples choose an anonymous donor even if they could have a known donor. The reasons for this choice vary. Often there is concern that an ongoing relationship with the donor could lead to confusion as to who is the "real" mother. This fear can be heightened because of the insecurities and inadequacies felt as a result of infertility.

In other situations the recipient may experience competition with the fertile donor. Such feelings could be intensified if the donor and the recipient had an ongoing relationship that could undermine the recipient's relationship with her child or create fears that the genetic mother might try to take the child away.

Couples often don't want to burden their relationships with family members or good friends with this request. They do not want to deal with the complications that a child created by using a known egg donor may create for their family or friendship. Being both the aunt and the genetic mother might well be difficult for some individuals and families to cope with. In addition, couples may not want to risk being turned down. They may also be concerned that an individual may not be able to say no even if she wanted to. Privacy may be another reason for choosing anonymous egg donation. Also, if there is a genetic problem, a relative may also have the same genetic problem, which would eliminate her as a donor.

In some situations a woman may select the donor procedure as a way to subtly deny her fertility problem and to avoid making her problem public. She may then continue to deny that the child is not genetically hers. This denial may make knowledgeable, sophisticated people appear naive, as in the case of one woman who stated during her evaluation that if she were to use egg donation, maybe her genes "would get mixed in" while the baby was in utero.

Choosing a donor can be extremely uncomfortable or overwhelming for some couples. They do not want to know the donor or even to think of her as a person, preferring to think of the eggs only, thus avoiding any feelings of indebtedness or obligation, even though they are deeply grateful. Such distancing is usually perceived as protective of their relationship with the child. They hope that this distance will make it clearer to them that the baby is theirs and that they are the parents. It also allows them more control over the information around the conception. They can decide when and if they are going to tell the child about his or her genetic heritage. These couples will not have to worry about the knowledge being a "family affair" or some relative making a slip before they are ready to disclose certain information to their child.

The decision to use an unknown donor is often a process. Many couples at the beginning of their infertility problems cannot imagine participating in a donor program, let alone using an unknown donor. After they have made the decision, the couple often feel grateful to the technology for making it possible for the wife to have a biological child with a genetic link to her husband. The fact that they are able to experience a pregnancy and provide good prenatal care brings back some of the control that they lost when their particular problem was diagnosed. For many women the possibility of a pregnancy helps them regain confidence in their body's ability to function normally.

When using an anonymous donor, it is useful for the couple to openly discuss what their expectations are about the donor. During this time the couple can describe what they hope their donor will be like and what kind of donor they hope to avoid. This discussion allows individuals and couples to look at and understand their fantasies about the donor and perhaps also to further grieve for the loss of the genetic connection. This intervention allows the couple to have more realistic expectations of the donor and the matching process. It also allows the team professionals to be more responsive to the couple's needs.

Couples vary in what they want or expect from a donor and how they ask for it. When egg donation first became available, couples were so grateful that they expressed few expectations. Simple hopes such as wanting the donor to be a nice person were all that patients asked for. As the procedure has become more popular and commonplace, couples' expectations have changed dramatically. Some requests reflect the individual's readiness or appropriateness for this kind of program.

During one couple's consultation the man stated his desire that the donor have a curriculum vitae and listed the features and characteristics that he wanted on it. They included high intelligence, attractive physical appearance, high energy, and the ability to use a computer (his wife was a computer programmer). By treating the donor as a job applicant rather than a provider of eggs for his future offspring, he was able to feel in control and keep distance from the process. He had not totally given up the genetic connection to his wife.

One woman seeking egg donation because of premature ovarian failure requested very specific physical characteristics that were the opposite of her own physical appearance. With further investigation it became apparent that infertility had worsened her preexisting feeling of inadequacy and unattractiveness. Her solution, to seek the opposite of self, was an attempt to give birth to an idealized child who would reflect favorably on her. Her unrealistic expectations required additional psychologic attention.

An important issue that is always addressed during the psychologic consultation is the question of openness. Questions that couples must ponder are: Do they plan to tell the child? If so, how and when? Whom have they told and whom do they plan to tell?

TABLE 5.3.   Donor Information Form

Name_____ Home Phone _____ Bus. Phone _____

Address _____

Characteristics

Age _____   Date of birth _____

Hair color_____
        Curly _____
        Straight _____

Eye color _____

Skin tone _____

Racial/Ethnic background _____

Religion _____

Height _____   Weight _____   Blood type _____

Education
        Highest grade completed _____

Occupation _____

Present place of employment _____

Do you have health insurance? _____

        Type _____

Have you ever participated as a donor in another program? _____

Social History

Do you use or have you ever used the following (check all that apply)

Alcohol _____   If yes, how many glasses per week on average

        Wine _____   Beer _____   Cocktails _____

Cigarettes _____   How many per day _____

Drugs (marijuana, cocaine, etc.) _____   Times per week _____

Previous pregnancies _____

Living children _____

        Ages _____

Married _____   Length of marriage _____

Continued

TABLE 5.3. *Continued*

Medical History

Current medications _____

Medications taken in the last five years and reasons for taking them

_____

_____

_____

Current medical problems

_____

_____

Hospitalized in the last five years

_____

_____

_____

Have you ever had the following:

Asthma _____

Diabetes _____

Seizure disorder _____

Counseling _____

Psychiatric treatment _____

Venereal or sexually transmitted disease _____ Date _____ Treatment _____

Last Pap smear was done _____

Are your periods regular? _____ Last period _____

How many days between periods? _____

Family History

	Alive	Age	Medical Status	Deceased	Cause of Death	Age
Mother	____	____	_____	____	_____	____
Father	____	____	_____	____	_____	____
Maternal grandmother	____	____	_____	____	_____	____

Continued

TABLE 5.3. *Continued*

	Alive	Age	Medical Status	Deceased	Cause of Death	Age
Maternal grandfather	___	___	_____	___	_____	___
Paternal grandmother	___	___	_____	___	_____	___
Paternal grandfather	___	___	_____	___	_____	___
Sisters	___	___	_____	___	_____	___
	___	___	_____	___	_____	___
	___	___	_____	___	_____	___
Brothers	___	___	_____	___	_____	___
	___	___	_____	___	_____	___
	___	___	_____	___	_____	___

Are there any congenital malformations known in the family?

Is there any psychiatric illness known in the family (e.g., alcoholism, depression), psychiatric hospitalizations, or suicides?

Do you have any of the known risk factors for HIV disease (bisexual partner or previous intravenous drug use)?

These can be difficult questions for infertile couples because it is difficult for them to imagine that there will be a child.

The issue of secrecy or privacy versus openness requires extensive discussion and is often unresolved even if the couple believe that they know how they wish to handle it. Some of the issues are similar to those discussed in the chapter on therapeutic donor insemination (TDI). The mental health sessions provide a forum for the couple to practice talking about this topic, as some couples find it difficult to discuss the subject. Having no one to talk to and no forum for discussion can cause isolation and can also be destructive to the relationship.

A common and central theme for most couples is that they want to do what is best for the child. Many would prefer to be open but are concerned about society's ability to handle this information and worry that their child will be stigmatized. Recipient women appear to be more comfortable with an "open approach" after egg donation than their counterpart men or couples in TDI. Scientific data to explain this finding is lacking, and research in the area is sorely needed.

It is possible that female recipients are less concerned about their ownership or ability to bond because they will still play the important biologic roles of carrying and delivering the baby. Women are also more open in our culture. They receive more support from other women and experience less of a stigma about their infertility problem. Women generally are more directly involved in the infertility workup and treatments and therefore may have more opportunity to mourn their loss and be more comfortable with this choice of treatment. The donor egg procedure also appears not to carry the sexual overtones that are often associated with TDI. Although the woman, like her male counterpart, may at times feel like less of a woman because her reproductive organs are dysfunctional, she does not describe any sexual feeling about the donation. The donated egg she is receiving is something that she/women produce normally. Receiving an egg is not associated with sexual intercourse as is receiving sperm. These differences in sexual connotation allow donor egg recipients to experience sadness about their loss of reproductive function that is segregated from their sense of sexual self-esteem.

Identifying and Evaluating Anonymous Donors

There are many similarities and differences among donor egg programs around the country regarding donor selection, screening, psychologic issues, and the matching process (Braverman, et al., 1993). Most donors are recruited through advertising and word of mouth. The advertising might be in local newspapers or on bulletin boards in academic settings or in local supermarkets and community gathering places. Some programs prefer to use medical settings because there is an assumption that prospective donors will already have an understanding of the scientific aspects of the procedure and that their proven interest in that area may be a motivating factor for them to be donors. Some potential donors have heard about the program through a friend or an acquaintance. These women are usually in their twenties and either have not had children or believe that they have finished their childbearing. The issues are quite different for these two groups.

During the psychologic interview, an individual and family history is taken to elicit infor-

mation about substance abuse, mental illness, medical and reproductive problems, and motivation for participating as a donor. It is important to understand how the donor thinks about her donation and whether she is comfortable with the particular program's protocol concerning disclosure. For example, some programs will not inform the donor if a pregnancy occurs, and most provide no information about the recipients. Information about the donor is saved and disclosed in an anonymous way to the recipients or put away for the future.

This psychologic screening has numerous and complicated goals. It must meet the needs of the donor, the recipient, and the medical team. Psychologic screening protocols vary from center to center and reflect the approach of the center. Some centers view the donors as their patients; others view them only as donors. The former allows more of a professional relationship to develop between staff and donor and allows the donor to experience more of a connection with the program. This connection may allow donors to make a more informed decision. Other centers try to remain distant from the donor through less personal contact. The emphasis in the screening is on standardized tests and short, structured interviews. Even though these women want to be donors, it is important that egg donation be appropriate for them. For potential donors who have not had children, professionals must try to help them understand what they are giving away and to comprehend the future meaning of such a gift. The interviewer should also try to anticipate with the donor whether she might later regret being a donor, how it might change her life, or whether it could be psychologically damaging. This is why it is important to rule out psychologically fragile women or women who are in the middle of life crises. Such crises could be the death of a family member or friend, termination of therapy, or ending of another significant relationship. Such losses tend to create turmoil in most people's lives and therefore interfere with their ability to make reasonable decisions. These interviews also help the donor to make an informed decision. The following is an example of how this interview can be an intervention:

Linda, a 25-year-old woman, answered an advertisement seeking potential egg donors. During her mental health interview, she stated that she was soon to be stopping her therapy because her therapist was pregnant. She had sought therapy to help with her difficulties in forming satisfying relationships. She was very sad and envious of her therapist's situation. She was single and convinced that she would never find a good relationship or have a family of her own. This made her extremely sad for historical reasons as well. Her mother had died suddenly when Linda was ten. Linda had a very close relationship with her now idealized mother. It was her feeling that her mother would want her to be generous and donate her eggs. She also thought that this would be a way for her mother's genetic material to be passed on and not stop with her. After conferring with the therapist, the consultant suggested that Linda wait several months after her therapist returned from maternity leave and that she give herself time to work through some of these feelings in her therapy. Linda reluctantly agreed and had a successful egg donation cycle six months later.

It is generally thought that most donors are not motivated solely by financial reasons and that most programs will eliminate anyone who seems only financially motivated. Donors often know someone who has been infertile and want to help some other individual in this population. They often have an idealized view of the desperate, infertile couple and immediately imagine them to be good parents. Some donors have had one or more abortions, leaving them with some residual negative feelings that they are hoping to let go of through the donation. Often, these are women who are not sure they want children but don't want their genetic material to go unused. They generally think of their donation as genetic material and not as a baby. At the time that they are involved in the program, they generally don't want to know whether a pregnancy occurs and usually assume that it will occur. Many times, they are women who are organ donors and have given blood and like to think of themselves as helpful to others. They also tend to be in transitional periods in their lives—students, beginning careers, between jobs, and so on.

Donors who go through the procedure seem to enjoy the attention that they receive from the medical staff but are surprised by the intensity and the amount of difficulty they have with the injections, medications, and procedure. The donors typically have a lower pain tolerance than infertility patients do. After the procedure the donor may feel a little low, perhaps because of the fluctuating hormones or the loss of attention from the medical staff. Some donors have had somatic complaints and have returned to be checked for various pains. Others have had pregnancy scares after their donation.

Rarely, there have been donors who have had problems completing a cycle because they have an undiagnosed fertility problem. Such women will need some attention to help them deal with their feelings of failure as well as the implications for their future fertility. To help donors talk about and work through any particular issues that may have come up during the egg donation cycle, we recommend meeting with each donor once before her discharge from the clinic's care. Questions to discuss include how she is feeling; who she talked to about her cycle; and how the medications, injections, retrieval, and post-operative phase went. It is important to ascertain whether she is comfortable with what she has done and with not knowing the outcome and to counsel extra attention to any wishes to act out sexually or make unexpected decisions.

There is also concern about donors who

apply but who are not selected. The mental health consultant must be prepared to deal with feelings of rejection as the woman probably feels that she is being quite generous only to feel badly that her offer is being turned down. The team's responsibility to this group of women remains uncertain but may need to include referral to a mental health provider.

The mental health evaluation for egg donors represents a striking difference from the usual screening done for sperm donors. Some question whether this dual standard reflects a sexist and paternalistic view that women are perceived as being incapable of making a good decision without the help of the mental health professional. However, it seems that the elaborate screening process for female donors evolved from concerns that have been raised about the process with their male counterparts. Society today is biased about the importance of the mother. It is felt that men are not as attached to, concerned about, or involved with their gametes or the subsequent biological offspring. This has led to problems for both male donors and their resulting offspring. It is also much easier for men to donate their gametes, a situation that may have contributed to the initial lack of psychologic screening and attention that men received. Many sperm donors have acknowledged that they now regret how lightly they handled the decision to donate their sperm, and many TDI children wish they had more information about and access to their genetic father. Sperm banks are beginning to develop a more elaborate psychologic screening process for men as well as providing recipients with much more background information about the sperm donor.

DONOR-RECIPIENT MATCHING

Methods of donor-recipient matching vary among centers. At one end of the spectrum, one person (either the nurse or the doctor) does the matching; on the other side, the entire medical team is involved in the decision. Often there are pictures of both the recipient couple and the donor so that physical characteristics can be attended to. We avoid matching individuals with large height and weight disparities. Attention may also be paid to talents and interests. We are especially careful to not load up potentially genetically linked diseases on both sides (i.e., the recipient husband and the egg donor). Toward that end, we ask for a similar medical questionnaire to be filled out by the husband or to obtain a "long form" medical history when a sperm donor is used. The staff should feel a tremendous sense of responsibility toward both parties. Not all recipients are as ideal as the donor imagines, and donors are not perfect people either. There are also limitations on what one can know, and what traits will be inherited by the offspring.

Some programs give recipients a tentative match and ask them to review a form that includes a particular donor's medical and physical attributes, interests, and talents. The recipient has the right to reject this donor. Some recipient couples fear that if they reject the donor, they will be penalized by having to wait longer. In some programs this is true; in others this is not the case. While the couple may have to wait for another appropriate donor, it should not be because they are being punished, but because there is a limited number of donors. Reviewing these forms gives the couple an opportunity to think in a realistic and tangible way about what it means to accept a donated gamete. They are able to decide together whether they prefer, for instance, a donor who has some family history of heart disease over a donor whose grandfather had alcoholism. Giving more control to the infertile population in this arena of donor approval is very important. Their infertility problem has taken so much control away. Participating in the process may also lead to a better adjustment and to realistic expectations about the procedure, the pregnancy, and, most important, their child. However, when a recipient or a couple have rejected 2 or 3 donors or when they are spending an inordinate amount of time with the staff asking more and more questions, the staff will usually refer them back to the mental health consultant to talk further about what is getting in the way of signing off on a particular donor. Perhaps they need a known donor or maybe they are not truly ready for egg donation despite their earlier conscious resolve.

CONCLUSION

Despite our attempts to provide ethical, thoughtful, and humane treatment to all the parties concerned, only long-term prospective studies will be able to show the social, psychologic, and emotional impact on our patients, our donors, and the children thus conceived. For this reason it is incumbent upon mental health professionals to continue to provide opportunities for social connections and emotional support (either individually or in groups) for all parties involved and for the subsequent families formed.

REFERENCES

1. Ethics Committee of The American Fertility Society. (1994) Vol 62, No 5, Fertility and Sterility, Supplement 1.
2. Braverman, et al. (1993) "Survey results on the current practices of ovum donation." Fertil Steril Vol 59, No. 6.
3. Dahlstrone WG, Welsh GS. (1960) MMPI Handbook: A guide to use in clinical practice and research: Minneapolis: University of Minnesota Press.
4. Schorer LR, et al. (1990) The psychological evaluation of oocyte donors. J Psychosom Obstet Gynecol 11:299–399.
5. Barran A, Panner R. (1989) Lethal Secrets. New York: Warner Books
6. Nickman S. (1994) Personal lecture at workshop on assisted reproductive technologies. Boston Psychoanalytic Society and Institute.
7. Klock S, Maier D. (1991) Psychological factors related to donor insemination. Fertil Steril 56:489–495.

6

Genetic Issues in Gamete Donation

MOSHE ZILBERSTEIN, M.D.
MARION S. VERP, M.D.

With the advent of assisted reproductive techniques (ART) and molecular genetics, gamete donation has rapidly evolved into a powerful modality for assisted reproduction. This chapter addresses genetic issues in gamete donation. We will look into the past at the experience gained with therapeutic donor insemination (TDI) to assess contemporary issues and to glimpse the imminent future.

TDI AS A PARADIGM

TDI has traditionally been used as the primary treatment for intractable male factor infertility. Criteria have evolved to evaluate sperm quality and to select appropriate couples for the procedure. Also using TDI are couples with longstanding infertility that is not amenable to various treatment protocols for the female or the male. TDI has become a mainstay of fertility treatment. However, before egg donation was initiated and TDI was the sole method of gamete donation, surprisingly few studies focused on genetic issues (Jalbert P, et al., 1989; Verp MS, 1987; Czeizel A, et al., 1979; Verp MS, et al., 1983; Fédération CECOS et al., 1983). Notwithstanding, the TDI paradigm is instructive for both sperm and egg donation in the contemporary era of multifaceted fertility technology (McCulloh DH, Wolf DP, 1993; Dean NL, Edwards RG, 1994; Shapiro S, 1992; Curie-Cohen M, et al., 1979).

The realization that both gametes contribute to the success or failure of fertilization expanded the use of TDI even to "normal couples" with longstanding infertility as well as couples with unexplained infertility. Such an approach encapsulates recent understanding of the intricate mechanisms involved in egg-sperm interaction (Zilberstein M, Seibel MM, 1994).

Advances in ART now allow donation of both sperm and eggs. These new developments allow couples to bypass obstacles to fertilization and embryo development that are inherent to either the egg or the sperm. In cases with intractable infertility despite correction and treatment of obvious or putative causes, gamete donation can be employed as an empiric therapy.

TDI is increasingly being performed for nontraditional indications. Because sweeping social changes allow and accept nontraditional families, notwithstanding the controversy, TDI has become an avenue for single women or nontraditional couples (lesbians, for example) to achieve parenthood (Knoppers BM, LeBris S, 1993; Jalbert P, et al., 1989). Egg donation may also extend the premise of establishment of various types of nontraditional families and parenting.

Genetic indications are the second major reason (other than infertility) for gamete donation. Although historically, TDI constituted the sole method of avoidance of transmission of a parental genetic trait, an equal opportunity currently exists to avoid transmission of genetic abnormalities conferred by either partner. Although relatively few TDI cases are performed for genetic indications (Verp MS, 1987), TDI can be used as a paradigm for understanding the important issues related to this mode of therapy. In an early multicenter study conducted by the Centre d'Étude et Conservation du Sperme Humain (CECOS), the authors found that only 0.77% of 15,238 requests for sperm donation were for genetic indications. Why are TDI and gamete donation (GD) so infrequently used as genetic therapy? Primarily because only a small number of couples have appropriate genetic indications for gamete donation. Also physicians and patients may not recognize GD as a viable option for such couples. In a later study when the CECOS centers employed a geneticist, pure genetic indication for TDI represented up to 3% of requests (Jalbert P, et al., 1989). From past experiences with TDI it appears that families with genetic disorders frequently perceive GD as an unsatisfactory solution, perhaps because it entails the elimination of genetic material from one of the partners. Both adoption and prenatal diagnosis with selective abortion are chosen more frequently (Verp MS, 1987).

In the original CECOS study, there were 117 requests for sperm donation specifically for a genetic indication. Specifically, 25 cases involved autosomal dominant conditions in the male partner, 59 cases were for autosomal recessive disorders in a previous offspring, 6 cases were for miscellaneous indications, and 16 others were for unspecified reasons (Fédération CECOS et al., 1983). Future indications for using gamete donation to avoid genetic disease must draw from past experience. However, events in this area are changing so rapidly that the relative importance of the past is limited. As issues and arguments evolve daily, "futuristic" issues may soon be current.

AUTOSOMAL DOMINANT INDICATIONS

If one parent has an autosomal dominant disorder, each offspring has a 50% chance of inheriting the gene and thus being affected with the disease at some time during his or her life. Many autosomal dominant conditions are expressed (the patient shows the symptoms of the disease) only after the age of reproduction (twenties and thirties). Therefore they may be transmitted to one's offspring before the determination that one has the gene. Examples of such autosomal dominant diseases include Huntington's chorea, a hereditary neurodegenerative disease with symptomatic onset at the fourth or fifth decade, and, more recently, possibly hereditary breast and ovarian cancer syndrome. These conditions should be evaluated in the context of two formidable issues. First, many members of the extended family and their offspring are threatened by the perception of being at risk. Adding to the psychologic devastation and despair of such an inheritance pattern is the fact that the individuals at risk feel that they are "sitting on a time bomb," waiting to either manifest the disease or find themselves disease-free.

The second issue is the devastating recognition that for many of these genetic disorders, prevention and management are imperfect and cure is unlikely at best. The dilemma confronting such an individual is therefore whether to take a chance and hope he or she is not a carrier, conceiving offspring into the same predicament, or to play it safe and avoid the risk by adopting or using gamete donation. The price paid for eliminating the gene from one's family is that in the process, one's genetic contribution to his or her family is lost forever.

Recently, for a limited number of autosomal dominant diseases, presymptomatic diagnosis has become an option. Diagnosis is usually based on the presence of DNA markers that can be detected rather than analysis of abnormal gene locus (indirect detection). This type of detection requires samples from several affected and unaffected family members to ensure that informative markers are present and are transmitted with the disease gene. Presymptomatic diagnosis thus is associated with the ethical problem of testing asymptomatic individuals (Andrews LB, et al., 1994). Also, indirect diagnosis always includes the possibility of erroneous predictor, with far-reaching psychologic and social complications.

Recently, the Human Genome Project has created the possibility of direct testing for particular mutations and thus presymptomatic detection. The state of the art in this field is in flux and still far from perfect, although the direction and the pace promise much. With increased ability to detect changes in DNA, we are beginning to realize that not every DNA change is expressed as a disorder.

To further complicate the issue, in many autosomal dominant disorders the severity of the disease varies substantially (variable expressivity) (Godfrey M, 1993). For example, neurofibromatosis is a fairly common genetic disorder. In a given family, some affected individuals may have only skin discolorations called "cafe au lait" spots. However others may have severe manifestation of the disease with large deforming tumors. The degree of manifestation of this gene in a family is unpredictable. Parents with mild expression may give birth to severely affected children. Parents must therefore be informed and counseled appropriately. This variable expressivity significantly limits the value of even direct testing, because having the mutation does not indicate the severity of the disease, which can range from almost normal to a severely affected individual. Because of these limitations in genetic testing, gamete donation will continue to be a relevant therapeutic method of prevention.

AUTOSOMAL RECESSIVE INDICATIONS

With autosomal recessive diseases, both parents of an affected child are phenotypically normal, although both possess the abnormal gene. Their future children face a 25% chance of being affected. Such couples may resort to gamete donation if other solutions such as amniocentesis and abortion are perceived as unacceptable. Alternatively, if accurate prenatal testing is available, couples may prefer to undergo prenatal testing and selective abortion of affected fetuses. GD may be seen as the best solution when prenatal testing is not available or when parents have already suffered through several induced abortions of affected fetuses. The advent of carrier testing for autosomal recessive disorders may affect the use of GD as a possible therapy. GD has already been used by couples who are at risk for more common disorders in which carrier screening has been available for some time (e.g., Tay-Sachs disease, cystic fibrosis).

Most autosomal recessive disorders are rare, and the frequency of carriers in the general population is low. Therefore, even for disorders in which carriers cannot be identified, the use of a donor who is unrelated to the couple and who has a negative family history for the disease in question converts the risk of another affected child from 25% to very low.

X-LINKED RECESSIVE INDICATIONS

Male fetuses always inherit their Y chromosome from their father and their X chromosome from their mother. Therefore males with an X-linked disorder never transmit the disease to their sons. Daughters always receive their father's X chromosome and one of their mother's two X chromosomes. Therefore fathers who are affected with an X-linked disorder (e.g., hemophilia) transmit the gene to 100% of their daughters. Their daughters are usually not affected but are obligate carriers and transmit the disease to 50% of their sons. In the past, few couples with X-linked diseases chose TDI, because of a lack of understanding either of genetics or of TDI. The emerging ability for preimplantation gender diagnosis and selection will bring additional solutions to couples who want to avoid the transmission of X-linked diseases and may lead to increased use of reproductive technology to help avoid such problems

Fragile-X is a disease that causes moderate mental retardation and dysmorphism in males and mild retardation in some females who carry the gene. The name comes from the appearance of the X chromosome that carries the abnormal gene (narrowing and breakage at a site on the distal end of the long arm of the chromosome). The genetic transmission of this disease is unusual in that some males are unaffected carriers and females are frequently affected if the gene was transmitted by a carrier mother but are usually not affected if the gene was transmitted through an unaffected male. The relevant issues with fragile-X syndrome is that selecting against males does not promise avoidance of the disease because some of the females in the family may be affected. Fragile-X may be an indicator for GD to avoid female, but not necessarily male, transmission.

CHROMOSOMAL ABNORMALITIES AS INDICATION

Chromosomal abnormalities can be either numerical (additional or missing chromosomes) or structural (rearrangement of pieces of chromosomes). Most chromosomally abnormal adults who are fertile and able to make repro-

ductive decisions are normal (balanced rearrangements) or only mildly affected (e.g., 47,XXX). However, they are at an increased risk of transmitting abnormalities of chromosome number or structure to their offspring, which may confer severe abnormalities resulting in recurrent abortion (Daya S, 1994), mental retardation, or birth defects. In very rare situations, parental chromosomal rearrangement (i.e., 45,XY, t [21q;21q]) will result in an obligate abnormal offspring. Then, gamete donation may be the only option. Prenatal diagnosis and selective abortion are an alternative for other couples if their moral and religious convictions so allow. If not, preimplantation diagnosis may be another option.

GAMETE DONATION AND THE GENE POOL

When gamete donation is done for fertility reasons without genetic screening of the donors, it will probably not affect the gene pool (all the genes that are present in the whole population). However in the face of the rapid unveiling of the human genome, the ability, the availability, and therefore the demand for genetic testing of the donor will likely increase. Under these circumstances, gamete donation could affect the gene pool. The effect of TDI on the gene pool has been discussed previously (Verp MS, 1987). These considerations can be extended to reflect the effects of GD in general. When the primary objective of GD is to prevent the propagation of deleterious genes through carriers, GD may or may not achieve this goal, depending on how the disorder is inherited.

First consider an autosomal dominant disease that does not decrease the ability to reproduce. If all individuals with this disease reproduce through GD, the gene frequency in the population will drop markedly within one generation, and the gene frequency will stabilize at a much lower level depending on the frequency of new mutations. In diseases in which new mutations are very rare (e.g., Huntington's chorea), the abnormal gene will be virtually eliminated from the gene pool.

In the case of an X-linked recessive disease and normal reproductive fitness, if all affected males reproduce by TDI, the frequency of the deleterious gene will be reduced by 33% (67% of the genes would be carried by females). In reality, however, many men with X-linked recessive diseases have reduced reproductive fitness, and the reduction by TDI would be less dramatic. Improvement in management and therapy is bound to increase reproductive fitness for many of these men. Theoretically, if obligate female carriers also chose to use GD, the deleterious gene frequency could be dramatically reduced in the population. Obligate carriers who make such reproductive choices may prefer to undergo gender selection; then, the theoretical reduction of the gene would be 33%.

In contrast, the use of GD by individuals with autosomal recessive disorders would have a limited effect on the gene pool frequency for that specific gene. That is because the recessive trait gene is maintained in high frequency in unaffected heterozygotes rather than in the rare affected homozygotes. It would therefore require hundreds of generations to reduce the gene frequency.

In the foreseeable future, genetic testing and early diagnosis coupled with the possibility for carrier testing will allow different ways to affect the gene pool. The limiting factor will be the excruciating ethical and social dilemmas associated with it. (Please also refer to Chapter 18 and later discussion.) However, even if all heterozygotes (carriers) can and will be identified and carrier couples use GD, the effect on the gene pool will still be small. This is because genes will be maintained in the population by heterozygotes who are reproducing with partners who are not carriers. GD would therefore not have a role in alteration of autosomal recessive gene frequency. If the testing of nonaffected carriers ever becomes prevalent (an issue that is extremely controversial) (Andrews LB, et al., 1994), other methods of avoiding affected offspring will prevail.

DONOR SCREENING

The production of a perfect child cannot be guaranteed in GD programs—or for that matter by any other current method of reproduction (Opinion in Nature, 1994a). Many times, GD is performed for nongenetic (infertility) or nontraditional indications. This "limitation" of the procedure might be overlooked by patients or misrepresented by caregivers. One can argue that when GD is performed for nongenetic reasons, the rule of thumb should be that donors ought to be tested only to the extent that traditional partners are tested. Some argue for more intensive testing of both donor and recipient (Jalbert P, et al., 1989).

The practical matter is that when GD is done for infertility therapy and, to an even greater extent when it is done for nontraditional reasons, the level of expectation is usually different. TDI, for example, is currently being done in this country from frozen sperm only. The days in which every practitioner had a list of "volunteering donors" from a nearby medical college are over. The process of preparing sperm and monitoring sperm for TDI is very tedious and time-consuming (McCulloh DH, Wolf DP, 1993). The practice of repeated testing of donors for infectious diseases was introduced. The process of such preparation has been taken over by commercial sperm banks, which sell the sperm samples to the recipient. Sperm donation therefore has been removed from the area of volunteerism and is now in the area of consumerism in which sperm is "packaged" and sold as a commodity. Sperm banks want their product to be commercially competitive. The consumer, on the other hand, expects guarantees and also expects to be able to examine the product in the package. A recent article (Rodrick S, 1994) in *The New Republic* entitled "Upward Motility (at the Ivy League sperm bank)" captures the contemporary interaction of sperm bank, donor, and customers (as they are touted):

"Wanted: brainy sperm nerds need not apply." So reads the ad in the Harvard University and MIT newspapers. The founder of the sperm bank makes a concerted effort to acquire superior specimens from the best and the brightest so that he can offer each client: a donor she would be proud to take home to her mother, a "twenty-five page donor profile, a novella-length questionnaire that asked about my academic achievements. . . . Additional facts were required about my relatives," states the potential donor. "Was my uncle balding? How about my aunt's bone structure: small, medium, large or very large?"

The bank also "boasts of a donor matching service." Stephen Rodrick, the reporter who went through the donor path, asked whether sperm banks market master race sperm, but the director "sniffs at the suggestion. This is a client driven market. While a college degree doesn't guarantee the child will be a good person, it does suggest a basic level of organization and a degree of integrity." Finally, Mr. Rodrick failed the screening. "Alas while my sperm was described as 'normal' I was not accepted as a donor." Mr. Rodrick asked a Harvard man who was accepted whether he was bothered by the bank's snobbish approach. The answer was "no way,

it's a business deal. If you pay top dollar, you should get top sperm. I'm pretty honored."

This perception is particularly prevalent and is being cultivated among nontraditional recipients. Sperm banks offer celebrity, genius, athletic, and Ivy League–derived sperm and try to supply any demand. In parallel, the media are flooded by information about recent discoveries in the field of genetics and the future prescribed by projects deciphering the human genome (Maddox J, 1993; Elmer-Dewitt P, 1994). This high level of expectation that visionary possibilities will become the reality of tomorrow are fueled by "the spate of information now flowing from human genetics and embryology engendering the illusion that everything is possible. (Triumphalist talk by some practitioners has not helped.) But everything is not yet possible, nor will it be" (Opinion in Nature, 1994a).

Traditionally, when donors were selected for TDI, attempts were made to match the donor's appearance with that of the recipient's partner. TDI programs were also trying to assess the fertility potential of the donor by choosing donors who had sired normal offspring. Recently records of fertilization, pregnancies, "objective" semen analysis, and measures of infectious diseases are employed. Historically, the level of sophistication in identifying genetic risk factors among sperm donors by practitioners of TDI was very low and was mostly limited to medical histories (Curie-Cohen M, et al., 1979). Only recently, with the recognition that open-ended self-assessment questions constitute inadequate screening for donors, have genetic questionnaires been developed (see Appendix 6-A, the questionnaire used for egg donors at the University of Chicago). This questionnaire requests information regarding the health of the donor and all her first-degree relatives (brothers, sisters, parents, and children); second-degree relatives, and third-degree relatives (mainly first cousins). Carrier testing for genes that exist in high frequency in specific ethnic groups may be necessary. People of African descent, for example, should be tested for sickle-cell anemia and β-thalassemia; those of Mediterranean descent for β-thalassemia; those of Asian descent for α-thalassemia; Ashkenazi Jews for Tay-Sachs disease, and southern European Caucasians for cystic fibrosis.

DONOR TESTING FOR CHROMOSOMAL DISORDERS

Potential gamete donors, male or female, who have had a trisomic offspring (including trisomy that was identified in a stillborn) should not be used because these individuals carry risk of recurrence. Similarly, a history of an unexplained stillborn, abnormal live born, or recurrent spontaneous abortions in an egg donor or the female partner of a sperm donor or their parent or sibling may indicate the possibility of a chromosomal abnormality and should exclude them as potential donors. Similarly, donors who have a balanced chromosomal translocation, low-level aneuploidy, or inversion should be excluded (Verp MS, et al., 1983). Alternatively, in some of these cases, cytogenetic studies of the donor could be performed with the use of the potential donor if no abnormality is found. However, routine cytogenetic studies on all donors is controversial because of the high cost and low yield. The common practice in anonymous egg donor programs is to use young donors below the age of 35. One must remember that even if chromosomal testing (as suggested by CECOS, for example) and younger donors are used, chromosomal abnormalities in the offspring are not precluded. Many TDI recipients are older women who themselves possess a higher

risk for chromosomal abnormalities and miscarriages. It is also possible that some couples with intractable infertility may themselves have chromosomal abnormalities that constitute an unrecognized contribution to their lower fertility. Also, older egg recipients may have reduced selective mechanism to elude chromosomally defective embryos. These latter considerations may encourage some programs to consider testing recipients as well as donors (Verp MS, 1987; Jalbert P, et al., 1989).

MENDELIAN DISORDERS

Donors are usually excluded from programs when their offspring are at risk for a serious Mendelian disorder. For example, donors who themselves have a serious autosomal dominant condition (e.g., Marfan syndrome) are excluded. In the case of autosomal dominant diseases with late onset, incomplete penetrance, or variable expression (e.g., Huntington's chorea, polycystic kidney disease), the likelihood that an apparently healthy donor with a positive family history carries the deleterious gene is high. Such donors should also be excluded. That notwithstanding, a genetic disorder with complete penetrance and early onset (e.g., achondroplasia) in which the disease is easily recognized in individuals who carry the gene should not preclude unaffected individuals from GD. For X-linked disorders the following guidelines apply. An affected male donor is excluded. However, there is no reason to exclude an unaffected male donor on the basis of a family history of Duchene muscular dystrophy. Historically, donors who were affected with serious autosomal recessive diseases were not used because all their offspring would be obligate carriers. Donors with a family history of an autosomal recessive disease for which carrier testing was unavailable were also excluded. Today, carrier status can be determined for Tay-Sachs, cystic fibrosis, and sickle-cell anemia. Exclusion of heterozygote carriers as donors is appropriate when the recipient is heterozygous for the same trait, but the same donor may be used for a recipient who does not carry the trait, especially if the donor is sufficiently desirable because of his ethnic background and if the recipient agrees.

More than half of the common congenital abnormalities (e.g., heart defects, cleft lip and palate, neural tube defect) result from the simultaneous involvement of several genes and environmental factors (polygenic/multifactorial). The risk to offspring or siblings (first-degree relatives) of affected individuals ranges from 2% to 15%. Donors who are affected by such disorders or who have affected children should therefore be excluded. Affected individuals who are second- or third-degree relatives of the donors have a much lower risk. It is very important to recognize that most of the desirable traits that potential recipients put in their "shopping list" when they choose a donor are inherited as polygenic/multifactorial traits (e.g., IQ, height, body structure). We understand even less about the inheritance of life interests or personality traits such as tenderness and love of music and arts. Examining the distribution of traits within families shows that even a child who resembles his or her parents (especially when racial phenotypes are examined) may differ markedly from both parents in appearance, psychic attributes, and abilities. It is therefore misleading to promise a given outcome on the basis of the level of matching between the donor and the recipient's partner or recipient's wishes.

Our increased ability to do more accurate genetic testing raises the false perception that in the near future it will be possible to identify the "ideal donor." Indeed, it will be possible to identify many of the individuals who carry one of the several thousand single-gene defects by DNA analysis. With imminent improvement in technology, carrier status for many rare autosomal and X-linked diseases will be detectable by multiplex technology (Andrews LB, et al., 1994; Check WA, 1993). How this technology should be used is a matter of bitter dispute (Elmer-Dewitt P, 1994). The detection or even the understanding of mode of inheritance of polygenic/multifactorial traits and defects is still far in the future. The controversy and the problems are apparent; however, it seems almost inevitable that the new technology will be used. It is conceivable, therefore, that such technology, albeit with its considerable costs, will be incorporated into GD programs. Practitioners of GD should recognize the impact of such testing and should be prepared to deal with it in the future.

Unlike sperm donation, egg donation programs have a limited supply of donors, and donor recruitment is a formidable task. This is because egg donation is a more involved and risky enterprise. Even just using family history as a source of exclusionary criteria puts a heavy toll on the availability of donors. These limiting factors apply to both egg and sperm potential donors; however, they are more critical to the already limited supply of egg donors.

It is feasible that introduction of directed DNA testing and identification and exclusion of specific disorders in donors will allow donors to be declared risk-free for a particular trait. However, from such an apparently beneficial role, testing can lead into the more controversial pursuit of the "perfect child." Such an extension of the technique may again threaten the size of the donor pool by excluding donors with proven "undesirable" traits or diseases.

Although in the past it appeared that TDI donors who were excluded from donation on genetic grounds did not seem to feel stigmatized (Czeizel A, et al., 1979), future testing may expose the donor to an undesirable risk (Allen W, Oster H, 1993). The use and moreover the possible prerequisite requirement of direct genetic multiplex testing of donors (which may reveal, for example, predisposition for late onset diseases such as breast or colon cancer) impose a heavy burden on the donor and on the GD program. This burden extends from the donor himself or herself to the donor's extended family. It is beyond the scope of this chapter to discuss the issue of testing healthy carriers, a category into which all tested donors fall. The results of a recent survey among directors of life insurance companies suggests that while "few insurers perform genetic tests on applicants," "most are interested in accessing genetic test information about applicants that already exist" (McEwen JE, et al., 1993). The problems of future insurability, discrimination in the workplace or in education, stigmatization, anxiety, and intrafamilial instability may all accrue following identification of a disease gene in a currently healthy donor (Holtzman NA, Rothstein MA, 1992; Opinion in Nature, 1994b). These problems have not been resolved for the issue of screening of the general population, and it is unlikely that there will be easy answers for the GD program. Historically, the responsibility of the GD program toward the donor was mainly in keeping his or her anonymity and providing an explanation when donation was rejected. This responsibility becomes manyfold increased and multifaceted when carrier testing is integrated. Genetic counseling is required for interpreting results of DNA testing. Short and long-term psychological and genetic counseling may be required for the carrier donor and members of his or her family.

The nature of GD is evolving and its indications widening. The use of known donors and ad hoc known donors, although controversial (because of intricate interpersonal and legal complications), is common in specific circumstances. In the face of extreme difficulty of donor recruitment in egg donation programs, many resort to using a member of the family, a friend, or an ad hoc volunteer whom they recruit on their own. In other circumstances a known donor may belong to the ethnic or racial group that is desired and not otherwise available. Under such circumstances, donor screening or testing may become even more problematic.

Previous statements that were made in this text regarding exclusion criteria for donors may not hold. Recipients may still insist on using a donor even when he or she has a predisposition for a severe disease or is actually an affected donor. This may be because the donor is a relative or has a specific rare ethnic background. Many practitioners may feel the need to put limits on their acceptance criteria, guided by their responsibility toward society. Ethical conflict therefore may arise between caregivers who refuse to use such a donor and the wishes of the couple. These sentiments may be construed by others as too paternalistic and eugenic. Traditionally, geneticists tend to be nondirective in their counseling. GD, however, involves multidisciplinary cooperation and professionals who may be less detached when acts of a selective nature are involved.

The Encyclopedia Britannica micropedia defines eugenics as "the study of human improvement by genetic means." Most of the genetic practice and counseling today are considered noneugenic owing to their nondirective nature. Therefore reproductive decisions and specifically participation in GD programs are made by the recipient or the recipient's family unit. Most of society believes that "the prevention of disease or abnormality is an important goal of counseling" (Wertz DC, Fletcher JC, 1993). In the context of the history of eugenics, negative eugenics programs in the world spawned monstrous social and political movements that culminated in genocide by the Nazis in Europe. Fear of such a eugenics comeback is prevalent (Garver KL, Garver B, 1994). Wertz and Fletcher suggest that "the basic fears appear to be (1) coercion into having prenatal diagnosis and abortion, (2) exploitation of women for the benefit of medical or social institutions, (3) excesses or misuses of prenatal diagnosis for 'frivolous' purposes such as sex selection, (4) discrimination against people with disabilities especially if their births could have been prevented." It is beyond the scope of this chapter to further discuss eugenics and its various definitions and dichotomies, which are summarized in excellent reviews (Paul DB, 1994; Wertz DC, Fletcher JC, 1993). All of these fears are summoned by the development of GD and especially the combination of GD and genetic testing. Despite the notion in some quarters that too little screening of donors is practiced, others voice the concern that GD donation may be used or misused for selective breeding of individuals who have desirable traits (positive eugenics). However, it appears that GD alone (despite the hopes of the proponents and the fears of the objectors) is far from being an efficient tool for positive eugenics. With the recognition that GD can be combined with the increased ability for accurate genetic testing, such fears and hopes are on the rise again (Garver KL, Garver B, 1994).

The rapid developments in ART and genetics necessitate serious considerations of genetic issues (Knoppers BM, LeBris S, 1993) that are also part and parcel of GD. As genetics affects society at large, its effect will specifically be felt in reproductive therapy and GD. It is our responsibility to explore these issues and to develop programs that avoid the mistakes of the past and meet the challenges and risks of the future.

REFERENCES

1. Allen W, Oster H. (1993) Anticipating unfair use of genetic information. Am J Hum Genet 53:16–21.
2. Andrews LB, Fullarton JE, Holtzman NA, Motulsky AG, eds. (1994) Executive summary assessing genetic risks implication for health and social policy. Committee on Assessing Genetic Risks, Division of Health Sciences Policy, Institute of Medicine. Washington, D.C.: National Academy Press.
3. Check WA. (1993) A coming together in genetics. CAP Today 7(12):15–24.
4. China's misconception of eugenics. (1994b) Opinion in Nature 367:1–2.
5. Curie-Cohen M, Luttrell L, Shapiro S. (1979) Current practice of artificial insemination by donor in the United States. N Engl J Med 300:585–590.
6. Czeizel A, Szentesi I, Horváth L, Shapiro S. (1979) Results of genetic screening of donors for artificial insemination. Clin Genet 24:113–116.
7. Daya S. (1994) Issues in the etiology of recurrent spontaneous abortion. Current Opinion in Obstetrics and Gynecology 6:153–159.
8. Dean NL, Edwards RG. (1994) Oocyte donation: Implication for fertility treatment in the nineties. Current Opinion in Obstet Gynecol 6:160–165.
9. Elmer-Dewitt P. (1994) The genetic revolution. Time Jan 17:46–53.
10. Fédération CECOS, Mattei JF, LeMarec B. (1983) Genetic aspects of artificial insemination by donor (AID): Indication, surveillance and results. Clin Genet 23:132–138.
11. Garver KL, Garver B. (1994) The Human Genome Project and Eugenic Concerns. Am J Hum Genet 54:148–158.
12. Godfrey M. (1993) Molecular heterogeneity: A clinical dilemma. Clinical heterogeneity: A molecular dilemma. Am J Hum Genet 53:22–25.
13. Holtzman NA, Rothstein MA. (1992) Invited Editorial: Eugenics and genetic discrimination. Am J Hum Genet 50:457–459.
14. Jalbert P, Leonard C, Selva J, David G. (1989) Genetic aspects of artificial insemination with donor semen: The French CECOS Federation Guidelines. Am J Med Genet 33:269–275.
15. Knoppers BM, LeBris S. (1993) Ethical and legal concerns: Reproductive technologies 1990–1993. Current Opinion in Obstet Gynecol 5:630–635.
16. Maddox J. (1993) Wilful public misunderstanding of genetics. Nature 364:281.
17. McCulloh DH, Wolf DP. (1993) Male factor and sperm preparation for assisted reproductive technologies. Infertility and Reproductive Medicine Clinics of North America 4(4):667–682.
18. McEwen JE, McCarthy K, Reilly PR. (1993) A survey of medical directors of life insurance

companies concerning use of genetic information. Am J Hum Genet 53:33–45.

19. More fuss about genetics and embryos. (1994a) Opinion in Nature 367:99–100.

20. Paul DB. (1992) Eugenic anxieties and social realities. Social Research (October issue).

21. Rodrick S. (1994) Upward motility (at the Ivy League sperm bank). The New Republic May 16:9–10.

22. Shapiro S. (1992) Strategies to improve efficiency of therapeutic donor insemination. Infertility and Reproductive Medicine Clinics of North America 3(2):469–485.

23. Verp MS. (1987) Genetic issues in artificial insemination by donor. Seminars in Reproductive Endocrinol 5(1):59–68.

24. Verp MS, Cohen MR, Simpson JL. (1983) Necessity of formal genetic screening in artificial insemination by donor. Obstet Gynecol 62:474–479.

25. Wertz DC, Fletcher JC. (1993) A critique of some feminist challenges to prenatal diagnosis. J Women's Health 2:173–188.

26. Zilberstein M, Seibel MM. (1994) Fertilization and implantation. Current Opinion in Obstet Gynecol 6:184–189.

Appendix 6-A

Pedigree

Name_____

Date_____

Genetic Screening Form for Egg Donor/Partner of Recipient

(Circle One)

**THE UNIVERSITY OF CHICAGO
DEPARTMENT OF OB/GYN**

1. Name _____   2. ID# _____

3. Date _____/_____/_____ (mm/dd/yy)   4. Birthdate _____

5. Age _____

6. How many of your (or your partner's) pregnancies have resulted in:

    1. _____ miscarriages at _____ weeks   4. _____ livebirths

    2. _____ elective abortions   5. _____ infant deaths

    3. _____ stillbirths

7. Family background (check one)   1. Black _____   2. Hispanic _____   3. Greek _____
   4. Jewish _____   5. Northern European Caucasian _____   6. Middle Eastern _____
   7. Italian _____   8. Southeast Asian _____   9. Other (specify) _____

8. If Jewish or French Canadian, have you been tested for Tay Sachs? _____

    If yes, where was test done? _____

    Results: _____

9. If Black, have you been screened for Sickle Cell? _____

    If yes, where was test done? _____

    Results: _____

10. If Greek, Italian, other Mediterranean, Hispanic, or Asian, have you been screened for Thalassemia?
    _____

11. If Northern European, have you been screened for Cystic Fibrosis? _____

12. Family Background

    Indicate if you, your siblings, parents, grandparents or other extended family members (blood relatives)
    have any of the conditions listed on the next page. Indicate which family member and age of onset.

    These are examples of some conditions that may be inherited in a family. Please list other inherited
    conditions or birth defects that are not mentioned. A negative family history does not guarantee a healthy
    baby.

Condition	Self Yes	Self No	Family Yes	Family No	Comments (Indicate which family member and age of onset)
Malformations:					
1. Cleft Lip					
2. Cleft Palate					
3. Spina Bifida					
4. Congenital Heart Defect					
5. Clubfoot					
6. Congenital Hip Dislocation					
7. Other (specify):					
Mendelian Disorders:					
8. Albinism					
9. Retinitis Pigmentosa					
10. Hemophilia					
11. Colon Cancer (before age 65)					
12. Breast Cancer (before age 50)					
13. Neurofibromatosis					
14. Marfan syndrome					
15. Tuberous Sclerosis					
16. Huntington Disease					
17. Muscular Dystrophy					
18. Cystic Fibrosis					
19. Sickle Cell Anemia					
20. Tay Sachs					
21. Other (specify)					

Condition	Self		Family		Comments (Indicate which family member and age of onset)
	Yes	No	Yes	No	
Familial Disease:					
22. Asthma					
23. Allergy					
24. Diabetes Mellitus					
25. Epilepsy					
26. Coronary Artery Disease					
27. Schizophrenia or Manic Depression					
28. Deafness (before age 60)					
29. Blindness					
30. Arthritis (before age 50)					
Chromosome Abnormality:					
31. Down Syndrome					
32. Other (specify)					
33. Mental Retardation					
34. Learning Delay					

Genetics Comments

Name_____

Date_____

PART II

LEGAL ISSUES

Seldom does the law lead the way into new arenas, and the field of assisted reproductive technology is no exception. Indeed, as the assisted reproductive technologies radically alter the ways in which we create families, these medical advances often stand in stark contrast to the judicial and legislative efforts to provide a framework within which to use them and with which to secure the families they help to create.

This section explores the legal aspects of the ARTs and ovum donation. Chapter 7 reviews the current laws that form the legal backdrop against which the reproductive technologies are emerging; Chapter 8 reviews legal issues of access, insurance coverage, and discrimination in this emerging field; Chapter 9 highlights specific legal issues that are raised by egg donation; and Chapter 10 addresses unique concerns that arise in drafting consent forms and recommended agreements for both donors and recipients. Legal guidance in establishing programs and guiding providers and participants through their use of these medical advances is desirable.

As medical advances continue to race forward, the challenge for both lawmakers and those seeking legal guidance in this area will be to create a thoughtful and consistent legal framework within which the rights and responsibilities of all involved will be recognized, defined, and protected.

Susan L. Crockin, J.D.

7

Laws Surrounding Reproductive Technologies

AMI S. JAEGER, J.D.

In our pluralistic society there is one issue on which most people can agree: Bearing and rearing children are fundamental to how we view ourselves and how we define ourselves in society. Yet for many people, having children is complicated by infertility. Thus couples and individuals turn to third parties to assist them in achieving their goal of being able to parent. The involvement of third parties alters the traditional notion of family structures formed around children. As it becomes clear that the old ways of structuring rights, duties, and responsibilities between individuals does not adequately deal with the issues raised by reproductive technologies, legal schemes are required to mediate the unique relationships created by these technologies.

BACKGROUND ON ASSISTED REPRODUCTIVE TECHNOLOGY AND THE LAW

New family dynamics are possible as a result of reproductive technologies. Originally intended to assist married couples, the new reproductive technologies can be used to facilitate single parenthood: Single men may hire a surrogate; single women may be artificially inseminated. The insemination of single women or women in lesbian partnerships or use of a surrogate by a single male or a gay male couple provides a new lens by which to view traditional notions of family. The increase in single parents and same sex couples as parents raises such issues as whether it is in the child's best interests to have two parents and whether a single parent can meet a child's physical and emotional needs, especially if the parent will have to work to support the child. These issues spark the debate about whether the quality and continuity of parental relationships, rather than a traditional lifestyle or a parent of either gender, are the primary factors contributing to healthy child development.[1]

As one thinks about how reproductive technologies affect our society and how the laws that regulate medically assisted reproduction affect behavior within society, it may be helpful to think about the overriding theme that has directed our notion of family. In a general sense, genetic links have defined the bounds (and boundaries) of family duties, obligations, and rights. Rules govern genetic relatedness in our society. As medical and scientific progress changes the way in which people can become a family and have a family, it has caused changes that stretch the traditional concept of genetic ties defining family structure. In addition to medical breakthroughs, changes in social relationships have also altered what society has come to accept as

113

a family. Now society accepts "blended" families created by divorce and remarriage.

How can we construct laws that are consistent and even-handed when the importance of the genetic link conflicts with different goals? For example, anonymous sperm donors want to relinquish all parental rights, but with surrogacy the sperm donor wants to retain all parental rights; or with gestational surrogacy the gestational mother who has no genetic link to the child may claim her biological link as being equal to or greater than the genetic component.

The media have caught our attention in troubling adoption situations in which biological parents change their mind about relinquishing their parental rights or claim that they never properly consented to the adoption and reassert the parental rights. The adopting parents claim that their bonding with the child outweighs the genetic link of the natural parents. What rights should the genetic parents have? At what time, and through what legal procedures, should they (or others) be able to sever or reassert these rights? Recent adoption cases speak to the importance of providing a loving, nurturing environment for our children and question the importance of the genetic connection among families as the sole indication of family ties. How should the law weigh these different measures and values of parenting? The legislation that is constructed around the issues reflects our values and priorities. We must carefully and thoughtfully consider what is best for the children of these families and devise legislative schemes accordingly.

CONSTITUTIONAL ISSUES

The law provides a legal basis for the protection of individual autonomy in reproductive decisions. Decisions about whether and when to have children are thought to be a matter of personal concern, not subject to government mandate. The U.S. Constitution protects reproductive decisions under the right to privacy. The right to procreate and reproductive autonomy is a fundamental right, meaning that the right to procreate is essential to our notion of liberty and justice.

The U.S. Supreme Court articulated the constitutional protection of reproductive decisions as early as 1942 in *Skinner* v. *Oklahoma*,[2] which struck down an Oklahoma statute authorizing the sterilization of habitual criminals convicted of crimes involving moral turpitude.[3] The Court stated, "we are dealing with legislation which involves one of the basic civil rights of man. Marriage and procreation are fundamental to the very existence and survival of the race."[4]

In a later series of cases involving contraception and abortion, the U.S. Supreme Court described an individual's decision about whether or not to bear or beget a child as constitutionally protected from governmental interferences.[5] The Court deemed childbearing and childrearing rights as "far more precious than property rights."[6] The Court wrote, "if the right of privacy means anything it is the right of the individual, married or single, to be free of unwarranted governmental intrusion into matters so fundamentally affecting a person as the decision whether to bear or beget a child."[7] For a governmental regulation that infringes on reproductive decisions to be upheld as constitutional, it must be necessary to further a compelling state interest, and it must regulate in the least restrictive manner possible.[8]

The U.S. Supreme Court reaffirmed the constitutional protection of reproductive decisions involving sterilization, contraception, and the creation of a family.[9] The Court wrote that the "Constitution places limits on a state's right to interfere with a person's most basic decisions about family and parenthood."[10] While the majority decision in *Casey* allowed the state of Pennsylvania to place some restrictions on a woman's access to abortion,[11] it affirmed that the state's regulations must not be an undue burden on a woman's liberty right. The liberty right is composed of the "private sphere of the family" and the "very bodily integrity of the pregnant woman."[12] A law or regulation creates an undue burden if the burden is too severe or if it lacks a legitimate, rational justification.[13]

It is hard to imagine a state interest strong enough to justify a law prohibiting a person from choosing to become a parent. "The decision ranks in importance with any other a person may make in a lifetime; an attempt to imagine state interests that would justify governmental intrusions amounting to a practical prohibition on procreation and childbearing takes us out of our experience and into an imaginary world of Malthusian nightmare."[14]

Various commentators and legislators have set forth particular state interests that they argue would justify regulating reproductive technologies. These include the fetus's interest in being free from pain; the potential child's interest in being physically and mentally healthy; the adult participant's interest in being free from undue physical and psychological risk; the individual's interest in making decisions about his or her body; the individual's and couple's interest in reproductive and parental autonomy; the donor's and surrogate's interest in being free from manipulation by other people; doctors' and researchers' interest in meeting their professional obligations to help patients and to further scientific knowledge; and society's interest in retaining values and maintaining institutions such as the family. Types of regulations that arguably would be permissible if they were narrowly tailored to accomplish the goal with minimal interference include governmental regulation to ensure quality of medical care, to ensure adequate disclosure of information to allow participants to make an informed decision, to protect gamete recipients from transmissible infectious diseases, and to

require record keeping and allow offspring access to nonidentifying medical information about their genetic and gestational parents.[15]

The constitutional right of privacy protects the decision to reproduce coitally because of the biological and social importance of being a parent.[16] The rationales that protect reproductive autonomy extend to decisions to reproduce noncoitally. One court recognized that "it takes no great leap of logic to see that within the cluster of constitutionally protected choices that are included within that cluster is the right to submit to a medical procedure that may bring about, rather than prevent, a pregnancy."[17] The New Jersey Supreme Court in the landmark *Baby M* case, dealing with a child conceived by artificial insemination of a surrogate mother, noted that alternative reproduction methods fall within the constitutional right of privacy.[18] Although the court's holding focused on the surrogate contract, the court carefully distinguished between reproduction, custody, and the use of money. Plainly, if one has the right to reproduce coitally, then one has the right to reproduce noncoitally. Not only is reproduction constitutionally protected, but the means of reproduction are protected as well. The values and interests underlying the creation of the family are the same.[19] Moreover, "the Constitution serves human values,"[20] regardless of any given moral opinion of assisted reproduction. The law and the judges who interpret the law have an "obligation to define the liberty of all, not mandate our own moral code."[21]

FAMILY LAW ISSUES: LEGAL AND BIOLOGICAL PARENTHOOD

One commentator argues that the right to procreate, which extends to coital and noncoital choices, should be characterized as the right to parent rather than the right to achieve and maintain a biological tie with a child.[22] This, the author argues, "could clear a conceptual path for a theory of family that turns on the existence of social relationships between individuals."[23] We do not need to look further than the Jessica DeBoer adoption struggles to appreciate that there is more to parenting than biological ties; however, the law has historically recognized biological ties as determinative of parental rights to ensure that children were cared for, to promote predictability in rights and responsibilities, and in part because medical technology (including DNA blood tests) was not sufficiently developed to assert parental rights outside of a traditional marriage.

One of the primary purposes of the law, besides to protect the parties' reproductive rights, is to clarify the parental rights of individuals with respect to the children who are created through alternative reproduction. As medical technologies have advanced, the legal and social definition of parenthood has lagged behind. Reproductive technologies make it possible for a child to have five parents: genetic mother, gestational mother, rearing (or social) mother, genetic father, and rearing (or social) father. The law is called upon to mediate the respective rights and duties of all parties involved. Until the introduction of advanced reproductive technologies, the law strove to provide a child with two parents—a father and a mother—allegedly to protect the best interests of the child.

The importance of a genetic connection between a father and child has been resolved in the law. A genetic connection between a man and a child will create financial and legal responsibilities, regardless of the man's intentions to produce or raise offspring, even without formal legal interventions such as adoption.[24] If the woman is married, however, the child is presumed to be genetically related to the woman's husband, regardless of the genetic reality. This presumption, in most states,

may be challenged. The legal presumption of paternity has made it easy to adopt therapeutic donor insemination (TDI) into the existing legal framework. The husband is presumed to be the father of the child. This is consistent with TDI, in which the sperm donor does not intend to maintain his parental rights. Courts have confirmed that when a sperm donor voluntarily agrees to relinquish his parental rights, he has no link to the resulting child, even if the donor changes his mind after the birth of the child.[25]

In most states, statutory responses to paternity issues have resolved the genetic and social aspects of fathering in the case of TDI.[26] In vitro fertilization and oocyte or embryo donation, however, raise novel issues, and the existing legal framework may not be sufficient to protect the parties' intentions. The gestational mother may or may not intend to raise the child. Likewise, the oocyte donor may not wish to relinquish her parental responsibilities. Statutory schemes addressing reproductive technologies, such as oocyte or embryo donation, must balance the social, genetic, and gestational aspects of paternity and maternity. In other words, the law must mediate between legal and biological parenthood.

Single Parenthood

The focal point of case law concerning the therapeutic donor insemination of single women has been paternity. Generally, single women choose TDI because they do not wish to establish future contact with the donor as a rearing parent; and men donating sperm share similar expectations.[27] Twelve states clarify that the sperm recipient is the sole parent of the child and the donor has no legal obligations or duties with respect to the child.[28] An Ohio law tries to clarify this issue by providing that if an unmarried woman is artificially inseminated, "the donor shall not be treated in law or regarded as the natural father."[29]

In contrast, a New Jersey case involving the home insemination of a single woman held that the man providing the semen was the legal father of the child.[30] This decision is based on a unique set of facts, and so it does not provide much guidance for other cases. The court held that the boyfriend who provided the sperm was the legal father and granted him visitation rights. In reaching its decision, the court distinguished this from previous artificial insemination cases because "there is no married couple [and because] there is no anonymous donor."[31] The court found that "If an unmarried woman conceives a child through artificial insemination from semen from a known man, that man cannot be considered to be less a father because he is not married to the woman."[32] The court also stated that the decision was consistent with judicial policy "favoring the requirement that a child be provided with a father as well as a mother."[33] This decision has been read narrowly. In another case, however, a known sperm donor is claiming parental rights to a child that he helped a lesbian couple father.[34] One court denied his claims, and noted the child already had a family and two psychological parents. An intermediate appellate court ruled in favor of the sperm donor having paternal rights and the case is on further appeal. There have been no cases in which an anonymous sperm donor has been held liable for child support against his wishes.

A majority of the TDI statutes assume that a married couple will be using the procedure, but none make it illegal for an unmarried woman to do so.[35] But many statutes either explicitly apply only to married women or could be interpreted as being inapplicable to single women. The Ohio and Oregon statutes specifically acknowledge that a single woman might use donor sperm.[36] No laws prohibit the insemination of unmarried women. Even if a state passed such a law, it is unlikely that it would be upheld as constitutional. The consti-

tutional protection of reproductive decisions extends to individuals as well as married couples.[37] As the U.S. Supreme Court noted, "It is the right of the *individual*, married or single, to be free of unwarranted governmental intrusion in matters so fundamentally affecting a person as the decision whether to bear or beget a child."[38] A single woman, denied TDI at a clinic affiliated with a state or federal institution that will inseminate only married couples, can claim that her privacy right to make procreative decisions and her equal protection rights are violated by the clinic's policies.

Social attitudes, including disapproval of nontraditional families, are not compelling reasons to prohibit the insemination of single women or to prohibit same sex couples from becoming parents. One court stated in a case involving an unmarried woman undergoing artificial insemination, "[w]e wish to stress that our opinion in this case is not intended to express any judicial preference toward traditional notions of family structure or toward providing a father where a single woman has chosen to bear a child."[39]

Laws have mandated physician involvement in procedures of assisted reproduction even when the medical complexity of the procedure is not great. To the extent that the law does not mandate that a physician provide assisted reproductive services, this can affect the ease of access to the technologies. What we are really calling into question is not the medical complexity of reproductive technologies, but the social issue of who should be allowed to parent and who should have the authority to decide who will parent. "Deputizing physicians to decide which women should become mothers" could be viewed as allowing physicians to make moral decisions about what makes a good parent.[40] Of course, if an individual physician is uncomfortable performing a particular procedure for personal or other reasons, another physician may be sought out.

If a woman wants to ensure donor anonymity and adequate semen screening, she must seek a physician who will perform the insemination. The physician as moral gatekeeper could be viewed as a capricious, unjust method of social control.[41] Society does not regulate or license conception through traditional intercourse, and so arguably it should not regulate who should become parents when the means of conception have changed.[42] However, conception through traditional intercourse, in contrast to donor gametes, is not anonymous or screened. Therefore the physician serves to ensure the medical, genetic, and infectious quality of the semen samples and to provide anonymity. As Daniel and Norma Wikler point out, involvement of the medical profession in artificial donor insemination has spared us "a troubling examination of our own values regarding reproductive freedom, the meaning of parenthood, and the interest of children."[43]

OVERVIEW OF CURRENT LEGAL STRUCTURE AFFECTING ASSISTED REPRODUCTION

There is a patchwork of laws governing assisted reproduction. These laws range from embryo and fetal research statutes, artificial insemination statutes, laws on in vitro fertilization, clinic success rate disclosure and laboratory regulation laws, surrogate parenting statutes, adoption laws, paternity statutes, medical practice statutes addressing confidentiality and record keeping, and uniform anatomical gift act governing donation. Not all states have passed laws in all of these areas; thus practitioners must be familiar with the laws specifically enacted in their state.

The statutes are an attempt to address the conflicting policy debate surrounding the moral status of the embryo and what ethical and legal duties are created with respect to the embryo. Society must balance the ethical and moral value of protecting the embryo with the potential scientific and social gains from such investigation.

Embryo Research

There are federal and state laws governing fetal research. Federal law defines "fetus" as a product of conception from implantation to birth;[44] thus it does not regulate techniques such as in vitro fertilization (IVF) or in vivo fertilization followed by embryo transfer. A further set of regulations prohibited federal funding of research involving IVF unless it was reviewed by the Ethics Advisory Board. The term of the board expired and was not reconstituted, so there has been a de facto moratorium on federally funded IVF research. On taking office in January 1993, President Bill Clinton signed an executive order lifting the ban on fetal tissue use for research.[45]

In response to the executive order, Harold Varmus, Director of the National Institutes of Health, created an advisory panel to recommend guidelines for reviewing applications involving human embryo research. The NIH Human Embryo Research Panel recommended that the federal government fund research on preimplantation human embryos as long as the research is conducted by qualified individuals, the research design is valid and promises significant scientific or clinical benefit, the research goals cannot be accomplished by using animals or unfertilized gametes, the number of embryos is kept to a minimum, and gamete or embryo donors have fully consented to the nature and purpose of the research. The report prohibits payment for gametes or embryos but allows reasonable compensation for the donor's expenses.

The panel recommended that research be conducted until the appearance of the primitive streak, or up to fourteen days. The panel specifically noted that cloning of preimplantation embryos followed by in utero transfer, nuclei transplant with in utero transfer, use of fetal oocytes with in utero transfer, research beyond onset of neural tube closure, preimplantation diagnosis for sex selection except for sex-linked genetic diseases, development of chimeras, transfer for extrauterine or abdominal pregnancy, nonhuman gestation of human embryos, and cross-species fertilization were unacceptable for federal funding.

The panel based its recommendations on three major premises: Human embryo research holds great promise for improving human health; preimplantation embryos, while worthy of serious moral consideration, do not have the same moral status as infants and children; and federal funding can provide more rigorous scientific and ethical review than current privately funded research can.

The final Panel Report was reviewed by the Advisory Committee to the Director, NIH, which approved the panel report in the fall, 1994 and presented it to Harold Varmus. In December, 1994, President Clinton issued a directive that federal funds may not be used to support creation of embryos for research purposes. That executive directive did not apply to research on "spare" embryos, those not created solely for research purposes. Congress could still pass substantive laws or funding restrictions which would go beyond those set forth by the President. The approved panel report is currently under review by the NIH.

State laws extend beyond federally funded research and could affect privately funded investigation and the clinical practice of a number of infertility techniques involving embryos. At least 25 states have laws specifically aimed at regulating fetal research.[46] Of these, 24 states impose some restriction on experimentation with live fetuses ex utero,[47] six prohibit or impose sanctions aimed at prohibiting any type of research on a live fetus,[48] and twelve prohibit nontherapeutic research on live fetuses.[49] The Louisiana statute prohibits an IVF embryo from being "farmed or cultured solely for research purposes or any other purposes."[50]

While federal law defines "fetus" as any product of conception from implantation to birth, states have adopted their own definitions. For example, only Utah has adopted the federal definition of fetus.[51] Other states have adopted a broader definition of "fetus," defining it from the moment of fertilization.[52] Many states do not define "fetus" or "embryo," which leads to confusion for medical practitioners, since their notion of embryo and fetus reflect scientific realities that the statutes do not take into account.[53] State laws that do not define "embryo" or conflate fetus with embryo, may erect barriers to useful procedures such as genetic screening of preimplantation embryos. Federal law, however, would not preclude such activities; such regulations apply only after the embryo is implanted.

Many genetic and reproductive technologies that are now available and under investigation were not contemplated at the time state fetal research laws were enacted. Most of the state fetal research statutes were passed as part of abortion legislation.[54] The constitutionality of existing fetal research laws should be considered in light of the context in which they were enacted. One state fetal research ban has already been ruled unconstitutional.[55]

The Federal Court of Appeals for the Fifth Circuit questioned the continued validity of the statutory bans on embryo and fetal research.[56] The court declared unconstitutional a Louisiana law that forbade experimentation on an aborted fetus unless the experimentation was therapeutic.[57] The court concluded that the word "experimentation" was impermissibly vague because physicians do not and cannot clearly distinguish between medical experiments and medical tests.[58] The court noted that "even medical treatment can be reasonably described as both a test and an experiment."[59]

Other courts have also found that "experimentation" and "therapeutic" are unconstitutionally vague terms.[60] In the federal district court case *Lifchez*, a group of physicians specializing in reproductive endocrinology and fertility counseling challenged an Illinois statute that prohibited experimentation on a fetus unless it was therapeutic to the fetus.[61] The court noted that even within the scientific and medical communities there is no single definition of "experimentation."[62] The court held that the statute was impermissibly vague. The court noted that what is an experimental procedure may change to an accepted procedure within six months.[63] This uncertainty would force physicians to guess which procedures were unlawful. Moreover, it could essentially freeze a given technique in time, thus preventing the development of procedures that are innovative, are less risky, or demonstrate an improved outcome.

In Vitro Fertilization

There are distinct federal and state regulations on fetal research that may affect in vitro fertilization (IVF), including federal requirements for reporting of pregnancy rates by clinics and state certification of embryo labs. Since federal law defines "fetus" as a product of conception from implantation to birth, IVF is not prohibited by federal law. State laws extend beyond governmentally funded research and could affect privately funded investigation and the private clinical practice of a number of infertility techniques involving embryos. Two states specifically address therapeutic IVF: Pennsylvania and Louisiana.[64]

A few states specifically address IVF in their fetal research statutes. For example, New Mexico defines "clinical research" to include research involving human IVF.[65] Illinois, on the other hand, in the statute reviewed by the court in *Lifchez*, specifically exempted IVF from the prohibition on fetal research.[66]

During IVF treatments a woman may produce more oocytes and embryos than she can safely use for reproductive purposes. Questions arise as to whether these embryos may be cryopreserved, discarded, donated or sold to another woman, or used for research. The answer depends on statutory regulation and the wishes of the couple. The laws regulating fetal research before or after a planned abortion would not affect cryopreservation after IVF, since neither procedure involves an aborted fetus.[67]

The Fertility Clinic Success Rate and Certification Act was enacted in October 1992 to take effect in October 1994.[68] The law requires reporting of pregnancy rates by clinics, specifically including clinics that perform IVF procedures, to the Centers for Disease Control. That same law provides for certification of embryo laboratories by requiring the Secretary of Health and Human Services to "develop a model program for certification of embryo laboratories to be carried out by the States."[69] States are permitted, but not required, to adopt the model program.

Cryopreservation of Embryos

One primary issue raised by IVF is the ownership of, and the right to control the fate of, the embryos that are created through IVF. Courts have recognized that the couple whose gametes were used to create the embryos have a property interest in those embryos.[70] In one situation a couple who underwent IVF treatment for infertility commenced a divorce proceeding. There were seven embryos that were cryopreserved pending implantation at the time the couple filed for divorce. During the divorce settlement the couple disputed the fate of the cryopreserved embryos. The trial court awarded custody of the embryos to the wife, Mary Sue Davis, and directed that she "be permitted the opportunity to bring these children to term through implantation."[71] The court reasoned that the cryopreserved embryos were children and that the best interest of the "children" was "that they be made available for implantation to assure their opportunity for live birth."[72] The trial court stated that issues of custody, support, and visitation were to be decided at the time an embryo resulted in a live birth.

The husband, Junior Davis, appealed the custody award. On appeal, the appellate court reversed the trial court's decision and vested "Mary Sue and Junior with joint control of the fertilized ova with an equal voice over their disposition."[73] The court found that there were significant scientific and moral differences between a cryopreserved fertilized ovum and an embryo in a woman's womb. Moreover, the court stated that it is "repugnant and offensive to constitutional principles to order Mary Sue to implant these fertilized ova against her will. It would be equally repugnant to order Junior to bear the psychological, if not the legal, consequences of paternity against his will."[74] The court cited Nazi Germany's Hereditary Health Courts as a grim reminder of the evils of state interference with reproduction. The embryos were ultimately returned to Junior Davis and allowed to expire amidst news coverage and further commentary.[75]

In another case that considered ownership of embryos, a couple undergoing infertility therapy had several embryos cryopreserved.[76] They moved from the East Coast to the West Coast and wanted to take the embryos with them for implantation by a West Coast infertility clinic.[77] The East Coast clinic refused to release the embryos. The court reviewed the consent form signed by the couple and the clinic. The agreement did not include a provision for interclinic transfer. The court noted, however, that the American Fertility Society Ethical Statement took the position that embryos are the property of the donors.[78] Under the theory of bailment, the court noted that the embryos were property of the couple; therefore the clinic, as bailee, was required to release the embryos to the couple.

Donation and Sale of Gametes and Embryos

A couple undergoing infertility therapies may wish to donate or sell excess embryos to another individual.[79] Fifteen states prohibit a woman from selling an embryo for experimentation;[80] nine states prohibit the donation of embryos or a fetus for research purposes.[81]

Following charges and investigations of some physicians' and programs' unauthorized use of excess eggs and embryos, in 1995 legislation was proposed in one state (California) which would provide civil penalties for the removal or use of eggs and embryos without the patient's consent. The proposed penalties are three times the value, defined as the amount of money, profit, or value the defendant gained, and never to be less than $10,000.

As embryo transfer after IVF or in vivo fertilization becomes standard clinical practice and no longer experimental, these regulations will no longer restrict donation, since the procedure falls outside the scope of the statute.

The restriction on the sale or donation of embryos for research must be distinguished from the bans in two states that restrict such sale or donation for any purpose.[82] The primary distinction between them is that even as in vivo fertilization followed by embryo transfer becomes standard clinical procedure, the latter laws would still restrict the sale or donation of embryos.

Although the Louisiana statute prohibits the sale of oocytes and embryos created through IVF,[83] it allows embryo donation.[84] It states, "[i]f the in vitro fertilization patients renounce, by notarial act, their parental rights for in utero implantation, then the in vitro fertilized human ovum shall be available for adoptive implantation in accordance with written procedures of the facility where it is housed or stored."[85] No payment will be made to either party. A further provision prohibits the culture of an in vitro fertilized human ovum for research "or any other purposes."[86] Thus it seems that excess embryos may be donated, but only for implantation in another woman, not for research purposes.

A Kentucky law seems to require public medical facilities to donate excess IVF embryos for implantation. The statute allows public medical facilities to conduct IVF "as long as such procedures do not result in the intentional destruction of a human embryo."[87]

A recent California legislative proposal that was defeated would have regulated egg donation.[88] The bill was intended to regulate surrogate and gestational surrogate parenting arrangements, but in the process it placed restrictions on egg donation. For example, it provided that an egg donor be at least 21 years old and already have borne at least one child. It also did not allow eggs to be donated for reasons other than implantation. It provided for a written egg donor contract in which the egg donor relinquished all parental or custodial rights to any child who is conceived with her egg. The proposal allowed for compensation to the egg donor.

The legislation and bills addressing egg and embryo donation seem oddly out of balance. Rather than paralleling public policy toward anonymous sperm donation, which places no requirement about previous children and does not prohibit payment for sperm, these provisions create restrictions on egg donors that seem unjustified from a policy perspective. There is an inequity in allowing payment to sperm donors but not allowing payment to egg donors. While not all states ban payment to egg donors, no state specifically prohibits payment to sperm donors. There is no moral or policy rationale for this disparity, and it is yet another example of gender-based dis-

crimination in the form of unequal compensation.[89] In fact, considering the medical risk and degree of invasiveness, egg donors should be more highly compensated than sperm donors.[90]

In contrast, at least two of three states that have recently passed legislation involving egg donation have simply tracked the language and scope of sperm donation statutes. Both Oklahoma (passed in 1990) and Texas (passed in 1993) have one-paragraph statutes[91] that state that a child born to a married woman as the result of egg donation is deemed to be the child of the marriage and the egg donor has no parental rights or responsibilities. The third state, Florida, passed a much more comprehensive statute[92] (also in 1993) that addresses gestational surrogacy as well as egg donation. The Florida statute also explicitly allows reasonable compensation for egg and embryo donation. (For a more comprehensive discussion and a copy of these laws, see Chapter 9, "Legal Issues in Egg Donation.")

Artificial Insemination

Unlike IVF when used by a couple to treat infertility, TDI introduces a person who will not have a continuing relationship with the child or the child's parent. The donor's involvement in the procedure is unrelated to rearing the child. Reasons for seeking TDI include male infertility, genetic background of the male partner (including carrier status), or absence of a male partner.[93]

Historically, TDI was the first reproductive therapy developed[94] and has been available as a therapeutic option since the early 1950s.[95] Early on, the courts were presented with the issue of defining who is the legal father of a child conceived with donated sperm and with the assistance of a physician.

Traditionally, children born to a married woman are presumed to be the children of the woman's husband, regardless of the biological realities. This "presumption of paternity" is common in many state statutes.[96] Early on, the courts recognized the consenting husband's legal parentage through a series of cases that established the child's legal identity. Usually, these cases arose out of a divorce proceeding. In one case the husband claimed that he should not have to support the child because they were not genetically related.[97] In another the wife tried to deny her husband visitation rights on the basis of the same rationale.[98] Sometimes, in the earliest cases, the courts declared the child born as a result of TDI to be illegitimate. It is well established, however, that the courts will protect the child financially and emotionally by finding the consenting husband to be the legal father, with support responsibilities and visitation rights.[99] All of the 35 states that regulate TDI clarify the paternity of a child by providing that the sperm recipient and her consenting husband are the child's legal parents.[100] The consenting husband is the legal father for legitimacy, inheritance, and support purposes.[101] Some statutes, such as those of Minnesota, Montana, Nevada, New Mexico, Virginia, Wisconsin, and Wyoming, require the husband's written consent to the procedure for him to be recognized as the legal parent.[102]

TDI is a relatively simple and common procedure. Yet semen donation presents the potential for transmitting communicable infectious diseases, including AIDS. Therefore adequate screening of donors and proper quarantine of samples with retesting of donors before release is essential. To promote and safeguard quality standards, federal regulations for semen banking have been proposed.[103] The regulation follows on the heels of American Association of Tissue Banks and American Society of Reproductive Medicine voluntary guidelines and would add federal regulatory enforcement authority to quality standards. The proposed rules would not address ethical or parental right issues.

Surrogate Parenting

When the female partner is infertile or unable to carry a child to term, a surrogate or gestational surrogate (also referred to as a gestational carrier) provides the missing component. This escalates the degree of third-party involvement in the process. No longer is there an anonymous donor, as with TDI, but a woman who contributes both the genetic and gestational component (if a surrogate) or the gestational component (if a gestational surrogate). The process of gestating and giving birth to a child raises serious questions about balancing the autonomy and bodily integrity of the surrogate or carrier while she is gestating a child for another person to rear. It also raises issues about what the appropriate legal response should be if she should change her mind and decide that she does not want to relinquish the child after birth.

The New Jersey Supreme Court in the landmark *Baby M* decision was faced with a surrogate who decided after the birth that she could not relinquish the child created though a surrogate parenting arrangement.[104] The New Jersey Supreme Court held that the man providing the sperm was the legal father and the woman providing the egg and gestating the embryo was the legal mother.[105] The court voided the surrogacy contract and thereby the parties' original intention to have the spouse of the man providing the sperm be recognized as the legal mother. The parties proceeded with a custody battle for the child between the surrogate and the genetic father. The court awarded custody to the father and his spouse but granted visitation rights to the surrogate.

Generally, parties seek the assistance of an attorney to draft a surrogate parenting agreement. The physician who agrees to participate in a surrogate arrangement would be well advised to consider whether he or she could comply with the terms of an agreement before agreeing to commence any procedures. For example, would the physician be comfortable if the contract afforded the intended rearing parents the final authority to consent to a cesarean section during delivery?

In addition to issues of bodily integrity of the surrogate and issues of remedies in the event the surrogate changes her mind and breaches the contract, payment to the surrogate raises issues of the legality of the surrogate arrangement contract. If payment to the surrogate is for the child, constitutional and likely state law prohibitions against baby selling are violated. If the contract is for services, that is, the service of providing a gamete or gestating an embryo, payment does not run afoul of baby-selling prohibitions.

Regulatory approaches that allow surrogacy contracts to be enforceable as long as the surrogate is not paid are arguably more coercive than allowing payment. Not allowing payment diminishes to zero the value added by the surrogate. People choose occupations that are physically and emotionally risky. Attorneys choose jobs that they know are stressful and demanding. Race car drivers and firefighters choose jobs that pose great physical risk. People freely enter into contracts and negotiate compensation for their services. While women should not be compelled to bear children they do not wish to raise, neither should they be prohibited from freely entering into contracts and negotiating compensation for services that are physically and emotionally risky. Prohibiting women from entering into contracts for money treats women as children and reinforces Victorian notions of women as weak and unable to navigate within society.

Arizona, Arkansas, Florida, Indiana, Kansas, Kentucky, Louisiana, Michigan, Nebraska, Nevada, New Hampshire, New York, North Dakota, Utah, Virginia, and Washington specifically regulate surrogate motherhood arrangements.[106] Of these sixteen states, only six specifically address paternity. The Arkansas statute presumes that the legal mother of a child who is conceived by artificial insemination and born to an unmarried surrogate mother is the intended mother. The Arizona statute presumes that the surrogate is the legal mother of the child; if she is married, her husband is presumed to be the legal father. The Arizona statute has been declared unconstitutional by an intermediate appellate court of that state.* [footnote cite: *Soos* v. *Maricopa County Sup. Ct.*, 1994 WL 682826 (AZ. App. Div.). The court found that the law was discriminatory by failing to provide a way for a woman to rebut the presumption of maternity, while providing a way for a man to disprove his paternity. In Florida, the intended parents are presumed to be the legal parents upon a determination that at least one intended parent is genetically related to the child;[107] otherwise, the woman giving birth is presumed to be the legal mother.[108] New Hampshire and Virginia laws provide that a judicial order signed before the pregnancy vests parental rights with the intended parents.[109] North Dakota presumes that the birth mother is the legal mother; her husband is the legal father if he was a party to the surrogacy agreement. The Arizona law bans surrogacy contracts. The Nevada and Virginia laws allow payment to a surrogate; Louisiana, Indiana, Kentucky, Nebraska, New York, North Dakota, and Utah void paid surrogacy contracts. New York also voids unpaid surrogate contracts. Florida, New Hampshire, and Washington limit compensation to payment of incurred expenses. If a dispute arose in states that void the contract or in those that have no surrogacy statute, the existing TDI, adoption, and parentage statutes would provide a framework for determining paternity. This statutory approach would not avoid parents having to go through formal adoption proceedings to establish parental rights, nor would it prevent potentially damaging child custody battles.

Gestational Surrogacy

Courts have placed importance on the genetic link to the child and thus have taken a different approach in cases involving gestational surrogates. Courts have adopted the position that the couple who provide the gametes and are the intended parents are the legal parents. In *Calvert* v. *Johnson*, a case involving a surrogate gestational mother who carried a couple's embryo, a district court recognized the genetic parents as the legal parents and granted them the right to have their names put on the birth certificate.[110] The gestational surrogate was not considered to be the legal mother, and the couple did not have to adopt the child. The California Supreme Court *upheld* the contract and found that the gestational surrogate had no parental rights to the child. It ruled that the law recognizes "both genetic consanguinity and giving birth as a means of establishing a mother and child relationship, when the two means do not coincide in one woman, she who intends to procreate the child—that is, she who intends to bring about the birth of a child that she intended to raise as her own—is the natural mother."[111]

Two New York courts reached contradictory conclusions. One, *In Re Andres,* refused to grant an Order of Maternity to the genetic mother of a child born to a gestational surrogate. Although the gestational and genetic parents were in agreement, that court found that there was no adequate provision in its state laws to recognize a genetic mother. It agreed to recognize the genetic father through an Order of Paternity but ruled that the genetic mother must proceed with a stepparent adoption to legitimize her parental status.[112] In contrast, a different New York court overruled a lower court that had refused to grant just such an order. In that case, *Arredondo* v. *Nodelman*[113], the intermediate appellate court granted a petition for maternity, ruling that the genetic tests performed excluded the gestational carrier as the mother of twins and granted the order for a declaration of maternity and paternity under existing New York law.

Judges respond to parental disputes by shaping outcomes that favor biological relationships over social relationships. Legislation reinforces the judicial and societal import that is placed on biological parent-child relationships. This view of parenting, however, may be too limited.[114] The best interest of the child may well be served by having legislation that avoids custody battles and provides a secure parenting arrangement.

INFORMED CONSENT, QUALITY ASSURANCE, RECORD KEEPING

Issues of informed consent, quality assurance, and record keeping are critically important and relate to all reproductive technologies. These issues touch on all areas of medical practice as well and should be familiar to medical practitioners. The practice of assisted reproduction poses unique considerations for informed consent, quality assurance, and record keeping.

Informed consent requires that a physician fully explain the risks and benefits of a procedure or treatment and alternative treatments to a patient before undertaking the treatment. In addition to obtaining consent to the procedure, professionals working with both gamete and embryo donors must pay careful attention to consent with respect to parental responsibilities. Donors must clearly relinquish parental responsibilities or specifically retain parental responsibilities to children created by using their gametes. If adoption is part of the legal process to clarify parental obligations (as in surrogacy and possibly in gestational surrogacy) and consent was not properly obtained, the adoption can unravel in extremely painful ways. In the case of sperm donors it is unlikely that anonymous sperm donors would change their mind later in life and wish to assert parental rights.[115] The best precaution is adequate, well documented, informed consent before the donation is made.

Additionally, the physician performing IVF should discuss the risks involved with egg or embryo donation with the donors. Women donating eggs should be counseled about the physical risks associated with egg donation, such as infection, permanent scarring, and other side effects. In addition to these physical risks, women who undergo infertility therapy must be counseled on the psychological risks of egg or embryo donation. First, the physician should make sure there is no coercion of the woman or the couple to donate an egg or embryo. Participation in an IVF program should not be limited to women or couples who agree to donate excess embryos.[116] Second, the physician must counsel the woman to consider the emotional risk of donation in case she herself does not achieve a pregnancy. Donors also should consider the risk of the resulting child's potential emotional reaction on learning of the existence a biological parent with whom he or she will have no contact.

Quality assurance issues for assisted reproduction include proper screening of donors and quarantine of donations. Donors should be screening for infectious diseases including HIV. Genetic screening may also be requested by the person (or couple) receiving donated gametes or embryos. This would especially be true for couples using donated gametes because both were carriers for a genetic disorder. Maintenance of proper clinic-specific information on pregnancy rates is advisable. A component of a quality assurance program includes continual monitoring and updating of practices and procedures.

Record keeping often becomes critical many years after the donation. Usually, the records contain information that is needed for the benefit of the child. The child may, for medical reasons, need to contact the donor to determine histocompatibility or to answer questions about his or her genetic history. Other reasons for maintaining accurate records on donors and recipients are to prevent further use of donated specimens if there is an unfavorable result, if the health of the donor changes dramatically, or if the recipient needs to be recontacted for other reasons. The record keeping requirement may seem burdensome to providers. However, they are in the best position to maintain accurate and irreplaceable medical information on donors, recipients, and resulting children.

IMPLICATIONS FOR EGG DONATION

As we look to the future of reproductive technologies, such as sperm injection,[117] preimplantation screening of embryos,[118] and fetal egg use,[119] we need to examine policies underlying the laws and consider how laws should be shaped or changed to meet scientific realities and ethical objectives. Women have been granted autonomy and constitutional protection in reproductive decisions, including deciding to obtain an abortion without consulting their spouse or the child's father.[120] We should not construct barriers to egg or embryo donation that threaten reproductive autonomy. Think how we would react to a statutory requirement that required sperm donors (most of whom are medical students) to have fathered a child and be responsible for it before they donated sperm. It seems ridiculous. Yet these restrictions have been proposed for egg donors.[121] It creates a troubling double standard for women. These technologies, while allowing women greater reproductive choices, can be subtly shaded to discriminate against and disempower women. Laws that allow payment for male gametes but not for female gametes are an obvious example of unfairness in reproductive laws.

In addition to regulating the donation of gametes, policy discussions may address who should receive donated eggs. Who should establish a priority, and how should the priority be established if there is a gamete shortage? Should researchers take priority over women or couples? Policies should consider the various reasons women seek donated gametes. These women may include women with genetic disorders, women who carry genetic disorders, women with other health problems, or women with infertility. Moreover, policies may consider issues of postmenopausal women receiving donated eggs.

Careful consideration of legislative action and vigilance to constitutional principles, including privacy and equal protection, are necessary as the law attempts to keep up with medical science and shape social and familial relationships. Ethical pitfalls abound, given the complexity of the issues and divergence of moral opinions in our society; the best approach is a political policy that protects individual autonomy and allows each person to be guided by his or her ethical values.

CONCLUSION

Laws mediate between parties with different intentions and different objectives but with a single purpose: to create a family. The laws must be shaped to protect the interests of the parties involved and of the children who are created as a result of using medically assisted reproduction. These technologies have created a new role for third parties, apart from rearing and caring for the child, which in turn has brought challenges to traditional social networks of families.

Early on, laws presumed that children born within a marriage were the children of the husband and wife. Thus therapeutic donor insemination and in vitro fertilization with donated gametes fit within traditional legal schemes. They did pose novel issues of ownership and control of extracorporeal embryos. Surrogacy and gestational surrogacy raised notions of how to structure and enforce complicated relationships between parties. It also brought to light issues of nontraditional families. As biological parentage and legal parentage become distinct because of medical breakthroughs, society will need to create schemes to provide a secure and nurturing environment for all children. Policies with respect to gamete donation are the core of any such scheme.

We all feel the reach of these laws, whether as patients, legal and health professionals, legislators, or judges. We should work in concert to ensure that the law protects parties involved, not that it unjustly prohibits people from the promise of creating and being part of a family.

ENDNOTES

[1] "Developments: Medical technology and the Law," 103 *Harvard Law Journal* 1519, 1535 (1990).

[2] *Skinner* v. *Oklahoma*, 316 U.S. 535 (1942).

[3] In this case the crime of moral turpitude was stealing chickens. The defendant in this case was sentenced to be sterilized because he was a chicken thief.

[4] *Skinner* v. *Oklahoma*, 316 U.S. 535, 541 (1942).

[5] See, for example, *Griswold* v. *Connecticut*, 381 U.S. 479 (1965); *Eisenstadt* v. *Baird*, 405 U.S. 438 (1972); *Roe* v. *Wade*, 410 U.S. 113 (1973).

[6] *Stanley* v. *Illinois*, 405 U.S. 645, 651 (1972).

[7] *Eisenstadt* v. *Baird*, 405 U.S. 438, 453 (1972).

[8] *Roe* v. *Wade*, 410 U.S. 113, 115 (1973).

[9] *Planned Parenthood of Southeastern Pennsylvania* v. *Casey*, 112 S. Ct. 2791, 60 U.S.L.W. 4795 (1992).

[10] *Casey* at 4779.

[11] Namely, it allowed a 24-hour waiting period and allowed parental consent for minors with a judicial bypass.

[12] *Casey* at 4812.

[13] *Casey* at 4819, J. Stevens, concurring.

[14]Karst, "The Freedom of Intimate Association," 89 *Yale L. J.* 624 (1980).

[15]Office of Technology Assessment, *Infertility: Medical and Social Choices* (1988) at 223. Hereinafter cited as OTA, *Infertility*.

[16]See Robertson, "Embryos, Families, and Procreative Liberty: The Legal Structure of the New Reproduction," 59 *So. Cal. L. Rev.* 939 (1986).

[17]*Lifchez* v. *Hartigan*, 735 F. Supp. 1361, 1377 (N.D. Ill. 1990).

[18]*In re Baby M*, 217 N.J. Super. 313, 525 A.2d 1128 (N.J. 1987); 109 N.J. 396, 537 A.2d 1227 (1988). See also *Lifchez* v. *Hartigan* 735 F. Supp. 1361 (N.D. Ill. 1990).

[19]Skoloff, "Introduction to Draft ABA Model Surrogacy Act," 22 *Fam. L. Q.* 119 (Summer 1988).

[20]*Planned Parenthood of Southeastern Pennsylvania* v. *Casey*, 112 S. Ct. 2791, 60 U.S.L.W. 4795, 4801 (1992).

[21]*Casey* at 4800.

[22]Harvard, *supra* n. 1.

[23]Harvard, *supra* n. 1 at 1532.

[24]OTA, *Infertility*, *supra* n. 15 at 239.

[25]Hevesi, "Court Rejects Sperm Donor in a Bid for Parental Rights," *New York Times* B3 (April 16, 1993).

[26]But realize that some states have required the involvement of physicians to ensure the relinquishment of the donor's parental interests. *Jhordan C.* v. *Mary K.*, 179 Cal. App. 3d 386, 224 Cal. Rptr. 530 (1986).

[27]Harvard, *supra* n. 1 at 1535.

[28]Arkansas, California, Colorado, Illinois, New Hampshire, New Jersey, New Mexico, Ohio, Oregon, Washington, Wisconsin, and Wyoming.

[29]Ohio Rev. Code Ann. §3111.37(B) (Baldwin 1987). The statute does not define "woman" as married woman.

[30]*C.M.* v. *C.C.*, 152 N.J. Super. 160, 377 A.2d 821 (1977).

[31]*C.M.* v. *C.C.*, 152 N.J. Super. 160, 377 A.2d 821, 824 (1977).

[32]*C.M.* v. *C.C.*, 152 N.J. Super. 160, 377 A.2d 821, 824 (1977).

[33]*C.M.* v. *C.C.*, 152 N.J. Super. 160, 377 A.2d 821, 824 (1977).

[34]*Thomas S.* v *Robin Y.*, 627 N.Y.S.2d 326 (1995).

[35]Kritchevsky, "The Unmarried Womans' Right to Artificial Insemination: A Call for an Expanded Definition of Family." 4 *Harvard Women's L. J.* 1 (1981).

[36]Ohio Rev. Code Ann. §3111.31 (Baldwin 1987); Or. Rev. Stat. §677.365 (1977). The Ohio statute applies to artificial insemination for the purpose of impregnating a woman so that she can bear a child that she intends to raise as her child. The Oregon statute requires the consent of her husband "if she is married." Or. Rev. Stat. §677.365 (1977).

[37]*Eisenstadt* v. *Baird*, 405 U.S. 438 (1972).

[38]*Eisenstadt* v. *Baird*, 405 U.S. 438, 453 (1972) (emphasis in the original).

[39]*Jhordan C.* v. *Mary K.*, 179 Cal. App. 3d 386, 224 Cal. Rptr. 530, 537-8 (1986).

[40]Wikler and Wikler, "Turkey-baster Babies: The Demedicalization of Artificial Insemination," 69 *Milbank Quarterly* 5, 31 (1991).

[41]Wikler and Wikler, *supra* n. 39 at 31-32.

[42]Perhaps that is why the debate around surrogate parenting including gestational surrogates is so troubling. We have not yet come to grips with the distinction between social and biological parenting, the degree of protection third-party participants need, and who is in the best position to ensure that all parties are protected.

[43]Wikler and Wikler, *supra* n. 39 at 35.

[44]45 C.F.R. §46.203(c) 1986.

[45]58 *Fed. Reg.* 7468 (Feb. 5, 1993). See Bianchi, Bernfield, Nathan, "Commentary: A Revived Opportunity for Fetal Research," 363 *Nature* 12 (May 6, 1993).

[46]Ariz. Rev. Stat. Ann. §36-2302 (1986); Ark. Stat. Ann. §§82-436 to 442 (Supp. 1985); Cal. Health & Safety Code §25956 (West 1984); Fla. Stat Ann. §§390.001(6), (7) (West 1986); Ill. Ann. Stat. ch. 38, para. 81-26(7) (Smith-Hurd 1986); Ind. Code §35-1-58.5–6 (1986); Ky. Rev. Stat. Ann. §436.026 (Baldwin 1985); La. Rev. Stat. Ann. §9:122, §14:87 (West 1991); Me. Rev. Stat. Ann. tit. 22, §1593 (1980); Mass. Ann. Laws ch. 112, §12J (Law. Co-op. 1985); Mich. Comp. Laws Ann. §§333.2685–.2692 (West 1980); Minn. Stat. Ann. §§145.421–.422 (West Supp. 1987); Mo. Rev. Stat. §188.037 (Vernon 1983); Mont. Code Ann. §50-20-108(3) (1985); Neb. Rev. Stat. §§28-342 to -346 (1985); N.M. Stat. Ann. §24-9A-1 (1981); N.D. Cent. Code §14-02.02-01 to 02 (1981); Ohio Rev. Code Ann. §2919.14 (Baldwin 1982); Okla. Stat. Ann. tit. 63, §1-735 (West 1984); Pa. Stat. Ann. tit. 18, §3216 (Purdon 1983); R.I. Gen. Laws §11-54-1 (Supp. 1992); S.D. Codified Laws Ann. §34-23A-17 (1986); Tenn. Code Ann. §39-4-208 (1982); Utah Code Ann. §§76-7-310 to -311 (1978); and Wyo. Stat. §35-6-115 (1977).

[47]Only Utah does not have such a restriction.

[48]Arizona, Indiana, Kentucky, Maine, Ohio, and

Wyoming. All these laws, except for Maine's, apply only to research on aborted fetuses.

[49] Arkansas, California, Florida, Missouri, Nebraska, Oklahoma, and Pennsylvania, which apply only to live aborted fetuses; and Illinois, Massachusetts, Montana, North Dakota, and Rhode Island, which apply to living fetuses.

[50] La. Rev. Stat. Ann. §9:122 (West 1991).

[51] Utah Code §76-7-301 (Supp. 1992).

[52] Arkansas, California, Ohio (a product of conception); Louisiana, New Mexico, Oklahoma (from the moment of conception to birth); Illinois, Kentucky, Minnesota, Pennsylvania (fertilization until birth).

[53] Arizona, Florida, Maine, Massachusetts, Missouri, Montana, Michigan, Nebraska, North Dakota, Rhode Island, South Dakota, Tennessee, Wyoming.

[54] L. Andrews, *Medical Genetics: A Legal Frontier* (1987) at 83. Andrews, "Regulation of Experimentation on the Unborn," 14 *J. Legal Medicine* 25 (1993).

[55] *Margaret S.* v. *Treen*, 597 F. Supp. 636 (E.D. La. 1984) *aff'd on other grounds, Margaret S.* v. *Edwards*, 794 F.2d 994 (5th Cir. 1986).

[56] *Margaret S.* v. *Edwards*, 794 F.2d 994 (5th Cir. 1986).

[57] *Margaret S.* v. *Edwards*, 794 F.2d 994 (5th Cir. 1986).

[58] *Id.* at 999.

[59] *Id.* at 999. The lower court held that there was no legitimate state interest in affording greater protection to fetuses than to deceased persons. *Margaret S.* v. *Treen*, 597 F. Supp. 636, 674-75 (E.D. La. 1984). The Fifth Circuit affirmed the district court's decision on the narrower grounds of the vagueness of the term "experimentation."

[60] *Lifchez* v. *Hartigan*, 735 F. Supp. 1361 (N.D. Ill. 1990).

[61] Ill. Rev. Stat. ch. 38, p. 81-26 §6(7) (Smith Hurd 1989).

[62] *Lifchez* at 1364.

[63] *Lifchez* at 1366.

[64] Pa. Stat. Ann. tit. 18, §3216 (Purdon 1983); La. Rev. Stat. Ann. §9:122 (West 1991).

[65] N.M. Stat. Ann. §24-9A01(D) (1986).

[66] Ill. Ann. Stat. ch. 38, para. 81-26(7) (Smith-Hurd Supp. 1987); *Lifchez* v. *Hartigan*, 735 F. Supp, 1361 (N.D. Ill. 1990).

[67] Arizona, Arkansas, California, Florida, Indiana, Kentucky, Missouri, Nebraska, Ohio, Oklahoma, Tennessee, and Wyoming.

[68] Pub. Law. 102-493, 42 U.S.C.A. 263a-1 (West Supp. 1994).

[69] 42 U.S.C.A. § 263a-2(a)(1) (West Supp. 1994).

[70] *Davis v. Davis*, 1989 WL 140495.

[71] *Davis* at 11.

[72] *Davis* at 11.

[73] *Davis* at 3.

[74] *Davis* at 3.

[75] "Embryos Destroyed", *National Law Journal* 8 (June 28,1993); Mansfield, "Destroyed Embryos Leave Legal, Social Legacy," *AP Wire Service* (June 21, 1993). Others expressed the opinion that the expiration would lead to the exploitation of embryos. "Geneticist Says Supreme Court Ruling Will Lead to Exploitation of Embryos," *AP Wire Service* (July 29, 1993).

[76] *York* v. *Jones*, 717 F. Supp. 421 (1989).

[77] The couple also alleged that the East Coast clinic fraudulently disclosed its pregnancy rate to be 38% when it actually was 15% and that the West Coast infertility clinic had a higher pregnancy success rate than the East Coast clinic.

[78] *York* at 426.

[79] Congress has expressly banned the sale of organs, including fetal tissue. 42 U.S.C. §VX (Supp. III 1985). See also Andrews, Medical Genetics, *supra* n. 53 at 165. The states that do not have a statutory framework regarding embryo and fetal tissue could be governed by the Uniform Anatomical Gift Act, which allows the donation of fetal tissue.

[80] Arkansas, Florida, Kentucky, Louisiana (only involves embryos created through IVF), Maine, Massachusetts, Michigan, Minnesota, Nebraska, New Mexico, North Dakota, Ohio, Oklahoma, Rhode Island, and Utah.

[81] Arkansas, Kentucky, Maine, Massachusetts, Michigan, Nebraska, North Dakota, Rhode Island, and Wyoming.

[82] Fla. Stat. Ann. §873.05 (West Supp. 1987); La. Rev. Stat. Ann. §9:122 (West 1991) (prohibits sale of IVF embryos).

[83] La. Rev. Stat. Ann. §9:122 (West 1991).

[84] La. Rev. Stat. Ann. §9:130 (West 1991).

[85] La. Rev. Stat. Ann. §9:130 (West 1991).

[86] La. Rev. Stat. Ann. §9:122 (West 1991).

[87] Ky. Rev. Stat. Ann. §311.715 (Michie 1990).

[88] Cal. S.B. 1160 (as amended) (May 26, 1993). The bill failed to pass the Senate and was dropped.

[89] See Mahar, "Special Report: The Truth About Women's Pay," *Working Woman* 52 (April, 1993). Even for nontraditional industries, such as biotechnology, women earn on average $27,000 *less* annually than men. 11 *Bio/Technology* 994 (September 1993).

[90] Seibel, "Compensating Egg Donors: Equal Pay for Equal Time?," 328 *N. Eng. J. Med.* 737 (1993).

[91]Okla.Stat.Ann.Tit. 10, Sec. 544 (1991); Tex.S.B. 512, 73rd Leg. R.S. (1993).

[92]Fla. Stat. § 742.14 (1994).

[93]Although the absence of a male partner is perceived as being a social problem, not a medical problem.

[94]Wikler and Wikler, *supra* n. 39 at 9-10.

[95]OTA, *Infertility, supra* n. 15 at 242.

[96]OTA, *Infertility, supra* n. 15 at 239.

[97]*Anonymous* v. *Anonymous*, 41 Misc. 2d 886, 246 N.Y.S.2d 1835 (1964).

[98]*N.Y.* v. *Dennett*, 15 Misc. 2d 260, 184 N.Y.S.2d 178 (1958).

[99]Harvard, *supra* n. 1 at 1533. In a recent custody case involving children conceived with IVF, the father made the argument that the children should be declared illegitimate, since they were not genetically related to the mother. The court rejected this argument. *McDonald* v. *McDonald*, 608 N.Y.Supp.2d 477 (2/22/94). This case is discussed more fully in Chapter 9, Legal Issues in Egg Donation.

[100]Similarly, laws of at least 16 of the 35 states explicitly provide that the man donating sperm to a woman who is not his wife is not the legal father of the child: Alabama, California, Colorado, Connecticut, Idaho, Illinois, Minnesota, Montana, Nevada, New Jersey (unless the woman and donor have entered into a contract to the contrary), New Mexico (unless the woman and donor have agreed in writing to the contrary), Oregon, Texas, Washington (unless the woman and donor have agreed in writing to the contrary), Wisconsin, and Wyoming. The statutes refer to the process as artificial insemination and not as therapeutic donor insemination.

[101]Alabama, Alaska, Arizona, Arkansas, California, Colorado, Connecticut, Florida, Georgia, Idaho, Illinois, Kansas, Louisiana, Maryland, Massachusetts, Michigan, Minnesota, Missouri, Montana, Nevada, New Hampshire, New Jersey, New Mexico, New York, North Carolina, North Dakota, Ohio, Oklahoma, Oregon, Tennessee, Texas, Virginia, Washington, Wisconsin, and Wyoming.

[102]Minn. Stat. Ann §257.56(1) (West 1982); Mont. Code Ann. §10-6-106 (1985); Nev. Rev. Stat. §126.061 (1986); N.M. Stat. Ann. §40-11-6(A) (1986); Va. Code Ann. §63.1-7.1 (1980); Wis. Stat. Ann. §767.48(9) (West 1981), §891.40 (West Supp. 1986); Wyo. Stat. §1402-103 (1985).

[103]57 *Fed. Reg.* 51320 (November 3, 1992).

[104]*In re Baby M*, 217 N.J. Super. 313, 525 A.2d 1128 (1987), 109 N.J. 396, 537 A.2d 1228 (1988).

[105]537 A.2d 1227 (1988).

[106]Ariz. Rev. Stat. Ann. § 25-21B (1991); Ark. Stat. Ann. §9-10-201 (1987); Fla. Stat. Ann. §§ 742.11 to 742.17 (West Supp.. 1994); Ind. Code Ann. §31-8-1-1 (Burns 1991); Kan. Stat. Ann §23-128 (1988); Ky. Rev. Stat. Ann. §199.590 (1991); La. Rev. Stat. Ann. §9:2713 (West 1991); Mich. Comp. Laws Ann. §§722.851 to .863 (West Supp. 1991); Neb. Rev. Stat. §25-21,200 (1989); Nev. Rev. Stat. Ann. §127.287 (Michie Supp. 1991); N.H. Rev. Stat. Ann. §§ 168-B:1–B:32 (Butterworth Supp. 1993); N.Y. Dom. Rel. Law §121 (McKinney Supp. 1993); N.D. Cent. Code §§ 14-18-01 to 14-18-07 (1991); Utah Code Ann. §76-7-204 (Michie Supp. 1991); Va. Code Ann. §§ 20-150 to 20-165 (Supp. 1993); Wash. Rev. Code Ann. §§ 26.26.210–.270 (West Supp. 1994).

[107]Fla. Stat.Ann. § 743.16(7) (West Supp. 1994).

[108]Fla. Stat. Ann § 743.11 (West Supp. 1994).

[109]N.H. Rev. Stat. Ann. § 168-B:23(IV)(Butterworth Supp. 1993); Va. Code Ann. § 20-158 (Supp. 1993).

[110]*Johnson* v. *Calvert*, 5 Cal. 4th 84, 19 Cal. Rptr. 2d 494, 851 P.2d 776, Cal. Lexis 2472 at 17 (1993).

[111]Id.

[112]*In Re Andres*, 156 Misc.2d 65, 591 N.Y.S.2d 946 (1993).

[113]622 N.Y.S.2d 181 (1994).

[114]See Harvard *supra* n. 1 at 1527.

[115]In reported situations in which sperm donors later tried to assert parental rights, the sperm donor had a relationship with the mother of the child or with the child.

[116]See Bonnicksen, "Embryo Freezing: Ethical Issues in the Clinical Setting," 18 *Hastings Center Report* (6) 26 (December 1988).

[117]Winston, Handyside, "New Challenges in Human In Vitro Fertilization," 260 *Science* 932 (May 14, 1993).

[118]Handyside, Lesko, Tarin, et al., "Birth of a Normal Girl After In Vitro Fertilization and Preimplantation Diagnostic Testing for Cystic Fibrosis," 327 *New England Journal of Medicine* 905 (September, 1992); Bishop, "Unnatural Selection," 73 *National Forum* 27 (Spring 1993).

[119]Dickson, "Use of Fetal Eggs in Research to Be Debated," 364 *Nature* 372 (July 29, 1993).

[120]*Planned Parenthood of Southeastern Pennsylvania* v. *Casey*, 112 S. Ct. 2791, 60 U.S.L.W. 4795 (1992).

[121]Cal. S.B. 1160 (as amended) (May 26, 1993). The proposal requires all egg donors to have previously given birth.

8

Insuring Infertility Treatment:
Legal Aspects of Insurance Coverage
and Discrimination

SUSAN L. CROCKIN, J.D.

INTRODUCTION

In an era of shrinking health care dollars, few would argue with the concept that medical treatments should be responsibly administered and fairly distributed. For many of the estimated 4.9 million infertile individuals (8% of the population) in this country,[1] however, obtaining access to affordable and appropriate treatment for this medical condition may be as arduous a process as undergoing some of the actual treatments. Physicians who deliver such care are also affected by widely varying practices and policies of insurance coverage, reimbursement, and denials, as well as by differing definitions of which infertility treatments are deemed "experimental." There may also be other obstacles hindering the infertile individual's efforts to gain access to care or to protect his or her job while obtaining such care.

Indeed, despite the growing acceptance and longevity of certain assisted reproductive technology (ART) techniques such as in vitro fertilization (IVF), resistance to comprehensive insurance coverage is common. Although infertility is now widely recognized as a medical disease,[2] and most infertility and ART treatments are not considered experimental by the medical profession,[3] insurance coverage for infertility or ART treatment has traditionally been denied on one or more of the following stated grounds:

1. Infertility is not an illness or disease.
2. The desired treatment either is not medically necessary or will not cure the underlying condition or disease.
3. The particular treatment is considered experimental.
4. Only specific procedures or treatments are covered, and others, typically ART procedures, are excluded.

Each of these arguments has been countered by proponents of coverage; and each is analyzed in this chapter in the discussion of particular legal challenges to denial of coverage for infertility.

This chapter reviews (1) the present status of state and federal laws surrounding insurance coverage for infertility and ART treatment and (2) the various legal challenges that have been brought largely on the basis of discrimination and job security issues as they relate to these treatments. Finally, the potential application of these laws and challenges to egg donation, as yet largely untested, will be discussed in detail.

STATE LEGISLATION

Because of the reluctance to voluntarily extend insurance benefits to infertility treatment, grass roots consumer organizations such as RESOLVE, Inc.©[4] have organized legislative efforts within some states to prohibit insurers from discriminating against infertility by passing laws that mandate insurance coverage for its diagnosis and treatment. Most commonly, such laws are drafted to require health insurance plans that cover pregnancy-related benefits, as most do, to either cover or offer to cover the diagnosis and nonexperimental treatment of infertility. As will be discussed further below, fully self-insured companies are exempted from such state laws and are governed solely by federal laws.

Ten states currently have laws that mandate varying degrees of coverage for infertility to individuals (Arkansas, California, Connecticut, Hawaii, Illinois, Maryland, Massachusetts, New York, Rhode Island, and Texas).[5] The laws vary widely and range from comprehensive coverage of nonexperimental procedures (including ART treatments) without limits on either numbers of cycles or lifetime benefit caps (Massachusetts) to coverage for IVF only (Maryland) to mandates that require insurers to offer coverage that employers then have the option of purchasing but are not required to purchase (California and New York). Most state laws have certain limits, such as limits on numbers of ART procedures or cycles or lifetime dollar amount caps. Some state laws apply to all commercial insurers; others apply only to group policies over a certain number of individuals. A few additional states have laws that require only certain entities, such as state employees or health maintenance organizations, to provide some coverage of infertility services.[6] Appendix 8-A at the end of this chapter includes a sample number of state mandate laws. Table 8.1 is a chart that outlines the basic provisions of the ten mandates.

Under the provisions of ERISA, the federal Employee Retirement Security Act of 1974,[7] federal law preempts any inconsistent state laws. Thus none of the ten state laws control entities that are fully self-insured and therefore are subject only to federal legislation.

Typically, legislation requiring insurance coverage for infertility has been opposed by insurance providers, largely on the basis of claims of prohibitive or disproportionate costs or claims of the "experimental nature" of various treatments and/or the "elective nature" of the condition. Proponents of such legislation counter each of these arguments with a number of counterarguments.

Although relatively little cost data exists, statistics that have been mandatorily reported to state licensing bodies or voluntarily provided by insurance companies appear to support consumers' arguments that the costs of including infertility coverage within an insured population are relatively minor. The Massachusetts law is illustrative; cost figures have been reported by commercial insurers to that state's Division of Insurance since 1988, the year following the law's passage. The most recent available figures for Blue Cross/Blue Shield of Massachusetts, from 1993, indicate that the percentage of health care premiums apportioned to comprehensive mandated infertility treatment was only 0.2% of a monthly family health care premium.[8] In Maryland, where since 1985 the law has required coverage for IVF only, state officials estimated in 1988 that the incremental cost attributed to mandatory IVF coverage was an additional $0.08 per family contract per month.[9]

Although ART procedures are costly on a per procedure basis, they appear to add negligibly to the total cost of insurance coverage. (In 1987, 0.1% of national health care costs were allocated to infertility.[10]) The explana-

TABLE 8.1. State Laws on Infertility Insurance Coverage

State	Date enacted	Mandate to Cover	Mandate to Offer	Diagnosis & Treatment incl. IVF	Diagnosis & Treatment excl. IVF	IVF Only
Maryland	1985	X				X
Arkansas	1987	X				X*
Texas	1987		X			X
Hawaii	1987	X				X+
Massachusetts	1987	X		X		
Connecticut	1989		X	X		
Rhode Island	1989	X		X		
California	1989		X		X**	
New York	1990		X		X++	
Illinois	1991	X		X***		

*Includes a lifetime maximum benefit of not less than $15,000.

+Provides a one-time only benefit for all out patient expenses arising from IVF.

**Excludes IVF, but defines IVF as "the laboratory medical procedures involving the actual in vitro fertilization process." Covers gamete intrafallopian transfer (GIFT).

++Provides coverage for the "diagnosis and treatment of correctable medical conditions."

***Limits first time attempts to 4 complete oocyte retrievals. If a child is born, 2 complete oocyte retrievals for a second birth shall be covered. Excludes businesses with 25 or less employees.

Prepared by: The American Society for Reproductive Medicine
The Society of Reproductive Medicine and Biology
Office of Government Relations
(202) 863-2494/2576

tion probably lies in the fact that a relatively small percentage (8%) of the population experiences infertility; of those who do experience infertility, only 31.4% seek any infertility treatment;[11] and, based on Center for Disease Control estimates, approximately 1.6% of women who seek infertility treatment undergo ART procedures.[12] Additionally, ART procedures often replace, at a lower cost and with a more effective outcome, costly in-patient surgical procedures such as tubal repair.[13]

The frequently made argument that costs will increase as more people seek treatment as the result of better insurance coverage would seem to be negated by the several years of relatively stable statistics in states such as Massachusetts. Blue Cross/Blue Shield of Massa-chusetts' mandatory filings with that state's Division of Insurance indicate that the following percentages for family premiums were attributed to infertility treatment: 0.2% (first quarter 1989[14]), 0.3% (fourth quarter 1990[15]), and 0.2% (1993).[16] It is likely that ART procedures in particular are so inherently intrusive that they are self-limiting.

The majority of states, however, do not require any insurance coverage for infertility treatment. In states without mandated coverage for infertility or ART treatments, coverage is inconsistent and varies widely from insurer to insurer. Although some insurers have voluntarily elected to cover some aspects of treatment, many deny all treatment for infertility or limit coverage to diagnosis or traditional therapies.

LEGAL CHALLENGES BASED ON INSURANCE CONTRACT ANALYSIS

Legal challenges have been brought against some insurers that have denied insurance coverage under a number of theories. Because these suits have usually been brought to enforce the specific terms of particular insurance policies and under a particular state's law, both of which vary widely, the results of these individual contractual challenges have been mixed.

In *Witcraft* v. *Sundstand Health and Disability Group Benefit Plan*,[17] an infertile couple successfully challenged an insurance claim denial for artificial insemination. The company's plan covered "illnesses," but the company claimed that "nonpregnancy" was not an illness and that artificial insemination was not a "treatment" because it did not change the condition of infertility. The court rejected the insurer's defense, ruling that infertility was an illness under the terms of that plan and artificial insemination was a treatment for it.[18] Nevertheless, nothing in the *Witcraft* court's decision would have precluded the company from simply excluding infertility as a covered illness had it seen fit to do so explicitly.

A similar case, *Egert* v. *Connecticut General Life Insurance Co.*,[19] was brought in Illinois by a patient with blocked fallopian tubes who was denied coverage for IVF before the passage of that state's mandated infertility law. The insurer, Connecticut General, denied the claim on the basis that the illness was the tubal obstruction and not infertility and that the only covered treatment would be tubal repair. Again, only because of the wording of the policy, which did not explicitly exclude infertility, was the insurer required to provide coverage.

These cases highlight the often-made argument that ART procedures do not really "treat" the illness because they are designed to achieve a pregnancy but not reverse the underlying disease. However, the same can be said about many treatments in other areas of medicine that do not cure the disease but simply treat symptoms of the condition. Heart bypass, kidney dialysis, and diabetes treatments are just three such examples.

In other cases, insurers have denied coverage on the grounds that certain forms of ART treatment are experimental. For example, one case brought by a successful IVF patient, *Reilly* v. *Blue Cross and Blue Shield United of Wisconsin*,[20] alleged that the insurer's refusal to cover the procedure, because it had determined that IVF was "experimental," was arbitrary and capricious and therefore illegal. The lower court agreed with the insurer, but the federal appeals court reversed the decision, first noting that the patient's numerous expert medical witnesses offered opinions that after 1992, IVF procedures were no longer considered experimental. Moreover, the court noted that the insurer used a "success ratio" only to justify exclusion of IVF treatments and not to determine whether treatments of other diseases should be covered by the policy. One commentator has suggested that the logical extension of applying a "success ratio" to all treatments would be to deny coverage to many sufferers of terminal illnesses, since the success ratio of curing their disease or condition would be 0.[21]

These and similar types of challenges are substantially dependent upon the language and interpretation of individual insurance contracts, policies, and manuals. For that reason, court rulings on such cases are likely to remain inconsistent. It is notable, however, that neither the policy language nor insurers' initial refusals to provide coverage are conclusive in this area. A close review of the policy and a legal challenge (threatened or actual) have frequently resulted in coverage for at least some portions of infertility diagnosis and treatment.

LEGAL CHALLENGES BASED ON FEDERAL LEGISLATION

Recently, infertile individuals have raised legal challenges that may have more widespread effects in the areas of insurance and job protection. One basis for such a challenge is the 1990 Americans With Disabilities Act ("ADA");[22] another possible basis is Title VII of the Civil Rights Act of 1978.[23]

The ADA is a comprehensive federal civil rights statute that provides a very broad range of protections for people with disabilities against discrimination by large employers (as of 1994, employers with fifteen or more employees). Being a federal law, its protections extend even to individuals in states without mandates or to those covered by self-insured employers.

Infertility that requires major medical intervention or infertility treatment of any significant duration may be subject to the ADA's protections. The relevant ADA definition of "disability" is "a physical or mental impairment that substantially limits one or more of the major life activities of such individual."[25] Regulations promulgated under the law explicitly list impairments of the reproductive organs as examples of qualifying physical impairments.[26]

The ADA may therefore provide grounds for individuals to sue their employer if, for example, they believe they have been discriminatorily fired because of their infertility or denied insurance coverage on the basis of their disability. At least three such lawsuits have been filed and are currently pending: *Pacourek* v. *Inland Steel Company*[27], *Krauel* v. *Iowa Methodist Medical Center*[28], and *Zatarain* v. *WDSU Television, Inc.* et al.[29] The *Pacourek* case has been described by at least one legal commentator as "ground-breaking" in terms of its legal theories.[30]

In *Pacourek*, the lower court has ruled that infertility falls within the ADA's definition of "disability." Charlene Pacourek alleged that her employer, Inland Steel Company, discharged her because of time she missed from work (and that she says she made up) for infertility treatments. The ADA defines discrimination to include an employer's failure to make "reasonable accommodations" for the employee unless making such accommodations would impose an "undue hardship" on the business.[31] The regulations make clear that such reasonable accommodations for the employee include "job restructuring and part-time or modified work schedules."[32] Thus the ADA may provide a significant protection to infertile individuals in the workplace who are undergoing treatment.

In an initial ruling on the legal issues, the federal district court denied the company's efforts to dismiss the case. It found that infertility was both a disability as defined by the ADA and a pregnancy-related condition protected under Title VII. In ruling that the protections of the ADA reached infertility, the court accepted the claim that infertility was a covered impairment under that federal law and that it substantially limits a major life activity. Regardless of the factual outcome of the case, this ruling is of legal significance because it is the first judicial recognition of infertility as a protected disability under that federal law.

In contrast, the initial court ruling in the *Zatarain* case reached the opposite conclusion. In that case, a female newscaster whose contract was not renewed after she requested alterations and a temporary reduction in work hours for infertility treatments sued the television station under both the ADA and Title VII. The federal district court in Louisiana, where the case was heard, granted the television station's request for summary judgment on the ADA claim. The court ruled that although infertility was a physiological impairment or disability under the ADA's definitions, it did not impair a "major life activity" and therefore did not run violate the federal law. The court concluded that reproduction is not like walking, seeing, learning, breathing, or working, the listed major life activities in the ADA regulations. The court ruled that, unlike those activities, "[a] person is not called upon to reproduce throughout the day, every day." Zatarain's appeal of the court's order which allowed summary judgment for the defendants is pending.

Burgeoning litigation that has been brought under the ADA, although not specifically relating to infertility, may also affect access to infertility treatment. In another federal court decision[33] an appellate court has ruled that insurers may be defined as employers within the employer provisions of the ADA. In that case a self-insured company had imposed a cap only on coverage for AIDS. The court ruled that this constituted discrimination in employee-related health care benefits, which it found was discrimination in violation of the employment provisions of the ADA. Although the appellate court did not touch on the merits of the case, its ruling supports an argument that the reach of the ADA's protections may extend to health benefits, even when they are provided by a self-insured company.

The ADA, as it relates to claims of denial of insurance coverage, also has its own specific language. In *Krauel* the plaintiff alleges that she is disabled because of her infertility and that her employer's health plan, established under ERISA, discriminates against her by excluding coverage for her disability.[34] The lawsuit charges that "said exclusion is not based on underwriting risks, classifying risks, or administering risks and is used as a subterfuge to evade the purposes of [the ADA]."[35]

The essence of a discriminatory insurance claim under the ADA lies in establishing "subterfuge," as that term is interpreted in the interim guidelines under the Act. Underwriting and other neutral limitations on policies are permitted, but the guidelines make clear that when a disability-specific exclusion from the employer's health plan is made, the employer will have to prove, on the basis of actuarial and financial data, that the exclusion is neutral and not a subterfuge for discrimination.[36] In light of studies and data about cost such as those cited in this chapter, such proof should be difficult to establish.

The ADA may also provide a basis for other forms of discrimination claims in the future, such as claims that state insurance laws may not be permitted to exclude, and thus discriminate against, infertility; that state insurance commissioners may not approve policies that exclude infertility coverage; that insurers or health care providers may not, as "public accommodations" covered under the ADA, discriminate against infertility patients; and that insurance companies may not exclude certain fertility treatments if they cover others that are not actually more cost-effective (e.g., tubal repair but not IVF).

One potential, and as yet untested, claim under Title III of the ADA may be of particular interest to medical providers: Title III prohibits the "imposition or application of eligibility criteria that screen out or tend to screen out an individual with a disability or any class of individuals with disabilities from fully and equally enjoying any goods, services, facilities, privileges, advantages, or accommodations."[37] Thus a provider who applies different criteria to his or her infertility patients than to patients in the rest of the practice, such as requiring patients to be married or excluding homosexual patients, could potentially be vulnerable to a claim of discrimination. Again, there has been no reported litigation under the ADA on this point.

Title VII of the Civil Rights Act of 1978 may provide additional legal protections for infertile individuals. Also known as the Pregnancy Discrimination Act (PDA), Title VII prohibits discrimination by employers to whom it applies on the basis of "pregnancy, childbirth or related medical conditions" for all "employment-related purposes."[38]

The argument has been made that infertility is a pregnancy-related condition and that employers violate federal law if they fire, demote, or discriminate against infertile individuals in the workplace because of their infertility or treatment thereof. In the *Pacourek* case, attorneys for the fired employee have claimed that her firing was illegal discrimination under the PDA as well as the ADA. The *Pacourek* court agreed that, if proven, such a firing would be a violation of that law. Whether that court will find the employee's claim to be proven is yet to be determined.

Finally, the recent federal health reform debate reflects the uncertainty and differences of opinion held by policy makers about the appropriateness of insuring infertility generally and ART treatments in particular. President Bill Clinton's initial plan excluded IVF treatment from coverage;[39] alternative plans varied widely on this issue.[40] It is still unclear precisely how the diagnosis and treatment of infertility will ultimately be viewed in the context of health reform. Depending on the ultimate scope of any federal health reform efforts, courts may still find or reject protections for infertility under previously enacted laws such as those discussed here.

COVERAGE FOR EGG DONATION

Because egg donation is still a relatively new procedure, insurance coverage for egg donation procedures is neither widespread nor uniform. In states that require coverage of nonexperimental infertility procedures, egg donation is not currently considered experimental, and therefore most aspects of egg donation are typically covered by the recipient's

policy.[41] This would include the donor's screening procedures, medications, stimulation protocol, and retrieval procedure. In general, notwithstanding the involvement of a third party, egg donation does not appear to present significantly different legal issues with respect to coverage, and court decisions and interpretations of existing laws for other infertility matters should continue to be relevant and applicable to egg donation.

Frequently excluded from such coverage, however, are fees paid to donors, which may reach or rarely exceed $2,500 per retrieval cycle. As one example, Illinois state law requires coverage of egg donation, but the regulations that were written to interpret and apply the law explicitly exclude donor fees from the requirement.[42] At least one commercial insurer covers ART treatment at a "global" or all-inclusive rate and includes within that rate a donor fee, which it states is intended to compensate a donor only for time, inconvenience, pain, and suffering. Although no figures are available for publication, the fee is specifically not intended as an inducement.[43] The exclusion starkly contrasts with sperm donation, in which the donor's fees, albeit much lower, are routinely included within the costs of the semen specimen that is frequently covered by the recipients' insurance.

One aspect of coverage that is of concern for those involved in egg donation involves the possibility of medical complications for donors undergoing drug stimulation and egg retrievals. For this reason, most programs require egg donors to carry their own health insurance. Some programs have considered purchasing group insurance for their egg donors. Others have made efforts to have egg donors temporarily added to a program's own health plan. To date, the author is unaware of any such efforts coming to fruition.

If an egg donor does not have her own insurance and a recipient or program chooses to bring and/or accept her into the program, the recipient, the provider, and donor all need to be extremely careful about allocating risk and responsibility for any uninsured medical complications. It is advisable to have the recipient(s) and donor execute, perhaps within a broader legal agreement drawn between themselves, an agreement to allocate these risks. A carefully worded provision might allocate these risks to the recipient, for a limited time period following the procedure and only for medical complications that are attributable to the procedure and are not otherwise covered. Recipients and donors might consider whether any risks assumed should also be "capped" at a dollar amount. Typically, consent forms for a program will disclaim any responsibility for nonnegligently performed medical complications or conditions that may result from an egg donor's participation in the program.[44]

Even in states with mandated coverage, however, egg donation procedures for recipient women beyond the normal childbearing years may not be covered. Thus insurers or HMOs may have criteria that reject women over a certain age (frequently 42) as candidates for their limited supply of donor eggs. Even in states such as Massachusetts, with mandated comprehensive infertility coverage, such cutoffs are routinely applied and have not been successfully challenged to date. A distinction is frequently made that women who are "normally infertile" as a result of age were not the intended beneficiaries of mandated coverage.

CONCLUSION

Insuring infertility treatment, particularly ART treatment, remains a challenging legal task for infertile individuals and providers. Individual court challenges, with the exception of still novel and broadly styled challenges under discrimination laws, will probably have only limited effect. Creative legal challenges may, however, have a major impact on the way in which society views and provides coverage for infertility treatment.

ENDNOTES

[1] Office of Technology Assessment Report of the U.S. Congress, 1988, "Infertility: Medical and Social Choices", Washington, D.C.: U.S. Government Printing Office, ("OTA Report"), ch.1, p.3. The OTA Report estimates that only 1 million, or 31.4% of that population, sought treatment in 1982. ch. 3, p. 56.

[2] The American Fertility Society Statement (1990).

[3] The American Fertility Society, "Policy Statement on Insurance Coverage/non-Experimental Procedures," July 1991.

The American College of Obstetricians and Gynecologists, "Ethical Issues in Human in Vitro Fertilization and Embryo Placement" (1986), Guidelines on gamete intrafallopian transfer (1989), and zygote intrafallopian transfer (1993).

[4] RESOLVE, Inc.©, 1310 Broadway, Somerville, Massachusetts 02144-1731.

[5] Tex. Ins. Code Ann. art 3.51-6 § 3A (West 1991); Conn. Gen. Stat. Ann. § 38a-536 (West 1991); Cal. Health & Safety Code § 1374.55 (West 1990), Cal. Ins. Code §§ 10119.6, 11512.28 (West 1991); Md. Ins. Code Ann. art. 48A, §§ 470W, 470EE (1991); Haw. Rev. Stat. § 431:10A-116.5(4)(B)(iv); Mass. Gen. Laws Ann., ch. 175, § 47H (West 1991); Ark. Code Ann. §§ 23-85-137, 23-86-118 (Michie 1991); R.I. Gen. Laws § 27-18-30 (1989); N.Y. Ins. Law § 3216(h)(12)(A), (B)(McKinney 1991); Ill. Legis. Serv. 87-681 amendment to the Illinois Insurance Code.

[6] Delaware (state employees); Ohio, West Virginia, Montana (HMOs); *Infertility and National Health Care Reform: A Briefing Paper*; joint publication of RESOLVE, Inc. and The American Fertility Society (Jan. 1993).

[7] 29 U.S.C. Sec. 1001 (1974).

[8] Joint Committee on Health Care for the Massachusetts State Legislature (telephone report by research analyst to S. Crockin, 1994).

[9] *Infertility and National Health Care Reform, supra* at p. 6.

[10] OTA Report, ch. 1, p. 3.

[11] OTA Report, ch. 3, p. 56, citing 1982 statistics.

[12] See n.9, Briefing Paper, p. 3.

[13]Holst et al. "Handling of Tubal Infertility After Introduction of In Vitro Fertilization: Changes and Consequences," Fertility and Sterility, Vol. 55, No. 1 (January 1991).

[14]Massachusetts Division of Insurance, letter of N. Turbull, Deputy Commissioner and Health Policy Director (2/8/89).

[15]Massachusetts Division of Insurance, letter of N. Turbull, Deputy Commissioner and Health Policy Director (12/31/90).

[16]*Supra* at n.8.

[17]*Witcraft* v. *Sundstrand Health and Disability Group Benefit Plan*, 420 N.W. 2d 785 (Iowa 1988).

[18]*Id.* at 790.

[19]*Egert* v. *Connecticut General Life Insurance Co.*, 900 F.2d 1032 (7th Cir. 1990).

[20]*Reilly* v. *Blue Cross and Blue Shield United of Wisconsin*, 846 F. 2d 416 (7th Cir. 1988).

[21]*The Status of Infertility Treatments and Insurance Coverage: Some Hopes and Frustrations*, Comment, South Dakota Law Review, at fn. 182 on p. 360 (1992).

[22]Americans With Disabilities Act, 42 U.S.C. § 1210.

[23]Pregnancy Discrimination Act, 1978 Amendment to Title VII, 42 U.S.C. §2000e.

[24]*Pacourek* v. *Inland Steel Co., Inc.*, U.S. Dist.Ct. (N.Dis.Ill. #4-93-CV-10815 1994). See also S.L. Crockin, "Legally Speaking," *Fertility News* (June, Dec. 1994).

[25]29 U.S.C. 794 (1988).

[26]See, for example, House Rpt. 101-485 Pt.III, Report of the House Judiciary Committee, 101 Cong., 2nd Sess., May 15, 1990 at 28; House Rpt. 101-485 Pt.II, Report of the House Committee on Education and Labor, 101 Cong., 2d Sess. (May 15, 1991) at 51.

[27]*Pacourek* v. *Inland Steel Company* U.S. Dist.Ct. (N.Dist.Ill #4-93-CV-10815 1994) See also S.L. Crockin, "Legally Speaking," *Fertility News* (June, Dec. 1994).

[28]*Mary Jo Krauel* v. *Iowa Methodist Medical Center*, No. 4-93-CV-10815, U.S.D.C.So.Dis.Iowa. (filed 12/7/93).

[29]Order granting Summary Judgment, 881 F.Supp.240 (E.D.LA 1995).

[30]Law Professor Jane Larson, Northwestern University, as quoted in "Pregnancy Law Covers Infertility, Suit Claims" by Stanley Holmes, *Chicago Tribune* (March 28, 1994).

[31]Sec 102 (b)(5)(A).

[32]29 CFR 1530.2.

[33]*Carparts Distribution Center, Inc.* v. *Automotive Wholesaler's Association of New England*, (1st Cir. 10/12/94).

[34]Complaint, paras. 2 and 10.

[35]Complaint, *supra* at para. 11.

[36]Interim Enforcement Guidance, Equal Employment Opportunity Commission (EEOC) (issued June 1993); "Exclusion of Infertility Coverage by Health Insurers May Violate the Americans with Disabilities Act," newsletter (Fall 1993), Resolve of the Bay State, P.O. Box 1553, Waltham, MA; and see "New Coverage Requirements and New Interpretations of Coverage Requirements for Self-Insured Plans," *The Health Lawyer*, vol. 7, no. 2, Spring 1994, pp. 10–11. The ABA Forum on Health Law.

[37]Sec. 302(b)(2)(A)(i).

[38]42 U.S.C. 2000e et.seq.

[39]Health Security Act of 1994, HR 3600.

[40]Senator Edward Kennedy (D-MA), The Chairman's Markup to Health Security Act of 1994 HR 3600; Congressman Pete Stark (D-CA), The Subcommittee on Health report, the Stark proposal, to the Committee on Ways and Means on HR 3600.

[41]Mass. Gen. Laws Ann., ch. 175, § 47H (West 1991); Ill. Legis. Serv. 87-681 amendment to the Illinois Insurance Code.

[42]"Permissible Exclusions," 50 Ill. Adm. Code, Ch. 1 Sec. 2015.60 (e).

[43]Blue Cross/Blue Shield of MA (telephone report to S. Crockin by [Wendy Monroe, Director of Contract Development, awaiting different name for attribution] 6/94).

[44]See Chapter 10, "Egg Donation Consent Forms."

Appendix 8-A

2 Texas Codes Annotated
§12.03A and §12.03B

§ 12.03A. Oocyte Donation

(a) If a husband consents to provide sperm to fertilize a donor oocyte by in vitro fertilization or other assisted reproductive techniques and the wife consents to have a donor oocyte that has been fertilized with her husband's sperm, pursuant to his consent, placed in her uterus, any resulting child is the legitimate child of both of them. The consent of each must be in writing.

(b) If a donor oocyte that has been fertilized with her husband's sperm implants in a wife's uterus, any resulting child is not the child of the donor of the oocyte.

Added by Acts 1993, 73rd Leg., ch. 666, § 1, eff. Aug. 30, 1993.

§ 12.03B. Embryo Donation

(a) If, with the consent of the husband and the wife, a donated preimplantation embryo implants in the uterus of the wife, any resulting child is the legitimate child of both of them. The consent must be in writing.

(b) If, with the consent of the husband and the wife, a donated preimplantation embryo implants in the uterus of the wife, any resulting child is not the child of the donor or donors of the preimplantation embryo.

(c) Subsections (a) and (b) of this section apply whether the donated preimplantation embryo is the result of separate egg and sperm donations or the result of donation of an embryo created for the purpose of assisting the reproduction of the donating couple.

Added by Acts 1993, 73rd Leg., ch. 666, § 1, eff. Aug. 30, 1993.

Appendix 8-B

10 Oklahoma Statutes Annotated §554

§ 554. Legal status of child or children born as result of heterologous oocyte donation

Any child or children born as a result of a heterologous oocyte donation shall be considered for all legal intents and purposes, the same as a naturally conceived legitimate child of the husband and wife which consent to and receive an oocyte pursuant to the use of the technique of heterologous oocyte donation.

Added by Laws 1990, c. 272, § 8, eff. Sept. 1, 1990.

Appendix 8-C

21A Florida Statutes Annotated §742.11

742.11. Presumed status of child conceived by means of artificial or in vitro insemination or donated eggs or preembryos

(1) Except in the case of gestational surrogacy, any child born within wedlock who has been conceived by the means of artificial or in vitro insemination is irrebuttably presumed to be the child of the husband and wife, provided that both husband and wife have consented in writing to the artificial or in vitro insemination.

(2) Except in the case of gestational surrogacy, any child born within wedlock who has been conceived by means of donated eggs or preembryos shall be irrebuttably presumed to be the child of the recipient gestating woman and her husband, provided that both parties have consented in writing to the use of donated eggs or preembryos.

Amended by Laws 1990, c. 90-139, § 5, eff. Oct. 1, 1990; Laws 1993, c. 93-237, § 1, eff. June 30, 1993.

9

Legal Issues in Egg Donation[1]

JOHN A. ROBERTSON, J.D.
SUSAN L. CROCKIN, J.D.

INTRODUCTION

One of the fastest-growing areas of assisted reproduction is human egg donation. Over 150 in vitro fertilization (IVF) programs in the United States and Canada now offer the procedure,[2] and thousands of women suffering from ovarian dysfunction or advanced reproductive age are potential candidates. Egg donation raises several ethical and legal issues that need attention if it is to be used in a productive and beneficial way.

Although the donor may be another woman going through IVF who donates extra eggs, the advent of cryopreservation of embryos has reduced the supply of donor eggs from this source. Egg donations increasingly come from friends or family members whom the recipient herself recruits or from anonymous donors recruited by the center providing the service. In the latter case the donors are extensively screened and are usually paid from $1,000 to $2,500 for their time, effort, and inconvenience, depending on their geographical location. Unless the egg donor is a friend or family member, the egg donor ordinarily has no contact with the recipient or the offspring.

Egg donation appears to be a medically safe and effective way to produce children for women who cannot themselves produce healthy eggs. Because there is a gestational link, it also replicates more closely than does donor sperm or surrogacy the biological ties that usually exist between parents and offspring. Although the female genetic connection is missing, egg donation enables each rearing parent to have a biologic connection with their offspring.

Because egg donation is still relatively new, a full assessment of its effects on offspring, donor, infertile couples, and society cannot now be made. Nevertheless, given the existing acceptability of in vitro fertilization (IVF) and of donor insemination, the combination of IVF and gamete donation in the form of egg donation should also be ethically and legally acceptable.

With the exception of five states, however, no legislation or court decision has directly addressed egg donation and thus clarified whether the parties' intentions to exclude the egg donor from all rearing rights and duties in offspring will be given legal effect. Some states have laws against buying and selling human organs and tissues that could restrict payments to egg donors. It is also unclear whether donors who are injured in the course of donation must bear those costs or whether other parties can be held responsible. In addition, a variety of other legal questions arise, from the offspring's right to have information about his or her genetic mother, to questions about whether egg donation to women who are past the normal age of childbearing can be banned, to concerns about the legal status of cryopreserved embryos created from donated gametes.

144

While these uncertainties present no insuperable barrier to performing egg donation, they do require that physicians, hospitals, couples, donors, and others involved in egg donation pay careful attention to how they conduct the practice. Until the law is clarified by legislation or judicial decision, egg donation programs should be conducted with a full understanding and disclosure of existing risks and uncertainties.

The following discussion identifies the main legal issues that need attention and suggests reasonable steps to deal with current legal uncertainty.

REARING RIGHTS AND DUTIES

A major legal issue with egg donation concerns rearing rights and duties in offspring. In almost all instances the intent of the parties is to have the sperm provider and the recipient be the rearing father and mother for all purposes and for the donor to have no rearing rights and duties at all. (Unique issues for single women who are recipients of donor eggs are discussed later in this chapter.) This goal will exist even if friends or family members act as egg donors. Egg donation thus attempts to replicate the situation that ordinarily occurs with donor sperm to a married couple, in which the consenting husband is the legal father for all purposes and an anonymous donor has no rearing rights or duties.

A problem for recipients and donors at the present time, however, is that only Oklahoma, Texas, Florida, North Dakota, and Virginia[3] have recognized such intentions as legally determinative of rearing rights and duties in offspring. Until legislators or courts address this issue, participants in egg donation in other states will lack certainty that their preconception intentions will be legally binding. Recipients and donors must be fully informed of this uncertainty and should execute consent forms, releases, and agreements that clearly state their intentions and acknowledge the legal uncertainty that they face.

The laws enacted in these five states provide desired clarity with respect to the legal status of the various participants. The Oklahoma and North Dakota laws define the legal status of both the child and the donor. Under Oklahoma's law, the child is defined as "the same as a naturally conceived legitimate child of the husband and wife," and the oocyte donor is deemed to have "no obligation or interest" to that child. The North Dakota law explicitly addresses the child's status and provides "[a] donor is not a parent." The Texas legislation reflects standard sperm donation statutes, stating that a child born to a married woman by virtue of egg donation shall be considered the legitimate child of the recipient couple for all purposes, and the egg donor shall not be considered the legal mother for any purposes. The Florida and Virginia laws are even more comprehensive. They seek to clarify and secure the rights of participants to gestational surrogacy as well as egg donation. All five statutes clearly relieve an egg donor of any parental rights or responsibilities. Copies of three of these laws are attached as appendices at the end of Chapter 8.

However, the absence of legislation does not mean that the express intentions of the parties will not be honored if a legal dispute arises over rearing rights and duties in children born of egg donation. In sperm donation, the intention of the parties to have the consenting husband assume all paternal rearing rights and duties and to exclude the sperm donor from any rearing role is recognized by statute or court decisions in over 30 states.[4] A court faced with a dispute over rearing rights and duties in children born of egg donation, whether between a divorcing couple over custody of children born of egg donation or between the donor and a couple that has received donor eggs, is likely to follow the donor sperm model and give legal effect to the intention of the parties to have the recipient of the donation recognized as the rearing mother.[5]

Thus in a New York case involving a dispute between a divorcing husband and wife over custody of twins born as a result of egg donation, the court rejected the husband's claims that the children were "illegitimate" and that he was entitled to sole custody of the children because he was the "only genetic and natural parent available"[6] despite the absence of egg donation legislation. On the basis of the couple's intention jointly to have and rear offspring, the court ruled that the recipient of the egg donation was "the natural mother of the children"[7] and was entitled to temporary custody as would be a woman who had given birth to children conceived with her own egg.

Consider two other types of disputes that could arise over rearing rights and duties in offspring in the absence of egg donor legislation. One would be a situation in which the donor as genetic mother later attempts to assert some rearing rights in the offspring. Since a sperm donor ordinarily would not have the legal right to play a parenting role, it is hard to see why an egg donor should have any greater claim. She explicitly waived or relinquished her parental rights in providing the egg, just as a sperm donor does, and a later change of mind should not give her any greater right of access to her genetic offspring than a sperm donor has. An argument could be made that she underwent a greater hardship of ovarian stimulation and surgical retrieval to provide the eggs; but she would not have had the experience of pregnancy and childbirth, which distinguishes the claim of surrogate mothers who in some states may retain rearing rights despite their promise to relinquish custody after birth. Fairness should require that the original intentions of the parties, on which all relied, be followed.

In the absence of a statute giving effect to consent or agreements to exclude the genetic mother from rearing, only a state that defined motherhood in genetic but not gestational terms might regard the matter differently. As was noted above, there is no litigation to date involving egg donation and disputed definitions of motherhood. However, a highly publicized case involving gestational surrogacy is instructive. In *Johnson* v. *Calvert*,[8] gestational surrogate Anna Johnson decided in the midst of her pregnancy that she wanted to play a rearing role after the child's birth, notwithstanding her preconception agreement to carry a child for its genetic parents, Mark and Chrispina Calvert. The intermediate court, the California Court of Appeals, ruled that motherhood, like fatherhood, was to be determined on genetic grounds.[9] That court therefore held that a gestational surrogate was not the "mother" of the child that she carried and gave birth to, because the egg was provided by another woman. If that rationale for the decision had been affirmed, an egg donor, like the woman providing the egg for surrogate gestation, would have been the "mother" under California law and thus would have standing to seek visitation or custody of resulting children.

However, this rationale did not survive the California Supreme Court's affirmation of the decision.[10] That court excluded the gestational surrogate from any rearing role and awarded sole custody of the child to the genetic couple on other grounds. It found that California laws were sufficiently ambiguous as to define either woman as mother, depending on which provision of the California laws one looked to. It recognized that the parties' preconception intentions were clearly to create a child for the Calverts and not for Anna Johnson and ruled that the parties' intentions, in light of other statutory provisions for defining parenthood, should be the deciding issue. The final decision explicitly did not apply to egg donation, thus removing the potential legal barrier to egg donation that the Court of Appeals decision appeared to create.

Even under a purely genetic definition of

motherhood it would not necessarily follow that the egg donor—the genetic mother—would be entitled to visit the child or have any other rearing role when she had agreed at the time of donation to relinquish all rearing rights and duties in offspring born of her donated eggs. Legal doctrines of waiver and best interests of the child should still control. If an egg donor had not asserted her claim before or shortly after birth, she would most likely be found to have waived it, as unmarried fathers who do not assert any rearing right soon after birth are held to do.[11] If she asserted her claim before the child's birth, it might be more difficult to establish waiver. However, even if waiver doctrines did not apply and the case was decided solely in terms of the child's best interests, in most cases it should be difficult to show that the child's interests are best served by having a nongestational, genetic parent involved in rearing a child when the parties had reached a contrary agreement at the time at which the eggs were donated.

In the final analysis the resolution of this issue will depend on society's view, as interpreted within a particular state, of the importance of genetic versus gestational motherhood and the importance of the parties' preconception intentions. In a state without egg donor legislation a very risk-averse couple could have the donor terminate her parental rights after the child is born and then have the recipient/gestational mother adopt her husband's child in a stepparent adoption. Just such a step was taken by a husband in Virginia whose wife gave birth to twins following donor insemination, even with a statute in that state to the effect that a sperm donor had no parental rights. In upholding the husband's right to bring such an action, the court ruled that the statute (which was subsequently amended) addressed only the status of the donor but not that of the husband.[12] As a general rule, however, such steps should be unnecessary unless and until there are court decisions that give the egg donor the right to assert parental claims after birth. Given the original intentions of the parties, the gestational role of the recipient, and established sperm donation practices, such court decisions are unlikely to occur.

A second type of dispute would arise if attempts were made to hold the egg donor liable after birth for child support or other rearing obligations toward her genetic child. Because egg donors ordinarily intend to be excluded from any rearing role, they will want legal protection from later rearing obligations. One can imagine a scenario in which one member of the recipient couple dies after the child's birth or the couple undergoes hardships that make it impossible for them to support the child. Either they or the state might then seek to hold the donor as genetic mother responsible for child support.

Until state law makes clear that egg donors have no rearing rights and duties, there is always some risk that such a duty could be imposed, but it is highly unlikely. The situation is unlike the situation of sperm donation to a single woman, in which the donor has occasionally been held responsible for child support when no rearing father existed.[13] Here the donation is from one woman to another with the recipient fully intending to gestate, rear, and be completely responsible for the child's welfare. Holding the egg donor liable for support in this situation would deter egg donation to married and single women alike. Followed to its logical conclusion, it would also make doctors who assist reproduction by a single woman potentially liable for child support.

Although it is highly unlikely that such a duty would be imposed on a donor, the donor needs to be fully informed of this uncertainty. If she is very risk-averse, she could demand that the recipient couple agree to hold her harmless for any financial obligation that might arise from the birth of such a child, but this guarantee might not be enforceable. Alternatively, a donor could terminate her parental rights at birth and have the recipient adopt the child to make clear that she has no parental obligations. However, depending on a given state's adoption laws, this procedure could require a waiting period of several months before an adoption is finalized. Except for the most risk-averse donors, this step should be unnecessary as a general rule unless and until a court decision holds an egg donor liable for later obligations, notwithstanding the original intentions of the parties.

Questions about rearing rights and duties could also affect questions of inheritance. Donor sperm legislation usually makes the consenting husband the legal father for all purposes and the donor the father for none, so devises to one's "children" or "heirs" or to children under intestacy statutes would, in the case of a deceased husband, go to the children born of sperm donation, while in the case of the deceased donor they would not.[14] A similar result might be reached in states without donor sperm legislation, though the question has not yet arisen. Of course, either party could make specific bequests to make sure that certain individuals did or did not take from their estate.

A similar result would probably be reached in legislation establishing rearing rights and duties in offspring of egg donation. The child would be the "heir" or "child" of the recipient and not of the donor unless a specific bequest were made. Until such legislation is passed, however, it is unclear whether the offspring of egg donation are children of the donor, of the recipient, or of both under intestacy statutes or general devises to one's "children" or "heirs." To avoid problems and make sure that intentions are honored, both recipients and donors should specify in their wills by name and relation the individuals whom they wish to share in their estate.

Finally, it should be noted that there may be rare instances of egg donation in which the donor and the recipient agree to share in parenting rights and duties.[15] While this will not be the usual case and may not even be known to the physician providing the service, individuals who plan such arrangements should execute written agreements that make very clear what their mutual rights and obligations are. There is no guarantee that their agreements will be honored, and they should understand both the risks and limitations in proceeding.

Dispute could also arise regarding future relationships in connection with cryopreserved embryos created from donated gametes. It is possible that an egg donor might have a subsequent change of mind and assert a claim to embryos, either to retrieve them for her own use or to destroy them to avoid any form of parentage. One can imagine a scenario in which a sister donates eggs to her sister and brother-in-law, embryos are created and cryopreserved, and the couple then separate or divorce without having depleted the store of embryos. The donor would have executed a consent form relinquishing all rights in the eggs. The recipient couple would have executed consent forms that, in addition to accepting all rights in and obligations to the embryos, should also have required that they elect options in the event of future changed circumstances such as death or divorce. If circumstances should change, there is the risk that the donor may disagree with the couple's agreed-upon disposition and make her own claim to the embryos. A similar result could occur if the donor later finds herself infertile and in need of embryos herself.

Ordinarily, the consent to egg donation would contain the donor's release of any rights in the donated eggs or in the embryos, fetuses, or offspring that result from donated eggs. In most instances this release would prevent the donor from successfully asserting any claim of dispositional authority over embryos resulting from her eggs, as well as claims to rearing rights and duties in resulting offspring. To minimize the possibility of disputes, the parties should execute a written agreement that confirms their understanding that the donor transfers and relinquishes any rights or duties she might have in embryos or offspring resulting from her participation to the recipient, in exchange for the recipient's undertaking to have resulting embryos placed in her uterus and carried to term and reared, as she chooses.

Such an agreement would serve two primary purposes. First, because it is in the nature of a legal contract, it runs directly between two or more parties. Thus one party could sue another if the promise or agreement is breached. The very fact of entering into an agreement, and intending to be bound by it, could serve to add security to the arrangement. For the donor and recipients to be forced to discuss and negotiate, and ultimately have drafted and execute, an agreement on issues such as future calamities or changed circumstances may avoid court battles altogether. One role of lawyers involved in drafting or reviewing such agreements for each party should be to counsel the participants about such future possibilities and aid them in reaching agreement on those possibilities. Examples that the authors have used include asking the participants to imagine the recipients divorcing and the donor disapproving of their disposition of embryos or their custody plans for any born child or how they might all feel sitting across the table from one another in ten years at a family Christmas dinner. This process has resulted in some potential donors and recipients reconsidering their initial plan; it has enabled others to move forward with a more secure understanding of their roles.

Second, because contract law is distinct from the law of informed consent and waivers, a program may gain additional protections if an agreement is in place. In a challenge brought under the doctrine of informed consent, the program would be a party to any lawsuit. A donor seeking to reclaim embryos created from her donation would likely sue the program and claim either that she did not understand the procedure or that she now simply wishes to withdraw her previously rendered consent. The issues would then revolve around whether she fully understood the situation at the time she consented and, more important, whether she had irrevocably waived any subsequent claim to the embryos if they are still cryopreserved. However, under contract law, one party to the agreement may sue the other directly for breach of their promises in that agreement, and the issues would be quite different. The litigation would focus on what the two parties negotiated with one another and what understandings they had reached. It is possible that the program might be able to avoid involvement in such litigation or have a more minor role in any litigation in which they were included. The overriding benefit, however, is that the act of creating an agreement may reduce the likelihood of a future change of mind or discourage litigation altogether.

DONOR AND PHYSICIAN LIABILITY

Another set of significant potential legal issues revolves around donors' and physicians' actions. A donor could be legally liable for intentionally hiding information about infectious disease or genetic history that pose risks to the recipient or offspring. Also, a donor who failed to meet her obligation to perform various steps as a donor and was not able to complete the process might be liable to a recipient couple, at least for their costs associated with the procedure.

Physicians and other professionals coordinating egg donations should also have a legal duty to screen potential donors who are not otherwise undergoing IVF so that risks to recipients and offspring are reduced. Care should be taken to disclose, and document such disclosure of, all relevant information to recipient couples. Intentional or negligent mishandling of eggs could lead to tort liability for destruction of reproductive possibilities, just as negligent destruction of stored embryos could.[16]

In a lawsuit brought by a traditional surrogate who claims to have contracted cytomegalovirus (CMV) during an insemination,[17] a federal appeals court ruled that a surrogacy "broker," the doctors who performed the insemination procedure, and the lawyers who participated in the arrangement were to be held to an affirmative duty, and a new and higher standard of care than mere negligence, where they had recruited a healthy woman for their program. The court found that the consent forms, which included CMV amongst the numerous listed risks, were alone insufficient to relieve the defendants from liability. To date, a jury has not yet determined whether or not that higher standard of care was breached.

RISKS TO DONORS

Egg donors face both psychosocial and physical risks of harm from participation in egg donation. A primary psychosocial risk is that they will wish to have more contact with resulting offspring than they are able to have and thus will feel cut off from their genetic offspring. In some programs, donors do not even learn whether or not their efforts resulted in a pregnancy or child. There is also the risk that women who wish to have no contact with offspring may later be faced with offspring seeking them out or with demands for child support. Donors should be fully informed (and counseled) that they might have different feelings about donation at a later point and about the legal uncertainties that, in the absence of legislation or court decision, exist about determining rearing rights and duties by preconception agreement. As noted, the most likely

scenario is that donors will be totally excluded from any contact or relationship with any offspring, no matter how much they desire it, if they had so agreed at the time of donation. In addition, even though they cannot be guaranteed that they will not have unwanted contact or later obligations, the chances of that occurring do not now appear to be significant.

Donors also face physical risks. Unlike sperm donors, who are asked to be abstinent and then masturbate into a jar, egg donors will have their ovaries stimulated with hormones to produce multiple eggs, which will then be surgically retrieved, either by transvaginal ultrasound-guided aspiration or by laparoscopy. Several days of injections will also be necessary. Risks of complications or infection, while small, do exist. They are the same risks that candidates for IVF undergo. These risks are elaborated on, and discussed more fully, in Chapter 10.

Although the known complication rate with ovarian stimulation and egg retrieval is very small, it is possible that some egg donors will be injured in the process. An important legal question is to determine who will be responsible for the medical and other costs of any such injuries. Potential donors need to be fully informed of the risks that they face and to be told who will bear responsibility for the costs of any injuries that occur.

One possibility would be to have the donor assume the costs of these risks. Just as human subjects of biomedical research bear the costs of any injuries sustained in the research process,[18] egg donors could also be asked to bear the cost. The risk of incurring these costs would then be part of the gift or service that the donor is donating to the infertile couple. If so, it should be made clear to donors that they are bearing that cost. However, the cost is limited to the cost of nonnegligently caused injuries, because donors cannot waive their right to recover for negligence that causes their injuries.[19] If donors clearly understand that they are bearing these costs, their assumption of that risk has a reasonable chance of protecting the program and recipient couple from liability for nonnegligently caused injuries that result from their participation as egg donors. However, programs should be mindful of the need to fully and fairly inform donors of the potential risks they are assuming in agreeing to participate. Some programs resolve this issue by refusing to take donors who are not already insured. An alternative solution is to have the program assume all or some portion of the costs of any nonnegligently caused injuries to donors. Because such costs would ultimately be passed on to recipient couples, the couples should also be clearly informed of the extent, if any, to which they will be responsible for the donor's medical and other costs. The program cannot hold couples liable unless they have specifically agreed to assume those costs. For their own protection they need to be informed of this risk and set limits on their exposure.

One solution to this problem might be to have the program that recruits the donor purchase a short-term health insurance policy to cover any medical costs that she incurs as a result of the donation. Programs that do not themselves recruit donors, but that retrieve eggs from donors identified by the recipient, may also wish to provide such insurance. The cost of this insurance would be paid by the program or the recipient and would be the extent of their responsibility for nonnegligently caused injuries. Such a limitation should be clearly explained to potential donors and recipients so that they are fully aware of their rights and responsibilities. Moreover, it would be prudent to limit the time period for which coverage is provided.

THE LEGALITY OF PAYING DONORS

Unless a couple seeking an egg donor has a friend or family member who is willing to donate, the main source of donor eggs is likely to be anonymous strangers who have been recruited for that purpose. Although they will have mixed motives, including altruism and the desire to have genetic offspring without gestational or rearing burdens, women may be unwilling to donate unless they are paid for their efforts, which are not inconsiderable. Thus without payment to donors, many women may be denied access to egg donation.

While some ethicists have objected to paying women for their eggs on the ground that it is exploitive and commodifies offspring, there is no clear consensus that such payments are unethical. Since sperm donors are paid, it would be discriminatory to ban payment to egg donors, who undergo greater burdens.[20] Nor is it clear that paying for eggs is exploitive or coercive of women. The amounts paid are not so large relative to the time and effort involved that they seem likely to induce women to undergo unacceptable risks. Experience also indicates that most women who volunteer are not poor or minority women. Finally, since the transaction should be structured as paying for the donor's physical services, time, and effort, rather than for the eggs themselves, as is recommended by the American Society of Reproductive Medicine, this should reduce the risk that the transaction will be viewed as one involving the sale of children.[21]

An important issue is whether federal and state laws that ban buying and selling organs for transplant also apply to paying egg donors. In response to fears that people would sell living or cadaveric organs for transplant, the federal government and several states passed laws making it a crime (with penalties ranging from felony to misdemeanor) to buy or sell organs.[22] Although the intent of these laws was not to apply to sperm and egg donation, and indeed predate the technological advances of egg donation, their language in some cases is so broad that the sale of eggs could be covered as prohibited.

The main concern is from state law, which

should be reviewed by legal counsel for a program before it initiates a program involving payments to donors. The 1986 Federal Organ Transplant Act, which prohibits the acquisition, receipt, or transfer of "any human organ for valuable consideration for use in human transplantation," defines "human organ" in such a way that sperm and ova are clearly excluded.[23] Only Louisiana expressly prohibits "the sale of a human ovum."[24] However, prohibitions in Texas, Ohio, California, and several other states are less narrowly defined than the federal law and leave open the possibility that the sale of ova and even sperm is criminally banned.

The Texas statute, for example, defines "human organ" to include "the human kidney, liver, heart . . . or any other human organ or tissue, but does not include hair or blood, blood components (including plasma), blood derivatives, or blood reagents."[25] The question turns then on whether ova are "tissue." Under a standard dictionary definition of tissue—"a collection of similar cells and the intercellular substances surrounding them"[26]—the contents of one follicle would not be tissue, even if cumulus and follicular fluid is also aspirated, because only the egg is donated. On the other hand, the legislature failed to exclude sperm and ova as it did blood and blood products, and in a broad sense ova could be viewed as tissue. The Ohio statute raises similar issues.[27]

A law in Nevada bans the sale of specified organs and "any other part of the human body except blood."[28] Are oocytes a "part of the human body," or are they products of the body? Either interpretation is possible. Still other states follow the federal model and authorize the director of the state department of health to add other "organs" to the list specified in the law (see Appendix 1-H, p.30).[29]

Another kind of ambiguity arises in California[30] and South Dakota[31] statutes that make it a crime to receive, sell, transfer, or promote the transfer of "any human organ, for purposes of transplantation, for valuable consideration." Human organ is defined as "the human kidney, liver, heart . . . or any other human organ or nonrenewable or nonregenerative tissue except plasma and sperm." Because the statute explicitly excludes sperm and plasma but not ova, and ova, strictly speaking, are nonrenewable and nonregenerative, one could conclude that ova are included within the definition of "human organ." However, one could also reasonably argue that ova are not tissue or that they are renewable tissue because a donor has a large supply of ova. One or more cycles of egg donation will not deplete the eggs available for the donor until she herself reaches menopause.

Finally, one can question whether California-type statutes ban payments to egg donors because egg donation is not for the purpose of "transplantation." Transplantation implies insertion of an organ or tissue in another person to replace a missing function. But eggs are not transplanted. Rather, they are fertilized in vitro, and then the cleaving embryo is placed in the uterus. Transfer of an embryo to the uterus followed by implantation and pregnancy is thus not "transplantation" of an organ or tissue. Indeed, in some cases the donated eggs will not produce embryos, and all embryos may not be transferred to the uterus, much less successfully implant therein.

These examples of state statutes banning the sale of organs show that the definition of organ as "tissue" or "any other body part" opens the door to the possibility that sale of ova is included in the statutory ban, particularly when it is not included in certain exceptions. However, an arguably more persuasive reading of these laws would exclude sperm and ova from them. They were written with sale of solid organs in mind. Sperm and ova are functionally renewable, and it is very doubtful that the donated ova and sperm are then "transplanted." Moreover, including the sale of sperm and ova would raise constitutional problems, of both vagueness and procreative liberty, and statutes are generally construed to avoid doubts about their constitutionality.

Despite these uncertainties, physicians, couples, and donors in states that have laws that could be interpreted to ban payment for egg donation may still determine that it is reasonable to proceed with paid egg donation when that is the only way to recruit suitable donors. While the risk of prosecution cannot be totally eliminated, it appears to be small. No prosecutions have yet been brought. Some states, such as Massachusetts, provide a mechanism for programs to file their protocols with the district attorney's office of the county in which they are located.[32] Where available, such a mechanism may provide programs with the opportunity and protection of an advance ruling from local authorities. If a prosecution did occur, the participants would have a strong defense that the statute is unconstitutionally vague in that a reasonable person could not tell whether ova are included in the prohibition.[33] In addition, if they honestly believed that ova were not covered, they would also lack the specific intent to violate the law required in most cases for criminal liability. They could also attack the law as an unconstitutional interference with the right of infertile married couples to form a family with the help of an egg donor.[34]

To reduce the risks of prosecution even further, the relationship between the donor and the program or recipient should be structured as one in which the recipient is paying for the services of the donor in undergoing the procedures necessary to produce eggs rather than the eggs themselves. Thus payment should depend on the number and kind of procedures undergone and not be calibrated to the production of eggs or of any number of eggs. The consent form and any agreement should state that payments are to compensate the donor for her time and effort and not for her eggs. Since payments may vary and change more frequently than the consent forms, it would be prudent to put this information into a separate fee schedule, which, together with the consent forms, would be reviewed and then provided to the donor.[35] The schedule might set out a series of escalating payments to reflect a donor's increasing time and effort, culminating in the largest payment being for the time, effort, and inconvenience of the retrieval procedure itself. Even if a donor were canceled or elected to withdraw, she would be entitled to the payments that correlated with her time, effort, and services to that point in time. The only exception might be if a donor was canceled because of her intentional or careless failure to adhere to the prescribed protocol and therefore failed to stimulate and produce eggs.

Skillful writing of the consent form and any agreement with the donor will reduce the risk, which may already be small, that the participants will be prosecuted for, much less found guilty of, unlawful sale of organs or tissue under state law.

In any event, even if these laws do apply, there would still be room to pay donors for their medical and other expenses. The statutes in question do allow for reimbursement of the donor's "expenses of travel, housing and lost wages."[36] Thus some fee to the donor would be possible if time off work were required, even if this did pose an upper limit. Also, such restrictions might still permit one couple to pay the expenses of another couple going through IVF with the understanding that they would share the resulting eggs harvested. This would seem to be the paying of expenses necessary to produce the donation, and not a payment for the eggs themselves.

ISSUES OF OFFSPRING WELFARE

Egg donation, like other assisted reproductive techniques, raises legal and ethical questions about the impact on offspring. A full discussion of these ethical issues is found in Chapter 15. Legal issues aside, there is a strong ethical obligation or duty to pay attention to how these procedures will affect the children who are produced as a result, and programs should be run and structured to minimize harm to offspring. This duty creates a paradox, however. But for the assisted reproductive procedure in question, the child would never be born. Of all collaborative reproductive arrangements, at least for married couples, egg donation is closest to the norm of two parents contributing genes, gestation, and rearing. Indeed, a ban on egg donation on the ground that it harms offspring because it splits genetic and gestational parentage should not rise to the level of compelling interest necessary to justify infringing the fundamental right to procreate.[37]

This is true even if eggs are donated to an unmarried woman or to a woman who is past the normal outer limit of menopause—say, to a woman in her fifties. Providing donor eggs to a single woman is not significantly different from providing her with donor sperm or, indeed, arguably different from a single woman engaging in coital reproduction. In each case a woman decides to conceive and give birth to a child knowing that there will not be a rearing male partner. Yet few people would now argue, particularly in the case of an economically stable woman, that birth to a single woman is such a detriment to the child that the child should not have been born at all.

Physicians treating infertility may choose whether or not to participate in such situations. Generally speaking, they will not be acting illegally if they select their patients, although a program's receipt of federal or state funds may limit its physicians' freedom to select patients in a discriminatory manner. Indeed, a law that outlawed assistance to unmarried women would be subject to attack on both equal protection and due process grounds, for it would deny an infertile unmarried woman the same rights that a married person has.

The use of donor eggs by a woman past the normal age of childbearing is not clearly harmful to the child either. To date, such cases have been rare, and although they will likely be relatively infrequent, they will occur and may garner wide media attention when they do, as occurred with the 1993 birth of twins in Britain to a 59-year-old recipient of donor eggs[38] and the pregnancy achieved that same year in a 62-year-old Italian woman after she and her husband lost their only (adult) child in an accident. Having an older mother does deviate from past practices and traditional views of motherhood, but men have been able to reproduce late in life. To deny women this opportunity when a technology permits it would seem arguably to be discriminatory on gender grounds. Even if the child's mother dies when the child is at an earlier age than usual, is the child so worse off that it would have been better that the child not have been born at all? A counterargument would be that older men achieve parenthood without medical intervention or assistance. Again, individual programs or practitioners may choose not to offer egg donation to older recipients, but it would not clearly be unethical to do so. ASRM Guidelines (IX) recommend potential recipients over the age of forty be thoroughly evaluated before being accepted as recipients. Given constitutional rights of equal protection and procreative liberty, it would be unlikely that such services could be legally banned in the United States.

RECORD KEEPING

Even though egg donation cannot itself be banned to protect offspring, it should be conducted in ways that will respect their interests. The most important measure here is to keep confidential records about donor identity and characteristics so that offspring may later, if the law or changes in social policy permit, learn the identity of their genetic mother and even have contact with her if that can be arranged in a mutually satisfactory way. Recognition of the child's right to have information about his or her genetic mother or even learn her identity at some later point does not also mean that the egg donor will have other rearing duties imposed against her wishes.

At present, there is no law that explicitly requires that such records be kept or that enables offspring of sperm or egg donation to ever learn who their genetic parents are. ASRM guidelines on sperm donation suggest that permanent confidential records be kept and that it is "highly desirable" that they be made available on an anonymous basis to recipient or offspring. While some state adoption laws allow the confidentiality of records to be pierced for good cause, there is no existing provision for offspring of gamete donation, and in some instances no records would be available if there were.[39] Whether and to what extent children should be informed of how they were born will have to depend on the families that raise them. It is unlikely that mandatory disclosure could or would be legislated. But should state law either permit or require disclosure or should the parties otherwise agree to disclosure, it will be necessary to have records of donors and recipients available. Legal counsel should be consulted about any applicable state laws with regard to creating or maintaining medical records.

It is thus essential that donors and recipients be clearly informed of the extent to which anonymity will be attempted to be preserved and records kept so that later contact or information, if mutually desired or otherwise required by state law, can be arranged.[40]

OWNERSHIP ISSUES

An important legal issue concerns ownership of eggs retrieved in the course of assisted reproduction. The key legal and ethical point is that persons own their gametes and embryos formed therefrom until they relinquish or transfer control of them to others.[41] In this context "ownership" means that they have dispositional authority: No one may take or use their gametes or embryos without their consent. The scope of their ownership or dispositional control will then depend on limits imposed by state law—for example, whether eggs and embryos may be bought and sold.

This issue has recently received national attention as a result of allegations that doctors at a California assisted reproduction program took eggs of couples undergoing IVF treatment without their consent or permission and inseminated them with donor or partner sperm of other women in the program.[42] Resulting embryos were transferred to the second woman's uterus and in some instances led to the birth of a child. In other cases the first couple's embryos may have been taken without permission and used to initiate pregnancy and delivery in other couples. The recipients of the misappropriated eggs and embryos were not aware that the eggs and embryos that led to their pregnancies and deliveries were taken without consent from other couples.

If these allegations are true, the persons who took eggs and embryos without the consent of the persons producing them have committed a serious violation of basic ethical and legal norms. Intentional or unintentional misappropriation of gametes or embryos will lead to civil damages for interference with persons' right to control disposition of their eggs and embryos. If the misappropriation has also been intentional, it will also support criminal charges of theft or larceny. A couple who has unknowingly had a child as a result of misappropriated eggs or embryos will also have a cause of action against the persons and program responsible for this result. The question of custody of resulting children in such cases raises complicated questions that will have to be settled between the parties involved or by the courts.[43]

Because of the potential for disputes or disagreements over disposition of donated eggs, it is essential that persons participating in egg donation understand very clearly when the donation legally occurs. This point is legally significant because once the donation has been made, transfer of ownership and dispositional authority over eggs and any resulting embryos, as well as rearing rights and duties in resulting children, passes from the egg source to the recipient.

Many consent forms are silent on this important point, while some state that the donation occurs at the time of retrieval and some that it occurs at the time of insemination. From the recipient couple's perspective, it would be most desirable to have the donation effective at the time of retrieval, so that they will be able to proceed with insemination and embryo transfer as planned. However, an approach that would protect the right of the donor to change her mind at this late stage would make the donation effective and thus transfer rights only at the point of insemination. This alternative would avoid a potential three-way dispute if the egg donor changed her mind at retrieval and a recipient couple demanded that the program proceed with insemination. However, if point-of-insemination is the point that effectuates the donation, it is likely that the donor would then be liable for the costs of the entire cycle and any payments advanced to her by the recipient for her costs as a donor. To avoid disputes and assure that participants are fully informed, the consent forms and agreements executed by the participants should specify precisely when the donation is legally effective and transfer of ownership and dispositional control over the eggs in question occurs.

CONCLUSION

Human egg donation is a promising technique for treating a major source of infertility, but it now lacks the legal infrastructure that is necessary to provide the participants with certainty about the legal consequences of this collaborative form of assisted reproduction. While only a handful of states have begun to address the legal issues that arise in egg donation, additional legislation and judicial action will be necessary to resolve the legal uncertainties that do exist.

Until that time, interested parties need not refrain from participation in egg donation but should be fully aware of the areas of uncertainty that currently exist and take steps to minimize undesired consequences. In the final analysis, full disclosure, free and informed consent, clear agreement, and respect for the interests of all parties will be the best protection for physicians, couples, and donors who participate in human egg donation.

ENDNOTES

[1]This chapter is an updated and expanded version, with assistance of Susan L. Crockin, J.D. of "Legal Uncertainties in Human Egg Donation," by John A. Robertson, J.D., which has been published in Cynthia Cohen, ed., *New Ways of Making Babies: The Case of Egg Donation*, Bloomington: Indiana University Press, 1995.

[2]M.V. Sauer and R.J. Paulson, "Understanding the Current Status of Oocyte Donation in the United States: What's Really Going on out There?," *Fertility and Sterility* 58 16–18 (1992).

[3]Okla. Stat. Ann. tit. 10, Sec. 544 (1991); Tex. Fam. Code Ann. Sec. 12.03A–.04 (Supp. 1995); Fla. Stat. Ann. Sec. 745.11 to .17 (Supp. 1995); N.D. Cent. Code Sec. 14-18-01-07 (Supp. 1995); Va. Code Ann. Sec. 20-156 to 165 (1995) and Sec. 32. 1–45. 3 (Supp. 1995).

[4]U.S. Congress, Office of Technology Assessment, *Infertility: Medical and Social Choices* 242-49 (1988). See also *Levin* v. *Levin*, Ind.Ct.App.1st Dist. (1993).

[5]S.L. Crockin, "Donor Oocytes, Once Given Can the Gift Be Taken Away?," *Clinical Consultations in Obstetrics and Gynecology* (September 1993).

[6]*MacDonald* v. *MacDonald*, 196 A.D.2d7, 608 N.Y.S.2d 477 (1994).

[7]Id.

[8]*Johnson* v. *Calvert*, 5 Cal.4th 84, 851 P.2d 776, 19 Cal.Rptr. 2nd 494 (1993).

[9]286 Cal.Rptr. 369 (Cal.App. 4 Dist. 1991).

[10]822 P.2d 1317, 4 Cal.Rptr. 2nd 170 (1992).

[11]*Lehr* v. *Robertson*, 463 U.S. 248 (1983).

[12]*Welborn* v. *Doe*, 394 S.E.2d 732 (1990); reviewed in S.L. Crockin, "Legally Speaking," *Fertility News* (March 1991).

[13]For example, *Jhordan C.* v. *Mary K.*, 179 Cal. App.3d 386; 224 Cal. Rptr. 530 (1986). A number of courts have refused to enforce agreements between a single woman and a man in which she attempted to release him from all parental obligations in exchange for his waiving any such rights he might be found to have. For a recent case collecting and citing earlier cases, see *OK Dept. of Human Services ex rel K.A.G.* v. *T.AD.G.*, OK Sup.Ct.(1993).

[14]Tex. Fam. Code Ann. Sec. 12.03 (Vernon 1986).

[15]J.A. Robertson, "Ethical and Legal Issues in Human Egg Donation," *Fertility and Sterility* 52:353–363 (1989).

[16]J.A. Robertson, "Ethical and Legal Issues in the Cryopreservation of Human Embryos," *Fertility and Sterility* 47:371 (1987).

[17]*Stiver* v. *Parker*, (Keane, Malonoff) 975 F.2d 2261 (en banc denied) (1992).

[18]President's Commission for the Study of Ethical Problems in Medicine and Biomedical and Behavioral Science Research, 1982, *Compensation for Research Injuries*, Washington, D.C.: U.S. Government Printing Office, 1982, pp. 81–98.

[19]*Id.*

[20]M. Seibel, "Compensating Egg Donors: Equal Pay for Equal Time," NEJM 328: 737 (1993).

[21]American Fertility Society, "Guidelines for Gamete Donation, 1993," Oocyte Donation Guidelines paragraph VI, *Fertility and Sterility* 62(5, Suppl. 1) (1994).

[22]Note, Regulating the sale of human organs. 1985. *Virginia Law Review*, 71:1015.

[23]42 U.S.C.A. #274(e) Prohibition of Organ Purchases.

[24]La. Civ. Code Ann. Art. 9:122 (Supp. 1987).

[25]Texas Health and Safety Code Ann., sec. 4802 (West 1989).

[26]*Stedman's Medical Dictionary*, 22nd Edition, 1972.

[27]Ohio Rev. Code Ann. S.2108.11, 2108.12 (Baldwin 1980).

[28]Nev. Rev. Stat. #201.460 (1991).

[29]New York Pub. Health Law, sec. 4307 (McKinney 1990).

[30]Cal. Penal Code, #367f (West 1988).

[31]S.D. Codified Laws Ann. S. 34-26-42.

[32]M.G.L. ch. 112 § 12J.

[33]*Margaret S.* v. *Edwards*, 794 F.2d 994 (5th Cir. 1986); *Lifchez* v. *Hartigan*, 735 F. Supp. 1361 (N.D. Ill. 1990).

[34]J.A. Robertson, "Technology and Motherhood: Ethical and Legal Issues in Human Egg Donation," *Case-Western Reserve Law Review*, 39:1–38 (1989). But see *Doe* v. *Atty General*, MI Ct.Apps (1992).

[35]M. Seibel, "Compensating Egg Donors: Equal Pay for Equal Time," NEJM 328:737 (1993).

[36]Texas Health & Safety Code Ann. #48.02 (West 1989).

[37]See n. 24 and 25 *supra*.

[38]William Schmidt, "Birth to a 59-Year Old Generates an Ethical Controversy in Britain," *New York Times* (Dec. 29, 1993). See also Associated Press, "53-Year-Old Grandmother Gives Birth to Premature Test-Tube Twins" *Austin-American-Statesman*, p. A18 (Nov. 11, 1992); *People Magazine* (May 8, 1992).

[39]J.A. Robertson, "Embryos, Families and Procreative Liberty: The Legal Structure of the New Reproduction," *Southern California Law Review*, 59:942-1039 (1986); J.A. Robertson, *Children of Choice: Freedom and the New Reproductive Technologies* Princeton, N.J.: Princeton University Press, 1994, pp. 123–125.

[40]See discussion in Chapter 10, "Egg Donor Consent Forms."

[41]J.A. Robertson, "In the Beginning: the Legal Status of Early Embryos," *Virginia Law Review* 76(3):437 (1990).

[42]S. Mydans, "Fertility Clinic Told to Close Amid Complaints," *New York Times* (May 29, 1995), p. A15.

[43]J.A. Robertson, The Case of the Switched Embryos, forthcoming, *Hastings Center Report* (November 1995).

10

Egg Donation Consent Forms

JOAN C. STODDARD, J.D.
JANIS FOX, M.D.

GENERAL REQUIREMENTS FOR INFORMED CONSENT

The doctrine of informed consent has developed from the recognition that a physician has both an ethical and a legal obligation to provide his or her patient with sufficient information to enable the patient to make an informed judgment whether to give or withhold consent to a surgical or medical procedure. In general, the information to be given to a patient includes the nature of the patient's condition; the nature and probability of risks involved; the benefits to be reasonably expected; the inability of the physician to predict the results, if that is the case; the likely result of no treatment; and the available alternatives, including their risks and benefits.

The requirements of informed consent are not satisfied merely by having the patient read and sign a consent form. Rather, the essence of informed consent is the dialogue between the physician and the patient in which the physician provides the information described above and the patient has an opportunity to ask any questions she or he may have. A signed consent form is not a substitute for this dialogue, but rather is evidence that the dialogue has taken place.

INFORMED CONSENT FORMS FOR OVUM DONATION

The consent forms that are necessary for an ovum donation program will likely be far more detailed and complex than standard surgical consent forms. As will be described below, a program's determination as to what information should be contained in ovum donation consent forms will need to reflect legal, ethical, and policy considerations.

Separate forms will need to be developed for the donor and the recipient. In addition, if a program uses both known and anonymous donors, separate forms will be necessary for each of these groups. Thus if a program accepts both known and anonymous donors, four consent forms should generally be developed: (1) donor consent form for known donors, (2) recipient couple consent form when a known donor is to be used, (3) donor consent form for anonymous donors, and (4) recipient couple consent form when an anonymous donor is to be used.

As a general matter, the donor consent form can be somewhat less comprehensive than the recipient consent form. It is essential that the recipient couple be fully aware of the entire procedure as it affects both them and the donor. The donor need only be informed about the procedure as it affects her. Of course, the risks to the donor, particularly with regard to fertility drugs, should be clearly spelled out, as described below.

One useful way to convey some of the information that donors and recipients need to know is to prepare an informational brochure or leaflet to be used in conjunction with the consent forms. This brochure can provide a general overview of the entire procedure from the standpoint of both the recipient and the donor. It can also discuss such topics as the background and history of ovum donation and any program restrictions or requirements, such as age limitations, health screening, and counseling requirements. The consent forms should include an acknowledgment by the patient that she has received this brochure and has read and understood its contents. A sample informational brochure is included at the end of this chapter in Appendix 10-A. The balance of this chapter addresses specific recommended provisions for consent forms and is divided into three sections: (1) a checklist for issues specific to recipient couples, (2) a checklist for issues specific to donors, and (3) issues that are applicable to both recipients and donors.

The discussion of information to be contained in consent forms for an ovum donation program is based on a review of consent forms developed by the Brigham and Women's Hospital of Boston, Massachusetts ("Brigham and Women's") (Appendices 10-C and 10-D) for use with known donors and recipients and by the Faulkner Centre for Reproductive Medicine of Boston, Massachusetts ("Faulkner") for use with recipients, known donors, and anonymous donors (Appendices 10-E, 10-F, and 10-G). Complete copies of these forms are included at the end of this chapter. A set of consent forms from Pennsylvania Reproductive Associates of Pennsylvania Hospital has also been included for comparison and reference (Appendices 10-I and 10-J).

CHECKLIST FOR THE RECIPIENT COUPLE'S CONSENT FORMS

Introduction

The consent form should contain a brief introductory paragraph indicating the recipient couple's desire to participate in the ovum donation program in order to achieve a pregnancy. This paragraph should also include a statement acknowledging that the pregnancy will be attempted with donated eggs and with either the husband's sperm or donor sperm, whichever the case may be.

Source of Donor

The consent form should clearly specify the program's policy as to how a donor will be obtained. The form should indicate whether the donor will be anonymous or known to the recipient couple or whether either approach is acceptable. The form should also state who is responsible for providing a donor, the couple or the program. If the recipient couple is to provide a donor, the form should specify any program limitations or restrictions, such as health or age, as to who is an acceptable donor. If the program is to provide a donor, the form should indicate how such donors are obtained. For example, donors might include women who undergo ovarian stimulation solely for the purposes of serving as a donor or IVF patients who produce excess eggs.

Screening

The form should indicate what type of screening will take place for both the recipient couple and the donor. Such screening might include (1) a physical examination including pelvic examination and a Pap smear for both recipient and donor, (2) a detailed social history including substance ingestion and sexual relationships, (3) screening for infectious diseases, (4) a detailed medical and family history focusing on possible familial and genetic diseases, (5) screening for inheritable diseases based on the results of the medical history and the ethnic background of the parties, and (6) psychological screening and counseling.

The consent form should also specify how information obtained from the screening process will be conveyed to the recipient couple, and in particular how problematic or potentially problematic information will be handled. This is an extremely sensitive issue in which the rights of both the donor and the recipient couple need to be balanced. Some information obtained during the screening may automatically disqualify a potential donor. Other information might indicate that a potential degree of risk exists. This type of information will need to be communicated to the recipient couple, who will be the ultimate decision makers (assuming that the donor still wishes to proceed). Clearly, if the donor does not wish screening information to be conveyed to the recipient couple, then the program cannot do so. However, the potential donor must then be disqualified. The recipient couple should be advised of this possibility. In addition, assuming that the donation is to proceed and the screening information is shared with the recipient couple, they should acknowledge in writing that they have had an opportunity to review the screening information and to discuss the information with a genetic counselor. At this time, some programs have the staff person who reviews the information with the recipient couple make a note in the chart to that effect. A more protective procedure, for both the recipient couple and the physician, is to have the recipient couple sign a written acknowledgment as to the exact information they have been given. This could be done by having them initial or sign the donor's (anonymous) screening form. Included at the end of this chapter is a donor screening form prepared by the Brigham and Women's Hospital that contains such an acknowledgment (Appendix 10-B).

Outline of the Steps to Be Followed in the Procedure

The recipient couple consent form should contain an outline of the procedure to be followed for the recipient. This section should include a discussion of all of the following that are applicable:

1. preparation of the recipient's uterus with estrogen and progesterone, if applicable;
2. synchronizing the menstrual cycles of the recipient and the donor;
3. blood samples and endometrial biopsy, if necessary;
4. fertilization of eggs retrieved from the donor by the husband's sperm or donor sperm; and
5. transfer of fertilized eggs to the recipient's uterus.

These steps should of course be described in more detail. See the descriptions contained in the consent forms included in the chapter appendices.

Risks and Discomforts Resulting from the Procedure

The consent form should also contain a listing of the risks and discomforts to the recipient that may result from the procedure. The risks and discomforts may be listed in the same section as the description of the procedure or may be contained in a separate section. Risks and discomforts to be specified may include the following:

1. Blood drawing: Mild discomfort and some risk of developing a bruise at the needle site.

2. Estrogen: Possible nausea, bloating, gall-bladder disease, abnormal blood clotting, migraine, darkening of the skin, growth of benign fibroid tumors, jaundice, breast tenderness, intolerance to contact lenses, and increased vaginal secretions.

3. Progesterone: Pain and swelling at the injection site, bloating, weight gain, breast tenderness, premenstrual-like syndrome, headache, fatigue, and mental depression. The progesterone is mixed in a peanut oil– or sesame oil–based solution and should not be used by patients who are allergic to these.

4. Leuprolide acetate or related drugs: Response may vary. Side effects include hot flashes, vaginal dryness, burning on urination, difficulty sleeping, bloating, headaches, hair loss, pain or numbness in extremities, local reactions at injection site, and temporary reduction in bone density.

5. Endometrial biopsy: Uterine cramping, small risk of infection or uterine perforation. A local anesthesia may be required.

6. Transfer of embryos: Minimal discomfort, minimal risks of developing infection that, in some cases, requires hospitalization and intravenous antibiotic treatment.

7. Psychological distress: Sometimes associated with assisted reproductive technology procedure.

8. Multiple births, miscarriages, ectopic pregnancies, congenital abnormalities: If a pregnancy is successfully established, multiple pregnancies (20–25% chance of twin pregnancy, 1–5% chance of triplet pregnancy, and a rare chance of a higher-order pregnancy), miscarriage, ectopic pregnancy, stillbirth, and/or congenital abnormalities may occur. The likelihood of multiple births, tubal pregnancies, and miscarriage is increased with ovum donation as compared to spontaneously occurring pregnancy. The risk of developing an abnormal fetus is no greater than the risk associated with a spontaneously occurring pregnancy (up to 5%, depending on the age of the donor).

9. Selective reduction: In the event of a multiple pregnancy, which places the woman and/or fetus at risk, selective reduction may be considered.

10. Sexually transmitted/infectious diseases: Although egg donors are screened for sexually transmitted diseases, there is a risk that HIV, hepatitis, gonorrhea, syphilis, cytomegalovirus, or other sexually transmitted diseases or infections may be transmitted. The long-term risks to an infant from such transmission can include mental retardation, developmental retardation, physical anomalies (abnormalities), and death. The woman and spouse are also at risk of contracting all such sexually transmitted diseases. This latter complication can include death as in the case of AIDS or hepatitis. A woman can require a hysterectomy if she develops a pelvic infection. It can cause such severe pain that intercourse is no longer possible. Daily life can also be affected.

Likelihood of Achieving a Successful Pregnancy and Obstacles to Success

It is strongly recommended that the recipient couple be given some type of information about the likelihood of success in achieving a pregnancy through ovum donation. This information may be contained in an informational brochure or in the consent form. The information conveyed can be very general, as provided by Faulkner in its consent form, or more specific by using statistics, as is contained in the Brigham and Women's brochure. When statistics are given, it is important that the source of any statistics are clearly stated and able to be substantiated. Any statistics provided should clearly indicate whether they are based on the particular program's experience or are statistics that reflect the procedures in general.

To aid the recipient's overall understanding of the process, it may be advisable to list some of the potential obstacles to success, including the following:

1. The donor may have a suboptimal response to the ovulation induction medications.
2. The attempt to retrieve the egg from the donor may be unsuccessful.
3. The egg or eggs may be abnormal.
4. The recipient husband may not be able to produce a semen specimen, or the specimen may not be normal. If frozen donor sperm is used, it may be of poor quality.
5. Fertilization may not occur or may be abnormal in some or all of the eggs.
6. Cell division in the fertilized eggs may not occur.
7. The embryo may not develop normally.
8. The embryo transfer may be unsuccessful.
9. Loss or damage to the fertilized or unfertilized eggs could occur.

Disposition of Fertilized Eggs

One extremely important and somewhat controversial issue that must be addressed in the consent form concerns the disposition of excess fertilized or unfertilized eggs. The number of eggs retrieved from a donor may be considerably more than what a recipient may use in a single cycle. All possible options available concerning excess eggs should be discussed with the recipient couple (and donor) in advance, and their choice or choices should be indicated on their consent form. Individual programs may have specific philosophies or approaches that limit the number of choices they will make available to couples. It is also important to review state law and hospital

policy, which may limit the use of certain of these options. The range of possible choices includes the following:

1. Inseminating all eggs retrieved and discarding all fertilized eggs in excess of the number that can be safely transferred to the recipient.
2. Inseminating all eggs retrieved and cryopreserving all fertilized eggs in excess of the number that can be safely transferred to the recipient.
3. Inseminating only a limited number of eggs (approximately five to seven) so that all eggs that fertilize can be transferred to the recipient and discarding the excess eggs.
4. Inseminating a limited number of eggs for the recipient couple and sharing the excess eggs with another recipient couple for fertilization by them and possible transfer to them.
5. Inseminating all eggs retrieved and donating to another couple all fertilized eggs in excess of the number that can be safely transferred to the recipient.

It is crucial that this subject, and the particular choices offered by the program, be discussed thoroughly in advance. Many individuals, providers as well as patients, have strongly held ethical and religious views concerning these issues, and not all of a couple's expectations may be met. Any limits on possible choices should therefore be very clearly conveyed. It is also crucial that the recipient couple's choice, and any alternative choice, be recorded in writing. Because circumstances may change and be difficult to predict, the consent form should also address potential changes of mind. It is recommended that the consent form explicitly address who may make such a change, what a program will do in the event of a future disagreement between the recipient couple, and how such a change is to be communicated. Any change should be required to be in writing.

Disposition of Other Bodily Fluids and Tissues

Information concerning the disposition of other bodily fluids and tissues should also be provided on the recipient couple consent form. This subject is typically not as controversial as the disposition of fertilized eggs and can be addressed briefly. It is generally sufficient to use a simple statement to the effect that the recipient couple authorizes the program to dispose of bodily fluids and tissues including unfertilized or abnormally fertilized eggs and, if applicable, that these materials may be utilized for diagnostic, research, or teaching purposes. Again, state law and hospital policy should be reviewed to determine the acceptability of using these materials for research purposes.

If, however, the program intends or desires to donate excess unfertilized eggs to another couple for insemination, the original recipient couple should be explicitly advised, and their express, written consent should be obtained. Failure to obtain their express, written consent would raise serious ethical concerns and subject a provider to potential civil, or even criminal, liability.

Financial Obligations and Insurance Coverage

Financial information and obligations should also be specified on the consent form. The recipient couple (or their insurance, if available) are generally responsible for all expected charges related to the ovum donation procedure. This includes the expected medical expenses for both the donor and the recipient. The issue that each program must resolve, however, is who will be responsible for the donor's medical expenses if unexpected complications occur.

The charges can be dealt with in a number of ways. Since there is no direct benefit to the donor from her participation, perhaps the fairest approach is to have the recipient couple be responsible for all of the donor's expenses, including those resulting from unexpected complications. This is the approach adopted by Faulkner. In programs in which a single donor's eggs are shared by two recipient couples, it may be possible to also share those expenses and reduce the cost to each recipient couple.

The difficulty with this approach, however, is that if serious unexpected complications occur to the donor, in the absence of insurance the recipient couple may be unable or unwilling to pay for these expenses. For this reason, some programs require donors to have medical insurance in place to cover the expenses of any complications. The donor consent form provides that the donor or her insurance is responsible to the hospital for any such costs, but the donor is free to make separate arrangements with the recipient for reimbursement of such expenses. An arrangement for reimbursement is likely to be feasible only in the case of known donors.

Regardless of the option selected by the program, the following topics should be covered in the consent form:

1. an outline of the types of charges and expenses the recipient couple will be responsible for;
2. an explanation as to whether the recipient couple or the donor will be responsible for the medical expenses of the donor, including expenses arising from an unexpected complication;
3. a statement as to who will be responsible for any charges not covered by insurance; and
4. if the donor is procured by the program, an explanation of any amounts due the donor from the recipient.

Risks of Complications During Pregnancy and Birth and Risks of Birth and Genetic Defects

A statement should be included that explains that during pregnancy and childbirth resulting from ovum donation, the same types of complications can arise as with pregnancy and childbirth resulting from sexual intercourse.

There should also be a statement indicating that a risk exists that a child resulting from ovum donation may be born with birth defects, medical problems, or learning disabilities and that the risk is similar to that for a child conceived by sexual intercourse.

Finally, there should also be a statement indicating that several risks may be unknown, despite the physician's best efforts to screen donors.

Use of Residents or Students

If residents, interns, or students will be observing or participating in the procedure, the consent form should so indicate.

CHECKLIST FOR OVUM DONOR'S CONSENT FORM

Introductory Paragraph

The introductory paragraph should include a statement expressing the donor's willingness to donate her eggs to another woman who is otherwise unable to have children. The consent form should indicate whether the donation is to be anonymous or to a known recipient. If the donation is nonanonymous, the name of the recipient should be indicated. (If potential recipients include single women, the consent form should encompass that possibility.)

Screening

The consent form should state what type of screening the donor is required to undergo. If the donor is married and participation by the donor's husband in the screening process is mandated, this should be indicated. Screening for the donor (and her husband, if applicable) might include (1) a physical examination including pelvic examination and Pap smear, (2) a detailed social history including substance ingestion and sexual relationships, (3) screening for infectious diseases, (4) a detailed medical and family history focusing on possible familial and genetic diseases, (5) screening for inheritable diseases based on the results of the medical history and ethnic background of the parties, and (6) psychological screening and counseling.

The donor must also be advised that if the donation is to proceed, the information obtained from the screening process must be shared with the recipient couple. If the donor does not want the information shared with the recipient couple, the program will not do so. However, the prospective donor is then disqualified. The donor screening form prepared by the Brigham and Women's Hospital and included at the end of this chapter (Appendix 10-B) contains the following acknowledgment to this effect:

> *Attention Donor:* Please read the statements below. After you have read them both, please sign your name under the *one* option you have selected.
>
> 1) I have carefully answered the above questions and my responses are true and correct to the best of my knowledge. I have had the opportunity to have my questions answered by a physician. I understand and agree that the information on this form will be provided to the recipient couple, and I consent to this disclosure.
>
> or

2) I have carefully answered the above questions and my responses are true and correct to the best of my knowledge. I have had the opportunity to have my questions answered by a physician. I do not wish the information on this form to be shared with the recipient couple. I understand that, as a result, I will not be permitted to serve as a donor.

Outline of the Steps to Be Followed in the Procedure

The consent form should contain an outline of the procedure for the donor and should include a discussion of the following topics:

1. Ovulation induction for the purpose of egg retrieval including (a) taking of fertility medications and antibiotics for a several-week period, (b) frequent blood samplings, and (c) daily transvaginal ultrasound examinations for approximately a one-week period.

2. Egg retrieval including (a) an injection of hCG (a natural hormone substance), which initiates the final egg maturation process, approximately 34 hours before the retrieval; (b) sedation and anesthesia used during the egg retrieval; and (c) the actual egg retrieval, which is accomplished by an ultrasound-guided needle.

These steps should of course be described in more detail. See the descriptions contained in the consent forms included at the end of the chapter.

Possible Risks and Discomforts to the Donor from the Procedure

The consent form should list the possible risks and discomforts to the donor that may result from the procedure. The risks and discomforts

may be listed in the same section as the procedure or in a separate section. Since the donor receives no direct benefit from serving as a donor, it is especially important that potential risks are clearly spelled out. Risks and discomforts to be specified may include the following:

1. Blood drawing: Mild discomfort and some risk of developing a bruise at the needle site.
2. Fertility drugs: Moderate weight gain, mood changes, stomach pressure, headaches, allergic reaction, and hyperstimulation of the ovaries (5% chance in any cycle). In very rare cases, hyperstimulation could lead to very enlarged ovaries and an increased susceptibility to develop blood clots necessitating hospitalization. Also, in very rare cases, hyperstimulation may lead to the development of fluid in the abdomen or lungs, kidney failure, stroke, or severe ovarian enlargement and possible rupture. In extremely rare cases, death may result. Ovarian rupture may also necessitate general anesthesia and major surgery, with all the inherent risks. Loss of one or both ovaries is possible. The risk of hyperstimulation is minimized if the follicles are aspirated as is planned to occur at the egg retrieval The risk increases if, after taking the fertility medications to stimulate the ovaries, the donor chooses not to undergo egg retrieval. There also exists an unlikely possibility of a lasting effect on the donor's pelvic organs, including pain, irregular menstrual function, or impairment of future fertility. Finally, an association between fertility drugs and ovarian cancer has been suggested but not proven.
3. Antibiotics: Possible allergic reaction that, in rare cases, may be severe.
4. Ultrasound egg retrieval: Many patients experience mild to moderate discomfort after the procedure. Potentially serious complications include bleeding, infection, and injury to the bowel or blood vessels. In extremely

rare circumstances, surgery may be necessary to repair damage to internal organs or to control significant internal bleeding (hemorrhage). Anesthesia will be necessary for the egg retrieval. (The risks associated with anesthesia will be explained during a consultation with an anesthesiologist.) If eggs cannot be retrieved by ultrasound, clear consent must be obtained from a donor before utilizing a laparoscopy and general anesthesia. There may be additional risks of donating eggs that have not yet been identified. Since it is theoretically possible that not all of the developed eggs will be recovered at the time of retrieval, there is a risk that the donor may become pregnant if she engages in unprotected intercourse during the egg donation cycle(s).

5. Ultrasound examinations: No known risks, minimal discomfort.

6. Psychological distress: Sometimes associated with assisted reproductive technology procedures.

7. Inconvenience: Monitoring procedures during the period of stimulation and the time needed to perform the egg retrieval itself will result in a certain amount of inconvenience and lost time.

Donor to Refrain from Unprotected Sexual Intercourse

The donor should agree to refrain from unprotected sexual intercourse from the time the fertility medications are begun until the egg retrieval is completed to guard against pregnancy and the transmission of infectious diseases.

Donor to Follow Medical Instructions

The consent form may request the agreement of the donor to follow, for an appropriate time period, medical instructions by agreeing not to smoke, drink alcoholic beverages, or use any illegal or prescription or nonprescription drugs without the consent of the program's doctor.

Disposition of Fertilized Eggs

An extremely important and potentially controversial issue that must also be addressed on the donor consent form concerns the disposition of fertilized eggs. All possible options available concerning excess eggs should be discussed with the donor in advance and her choice(s) clearly indicated on her consent form. A donor may agree to donate eggs to any recipient individual or couple. Alternatively, she may make restrictions on her donation, such as limiting her donation to a selected individual or couple. In the case of a known donor, for example a sister of the female recipient, she may wish to restrict her donation to the couple only; and may even wish to exclude use of any cryopreserved embryos by the recipient husband in the event of a subsequent divorce or her recipient sister's death. All such choices should be indicated on the donor's consent form and parallel provisions should be contained in the recipient consent form. Failure to obtain a donor's express, written consent to potential uses of her fertilized eggs could raise serious ethical concerns and subject a program to potential civil, or even criminal, liability.

Disposition of Unfertilized Eggs and Other Bodily Fluids and Tissues

Information concerning the disposition of unfertilized eggs and other bodily fluids and tissues should also be provided on the donor consent form. It is generally sufficient to use a simple statement that the donor authorizes the program to dispose of bodily fluid or tissue, including, if any, unfertilized or abnormally fertilized eggs, and, if applicable, that these materials may be utilized for diagnostic, research, or teaching purposes. As was noted above, state law and hospital policy should be reviewed to determine the acceptability of using these materials for research purposes.

Financial Obligations and Insurance

The donor consent form should specify any financial obligations of the donor and how the donor's medical expenses, including expenses arising from unexpected complications, will be paid. As was discussed more fully in the recipient couple section above, the donor's medical expenses can be addressed in a number of ways. Regardless of the option selected, however, information on the following topics should be included on the donor consent form:

1. a listing of any charges or expenses that will be the responsibility of the donor;
2. an explanation as to whether the recipient couple or the donor will be responsible for the medical costs of the donor, including expenses arising from unexpected complications; and
3. if the donor is procured by the program, a detailed explanation of any amounts due to the donor from the recipient or the program, as well as a clear explanation of when any amounts are due and under what circumstances, if any, payments are not made.

Because some of these items may change more frequently than the consent form, some programs may wish to consider a separate compensation schedule that may be attached and incorporated into the consent form by reference. The consent form and any schedule should state that the donor is being compen-

sated for time, inconvenience, and effort for screening, ovulation induction, and egg retrieval and that the donor will be paid in accordance with the attached payment schedule. Payment may then vary depending on whether a cycle is completed or length of participation in the program. Any compensation payments should adhere to the Faulkner Centre for Reproductive Medicine's "Guidelines for Oocyte Donation" (see Appendix 4-A). Those guidelines recommend that payments be made not for number or quality of eggs, but for time and inconvenience.

CHECKLIST OF PROVISIONS APPLICABLE TO DONORS AND RECIPIENTS

There are a number of provisions that apply to both a donor and a recipient couple that a program or its legal counsel will want to include or consider when preparing consent forms. Some of these provisions may be found in the forms at the end of the chapter. Others are mentioned as possible issues that may be appropriate depending on the specific program.

Explanation of Ownership of Eggs and Embryos and Parental Rights to Offspring

This section may be the single most critical provision in either the donor's or the recipient couple's consent form.

First, the consent form should indicate at what point ownership of the eggs passes from the donor to the recipient. This is very important, since, particularly with a known donor, disputes may arise between the donor and the recipient couple over the ownership of the eggs or resultant embryos.

As discussed below, the consent forms should also allow for the possibility that either the donor or the recipient couple may wish to change their minds either before or during the procedure. Any withdrawal, if permissible, should be required to be in writing.

The form should also state whether the recipient couple or the donor has authority to make decisions regarding donating, discarding, or cryopreserving excess eggs and/or embryos as applicable.

Different consent forms address the time of ownership transfer differently. Some state that the donor may change her mind about proceeding with the donation up to the point at which the retrieval is completed, but once the retrieval is concluded, she loses all rights to the eggs. Others transfer ownership upon insemination. A program may want to consider having ownership transfer at insemination, thereby reducing the risk of a legal challenge by the intended recipient couple in the event that the donor changes her mind following retrieval but before insemination.

Additionally, the consent form should state that all ownership and decision-making authority with regard to any resulting embryos belong to the recipient couple or, at their election, to the survivor of the couple, in the event that one of them dies. An exception to this rule may be made by a known donor and couple where, as discussed above, the donor wants her eggs used only by the couple. Any such exception should be documented thoroughly. The form should also contain a statement indicating that the recipient couple will accept any resulting offspring as their own and will care for and support such offspring. It would be prudent to explicitly state that the donor has no parental rights or responsibilities to any resulting offspring, that she agrees not to seek a court order or institute any adversarial proceedings to establish parental or other rights to any resulting embryos or offspring, and that she relinquishes

any right or claim to such offspring as she might be deemed to have.

In the event that any dispute should arise between the donor and the recipient couple over ownership of or control over the donated eggs or resultant embryos, it is very important that the consent form specify the point at which the donor relinquishes rights to and control over her eggs. Both the donor's and recipient's forms therefore should state the point at which ownership of the eggs passes from the donor to the recipient, that is, whether upon retrieval or upon insemination, and should also indicate whether the recipient couple or the donor has the authority to make decisions regarding donating, discarding, or cryopreserving excess eggs and/or embryos, as applicable. The situation is more complex if donor sperm is used.

A program is advised to consult legal counsel before proceeding further in a situation in which a donor changes her mind after her eggs have been fertilized with donor sperm but before their implantation in the recipient.

Signature and Acknowledgment

The consent forms should contain acknowledgments similar to the following:

[For Recipient Couple]

We have read this consent form and the information packet provided by Brigham and Women's Hospital, and have had the opportunity to discuss this decision with a physician and social worker/ psychologist. All of our questions have been answered to our satisfaction.

Our signature below constitutes our acknowledgement: (1) that we have read, understood, and agreed to the foregoing; (2) that the proposed operation(s) or procedure(s) have been satisfactorily explained to us and that we have all the information that we desire; (3) that we received a copy of the form; and (4) that we hereby request the procedures described above and give our authorization and consent.

The consent form should be signed and dated by both members of the recipient couple. The signature of a witness is advisable. The recipient couple should be given a copy of the form, and the original should be placed in the recipient's medical record.

The donor consent form should contain an acknowledgment similar to the following:

[For Donor]

I have read this consent form and the information packet provided by Brigham and Women's Hospital, and have had the opportunity to discuss this decision with a physician and social worker/psychologist. All of my questions have been answered to my satisfaction.

My signature below constitutes my acknowledgement (1) that I have read, understood, and agreed to the foregoing, (2) that the proposed operation(s) or procedure(s) have been satisfactorily explained to me and that I have all the information that I desire, (3) that I received a copy of the form, and (4) that I hereby request the procedures described above and give my authorization and consent.

The consent form should be signed and dated by the donor. The signature of a witness is desirable. The donor should be given a copy of the form, and the original should be placed in the donor's medical record.

A remaining issue to be addressed in this section is whether to require the signature of the donor's husband if she is married. The arguments against such a requirement are that a woman may donate eggs without her husband's

consent, a woman may have any number of valid reasons for not wanting her husband to know about the donation, and the requirement may hinder someone from serving as a donor. On the other hand, requiring the husband's signature reduces the possibility of any claims by the husband against the program. Faulkner and Brigham and Women's both require the signature of the donor's husband.

Confidentiality

The donor and recipient consent forms should contain essentially the same information on how confidentiality will be maintained and any exceptions to this confidentiality. It is recommended that at least the following information be included:

1. No entry will be made on the donor's medical records as to the disposition of any eggs that may be retrieved.
2. No entry will be made on the recipient's medical record as to the source of the donated eggs.
3. A separate record may be kept by the physician indicating the source and disposition of donated eggs.
4. It is possible that the identity of one or both parties may be inadvertently revealed through insurance claims or similar records or if required by a change of law or future court order, and the recipient and donor bear the risk of such disclosure.

Consultation with Attorneys

The donor and recipient couple should each be advised to consult independent legal counsel of her or their own regarding the complex issues surrounding ovum donation and whether a written agreement between the recipient and the donor (if known) is advisable.

This topic is covered in the attached informational brochure and is discussed more fully in Chapter 9.

Use of Residents or Students

If residents, interns, or students will be observing or participating in the procedure, the consent form should so indicate.

Waiver

Programs may wish to consider language that releases them from any future claims by either the donor or the recipient couple. The language should indicate that, to the extent permitted by law, the donor/recipient couple waive(s) the right to pursue any claims, demands, or actions for damages against the program, including, but not limited to, claims for pain and suffering, loss of consortium, and loss of time from work. Since many states prohibit waivers of the right to recover damages for negligence by health care professionals, any program that wishes to consider this language should first consult their attorney.

Future Contact/Information

If the donor is anonymous, the consent form should reference whether the donor will be informed of whether any offspring result from her egg donation. The program may also wish to consider asking donors whether they would be willing to update their permanent address and be contacted in the event that any offspring resulting from the egg donation should develop a serious or life-threatening illness for which the donor may be uniquely able to offer assistance. Should a program wish to offer this service, the recipient couple should be made aware of the risk that if their donor has agreed to keep an address on file, the program is not responsible or liable if the information is not actually provided or, if provided, is not updated or kept current.

Appendix 10-A

Ovum Donation Information

**BRIGHAM AND WOMEN'S HOSPITAL
KNOWN DONOR PROGRAM**

The IVF Program at Brigham and Women's Hospital is pleased to offer ovum donation.

WHO MAY BENEFIT FROM OVUM DONATION?

Ovum donation* provides many couples previously considered "incurably sterile" with the chance for a pregnancy. The most common condition motivating infertile couples to request ovum donation is premature ovarian failure (also known as premature menopause), which is defined as permanent ovarian failure before the age of 40 years. Now, even women who have entered menopause after age 40 have become pregnant and successfully delivered babies through the use of ovum donation.

Ovum donation can also be used to treat infertility arising from either congenitally or surgically absent ovaries, or from ovaries which have stopped functioning due to chemotherapy or x-rays. It can also be an option when ovaries are present but do not produce healthy eggs, or when the eggs produced are "unfertilizable." Women who carry genetic abnormalities in their own eggs can safely become pregnant with eggs donated by a woman who doesn't have such genetic abnormalities.

Candidates for ovum donation must be in good physical health and must have a uterus with a normal endometrial cavity. Their husband's semen analysis should be normal or close to normal (unless they plan to use donor sperm as well). A potential recipient of donated eggs requires medical clearance for estrogen and progesterone replacement, and must be considered to be an acceptable risk for carrying a pregnancy. Except in unusual cases, the recipient must be 45 years of age or younger. A screening interview with a social worker (similar to one routinely employed in cases where donor sperm is utilized) will also be conducted for all recipient couples, as well as for all donors.

BACKGROUND

Although medical technology has only recently allowed us to utilize donor eggs, sperm donation has been an accepted treatment for male infertility for many years. Although many of the philosophical and legal considerations regarding egg donation are logically similar to those of sperm donation, there are some obvious differences. The relative inaccessibility of a woman's eggs and the need to synchronize all the elements of the reproductive cycle in both donor and recipient make the process technically more difficult and more complicated. Furthermore, there is no well developed technology for cryopreserving eggs as there is for sperm (although intensive research is currently underway).

Nonetheless, ovum donation in the human has been used quite successfully and has provided many couples with a previously impos-

---

*The terms "ovum" and "egg" are used interchangeably throughout this material.

sible opportunity to experience pregnancy, childbearing, and nursing. The Society for Assisted Reproductive Technology (SART) published in the January 1992 issue of *Fertility and Sterility* the *nationwide* success rates for all ovum donation cycles initiated in the United States in *1990*. Pregnancies were followed until October of 1991 to determine outcomes. In 1990, 29% of donor transfers produced a clinical pregnancy, with a 22% live delivery rate. Statistics can be misleading, since they apply to groups and not to individuals. You should discuss with your physician how these figures apply to your specific case.

WHO ARE POTENTIAL OVUM DONORS?

While similar in principle to sperm donation, ovum donation is more difficult and complicated. The donor will experience considerable inconvenience and some discomfort, and will be subject to some risk. She will take daily injections, submit to frequent pelvic ultrasound examinations and blood tests (both of which are performed at the hospital), and undergo an aspiration of her eggs (which is performed under ultrasound but generally requires heavy sedation or spinal anaesthesia). All ordinary medical and hospital expenses related to the ovum donation including medical evaluations, social services screening, psychological evaluation, medications, blood tests, and surgical procedures will be the responsibility of the recipient.

The BWH ovum donation program provides for the following two sources of donors to be utilized:

1. *Donors who are close relatives of the recipient:* For example, sister to sister donations have been frequently used with much satisfaction. Some recipients feel most comfortable with this donor source due to the fact that there is a close genetic relation-

ship between the donated eggs and the recipient. Less frequently other relatives (i.e., niece, cousin) have donated eggs.

2. *Other donors recruited by the recipients:* These may be friends, distant relatives, or other individuals who are recruited via word of mouth or advertising.

Ovum donation presents a number of unique legal and emotional issues, which need to be carefully considered. Brigham and Women's Hospital will be happy to offer assistance in resolving some of the emotional issues. It is also strongly recommended that the parties consult independent legal counsel to discuss, among other things, whether a written agreement between the recipient and the donor is advisable. In addition, both the donor and the recipient couple will be required to sign BWH consent forms.

PREPARATION OF OVUM RECIPIENTS

After a thorough screening which includes careful review of medical records, physical examination, blood testing, screening for familial, genetic, and infectious diseases, evaluation of the endometrial cavity, and a screening by social services, a preparatory cycle will be performed. This cycle will mimic the actual transfer cycle and is performed (1) to ensure that an endometrium which is suitable to allow for embryo implantation and pregnancy can be induced in the recipient and (2) to determine the recipient's hormone requirements.

During the preparatory cycle, estrogen and progesterone will be administered in a sequential fashion. The estrogen is usually given as transdermal skin patches, while natural progesterone is given in an oil base as an intramuscular injection. Repeated blood sampling is needed to assess the adequacy of the hormone replacement. A timed endometrial biopsy with a uterine sounding is performed to confirm proper morphological changes compatible with embryo implantation. In patients whose ovaries continue to function, even intermittently, an additional hormone (Leuprolide acetate or related drug) may be used to suppress endogenous ovarian function. Preparatory cycles may need to be repeated before a treatment cycle is scheduled. During the actual treatment cycle (in which embryos are to be transferred), the same sequential estrogen and progesterone replacement and frequent blood sampling are necessary.

PREPARATION OF OOCYTE DONORS

Potential donors will be carefully screened by our doctors for any medical conditions which would make them an unsuitable donor. A thorough family history will be taken to identify any risks or known familial genetic diseases. A battery of tests to screen for infectious and sexually transmitted diseases (e.g., HIV, hepatitis, syphilis) will also be performed. Potential donors will be screened by our staff social workers, with additional psychological evaluation if recommended, in order to assess their emotional stability and attitudes regarding donating their eggs.

If the donor is considered to be appropriate by the IVF Team, she will need to undergo controlled ovarian hyperstimulation. At this time, injections of hormones are given in order to stimulate the ovary to produce multiple mature eggs. She will be closely monitored with blood tests and ultrasound exams in order to assess response to the hormones and the maturity of the developing eggs. Once the eggs are mature, an egg aspiration is performed. This is done under endovaginal ultrasound guidance, and the donor receives intravenous sedation or spinal anaesthesia for this procedure. Once the retrieval procedure is over, the egg donation is considered complete.

AFTER THE RETRIEVAL

On the day of the donor's egg retrieval, the recipient's husband will need to come to the hospital to provide a sperm sample. The sample will be carefully prepared and placed in a dish containing the donated eggs, and the dish incubated overnight. The eggs will be checked the next day for evidence of fertilization. If one or more of the eggs has fertilized, an embryo transfer is scheduled for the following day.

The recipient, who will have started her progesterone replacement, does not require anesthesia for the embryo transfer. A thin catheter is placed through the cervix into her uterus, and the embryos are passed through the catheter using gentle pressure. If there are any surplus embryos suitable for freezing, they can be cryopreserved for future use if the recipient couple so chooses.

After the transfer, the recipient remains supine for about an hour before going home. She continues to take estrogen and progesterone replacement until a pregnancy test is done two weeks after the procedure. If pregnant, the medications are continued for approximately 10 weeks. If the pregnancy test is negative, the medications are discontinued. The cycle will then be reviewed by the IVF Team, and recommendations made for the future.

CONCLUSION

Pregnancy through the donation of eggs is a relatively new procedure. Although not for everyone, ovum donation may be the answer to a couple's dream of achieving a pregnancy. We are delighted to be able to offer this technology to interested patients. Please contact the IVF Office (617-732-4239) if you have any questions or if you wish to schedule a consultation.

Revised July 7, 1992

Appendix 10-B

Known Donor Screening Sheet

BRIGHAM AND WOMEN'S HOSPITAL
IVF-ET/GIFT PROGRAM

You have an appointment to be screened by a physician, to determine if you will be a suitable ovum donor. In addition to evaluating your general health and past medical/surgical history, and performing a physical examination, a thorough screening for familial and genetic diseases is important.

Please complete the enclosed questionnaire, and please be completely candid. A "yes" response will not necessarily eliminate you as a potential donor. Many women will have at least one of these conditions in herself or a family member.

The physician will review this form with you. With your permission, the information on this form will be provided to the intended recipient so that she may have any relevant questions answered and obtain genetic counseling if she wishes.

If you do not wish the information on this form to be made available to the intended recipient, please let us know. This information will not be divulged without your permission. If you choose not to share this information with the intended recipient, you will not be allowed to donate. The recipient will simply be told that you were not considered to be a suitable donor; no further explanation will be provided.

To reiterate, this information will remain a confidential part of your medical record unless you agree to allow us to share it with the intended recipient. Please answer all questions candidly.

Ia.   Some people cannot provide a complete family history (including grandparents). For example, if you are adopted, or do not know one side of your family, your ability to provide a complete family history may be compromised. Is there any reason you cannot provide a complete family history?   No   Yes

If yes, please explain: _____

_____

b.   Please list the members of your immediate family (mother, father, brothers, sisters), their age (or age at death) and any medical problems they may have (and/or their cause of death). Be sure to list any siblings who may have died in infancy.

	Age	Medical Problems	Age of Death (if applicable)	Cause of Death (if applicable)
Mother				
Father				

	Age	Medical Problems	Age of Death (if applicable)	Cause of Death (if applicable)
Sister 1.				
2.				
3.				
Brother 1.				
2.				
3.				
Additional Sibs 1.				
2.				
3.				

IIa. What is your ethnic background? (Check where applies)

_____ Caucasian   _____ Mexican

_____ Northern European   _____ South American

_____ African   _____ Mediterranean (Italy, Greece)

_____ African American   _____ Middle Eastern (Iran, Israel, Turkey)

_____ Southeast Asian (Cambodia, Viet Nam)   _____ Spanish

_____ Far Eastern (China, India, Philippines)   _____ Portuguese

_____ Ashkenazi Jewish   _____ Native American

_____ Sephardic Jewish   _____ Other _____

_____ Caribbean

b. Have you ever been pregnant?   No   Yes

If yes, how many times? _____   How many livebirths? _____

If yes, how many stillbirths? _____   How many miscarriages? _____

III. Below is a list of diseases and conditions. Please indicate if you or a family member has ever had any of these. If you have any questions, ask the physician at the time of your consultation.

(Continued . . . next page)

Disease/Condition	Self		Family Member [specify mother, father, sister, brother, son, daughter, aunt, uncle, cousin, etc.]	
1. cleft lip	No	Yes	No	Yes _____
2. cleft palate	No	Yes	No	Yes _____
3. spina bifida	No	Yes	No	Yes _____
4. congenital heart disease	No	Yes	No	Yes _____
5. congenital hip dislocation	No	Yes	No	Yes _____
6. club foot	No	Yes	No	Yes _____
7. other birth defect (specify) _____	No	Yes	No	Yes _____
8. albinism	No	Yes	No	Yes _____
9. hemophilia	No	Yes	No	Yes _____
10. hemoglobin disorder	No	Yes	No	Yes _____
11. hereditary hypercholesterolemia	No	Yes	No	Yes _____
12. neurofibromatosis (von Recklinghausen's Disease)	No	Yes	No	Yes _____
13. tuberous sclerosis	No	Yes	No	Yes _____
14. asthma	No	Yes	No	Yes _____
15. juvenile diabetes	No	Yes	No	Yes _____
16. epilepsy	No	Yes	No	Yes _____
17. hypertension	No	Yes	No	Yes _____
18. psychiatric disorders	No	Yes	No	Yes _____
19. rheumatoid arthritis	No	Yes	No	Yes _____
20. severe refractive disorder	No	Yes	No	Yes _____
21. early coronary disease	No	Yes	No	Yes _____
22. cystic fibrosis	No	Yes	No	Yes _____
23. G6P deficiency	No	Yes	No	Yes _____
24. thalassemia	No	Yes	No	Yes _____
25. sickle cell anemia	No	Yes	No	Yes _____
26. Tay Sachs disease	No	Yes	No	Yes _____

Disease/Condition	Self		Family Member [specify mother, father, sister, brother, son, daughter, aunt, uncle, cousin, etc.]	
27. balanced translocation	No	Yes	No	Yes _____
28. mental retardation	No	Yes	No	Yes _____
29. Huntington's chorea	No	Yes	No	Yes _____
30. fascioscapulohumeral muscular dystrophy	No	Yes	No	Yes _____
31. adult onset polycystic kidney disease	No	Yes	No	Yes _____
32. hypertrophic idiopathic subaortic stenosis (HISS)	No	Yes	No	Yes _____
33. Amyotrophic Lateral Sclerosis (AMLS)	No	Yes	No	Yes _____
34. hereditary spherocytosis	No	Yes	No	Yes _____
35. myotonic dystrophy	No	Yes	No	Yes _____
36. Duchene's Muscular Dystrophy	No	Yes	No	Yes _____
37. Becker's Muscular Dystrophy	No	Yes	No	Yes _____
38. aquaductal hydrocephalus	No	Yes	No	Yes _____
39. fragile X syndrome	No	Yes	No	Yes _____
40. retinitis pigmentosa	No	Yes	No	Yes _____
41. multiple polyposis of the colon	No	Yes	No	Yes _____
42. Marfan syndrome	No	Yes	No	Yes _____
43. retinoblastoma	No	Yes	No	Yes _____
44. Alport's disease	No	Yes	No	Yes _____
45. breast cancer	No	Yes	No	Yes _____

IV. Have you ever been screened for:

	Self	
Tay Sachs	No	Yes
sickle cell	No	Yes
thalassemia	No	Yes
G6P deficiency	No	Yes
cystic fibrosis	No	Yes

If yes, please bring result/documentation to your consultation.

(Continued . . . next page)

V. Attention Donor: Please read the statements below. After you have read them both, please sign your name under the <u>one</u> option you have selected.

1) I have carefully answered the above questions and my responses are true and correct to the best of my knowledge. I have had the opportunity to have my questions answered by a physician. I understand and agree that the information on this form will be provided to the recipient couple, and I consent to this disclosure.

_____

Known Donor's signature   Date

* * * OR * * *

2) I have carefully answered the above questions and my responses are true and correct to the best of my knowledge. I have had the opportunity to have my questions answered by a physician. I do not wish the information on this form to be shared with the recipient couple. I understand that, as a result, I will not be permitted to serve as a donor.

_____

Known Donor's signature   Date

VI. Attention Recipient: Please read and sign your name.

I have been given the opportunity to review the information on this form and have been offered the opportunity to discuss this information with a genetic counselor.

_____

Recipient's signature   Date

_____

Recipient's husband's signature   Date

The following questions pertain to HIV risk factors and your sexual history. The results will not be released to anyone without your written consent. Please be completely candid and forthright.

1. Have you ever been tested for HIV?   No   Yes

    If yes, please bring documentation of the results (if available) to your consultation.

2. Have you had more than one sexual partner within the past six months?   No   Yes

3. Have you ever used IV drugs?   No   Yes

    If yes, when was the last time? (month/year)_____

4. Have you ever had a blood transfusion?   No   Yes

    If yes, when? (month/year)_____

5. Have you ever had sexual relationships with someone who is bisexual,
    has used IV drugs, or has had a blood transfusion prior to 1985?   No   Yes

6. Have you ever had:

    chlamydia   No   Yes

    genital herpes   No   Yes

    genital warts   No   Yes

    gonorrhea   No   Yes

    syphilis   No   Yes

    If yes, when? (month/year)_____

Appendix 10-C

Recipient Couple Consent

BRIGHAM AND WOMEN'S HOSPITAL
IVF-ET/GIFT PROGRAM

PART ONE

I. My husband and I wish to participate in the ovum donation* program in order to achieve a pregnancy. We are candidates for this program because I do not have ovaries, or my ovaries do not produce viable eggs, or the eggs are genetically abnormal, or (due to disease) the eggs are not available even by surgical procedure such as is ordinarily used in an in vitro fertilization program. A pregnancy attempt will be accomplished by providing us with embryo(s) originating from egg(s) donated by another person for this purpose. These eggs will be inseminated in the laboratory by my husband's sperm (or donor sperm, if my husband's sperm is not suitable). If fertilization takes place, the fertilized eggs will then be transferred into my uterus with the hope that a pregnancy will ensue.

II. Procedure

We understand that the following is an outline of the steps for this procedure:

a. We understand that we are solely responsible for providing an acceptable ovum donor for ourselves, and that this donor will need to be approved by the IVF Team as an individual medically and emotionally suitable to serve as an egg donor. In order to assess her suitability, the donor we provide will be questioned by members of the IVF Team about familial and genetic diseases. She will also be asked about high risk behavior for HIV infection, and will be screened for infectious diseases including HIV, hepatitis, gonorrhea, syphilis, and chlamydia. We understand that our physician and Brigham and Women's Hospital cannot guarantee the reliability of the history the donor gives. A thorough psychosocial assessment will be conducted on the donor as well as on us.

b. If I am not having menstrual periods due to absence or complete failure of my ovaries, I understand that it will be necessary to prepare my uterus with estrogen and progesterone. This will require one or more artificial "preparatory" cycles prior to the actual embryo transfer cycle. This is done to ensure that my endometrium (uterine lining) can be adequately prepared to allow for embryo implantation and pregnancy. This treatment will utilize estrogen (taken orally or through the skin patches), and progesterone (taken as injections into a muscle or as vaginal suppositories).

c. If I am having menstrual periods, even intermittently, they will most likely need to be regulated in order for me to be synchronized with the donor. This may involve addition of the drug Leuprolide acetate (or related drug) to the above mentioned hormone therapy. Related drugs may be taken subcutaneously or intranasally.

d. The preparatory cycle (lasting about four weeks) will require blood samples (1-2 X week,

---

*The terms "ovum" and "egg" will be used interchangeably in this consent form.

up to 2 tablespoons/day). The cycle may possibly also require ultrasound examinations. A biopsy and sounding of the endometrial cavity will be performed at the end of the preparatory cycle, to determine endometrial adequacy. These are office procedures.

e. On the day of the donor's egg retrieval, sperm will be provided by my husband (or, if necessary, donor sperm will be obtained) and used to fertilize the egg(s) by incubating them in a suitable culture medium.

f. If any of the eggs fertilize an embryo transfer will be planned for two days after the retrieval. This procedure is performed at the hospital using no anesthesia. I will have a thin catheter placed through my cervix into my uterus, and the embryos will be deposited there. Up to five embryos will be transferred. We also understand that if more than five embryos result from the process, we have the option of cryopreserving them for any future attempts to achieve pregnancy. (Additional information and consent forms regarding disposition of eggs and cryopreservation will be provided.)

III. I also understand that any of the following may occur which would prevent the successful completion of these procedures and preclude the establishment of a pregnancy:

1. There may be a suboptimal response in the donor to the ovulation induction medications, thus precluding any attempt at obtaining an egg.
2. Attempted obtaining of an egg or eggs may be unsuccessful because of undetected ovulation, abnormal follicle development, or technical problems with retrieval.
3. The egg or eggs may not be normal.
4. My partner may be unable to produce a semen specimen or the sperm specimen may not be normal. In couples using frozen donor sperm, donor sperm may be of poor quality and not usable.
5. Fertilization may not occur or may be abnormal in some or all of the eggs.
6. Cleavage or cell division of the fertilized egg may not occur.
7. The embryo may not develop normally.
8. The embryo transfer may be technically difficult.
9. Implantation may not occur.
10. Loss or damage to the fertilized or unfertilized eggs could occur.

IV. Potential Risks and Discomforts

I understand that the following are some of the risks and discomforts associated with these procedures:

a. Blood drawing - mild discomfort and some risk of developing a bruise at the needle site.
b. Estrogen - possible nausea, bloating, gallbladder disease, abnormal blood clotting, migraine, darkening of the skin, growth of benign fibroid tumors, jaundice, breast tenderness, intolerance to contact lenses, and increased vaginal secretions.
c. Progesterone - pain and swelling at injection site, bloating, weight gain, breast tenderness, premenstrual-like syndrome, headache, fatigue, and mental depression. The progesterone is mixed in a peanut or sesame oil-based solution and should not be used by patients who are allergic to these.
d. Leuprolide acetate or related drugs - Response may vary. Side effects include hot flashes, vaginal dryness, burning on urination, difficulty sleeping, bloating, headaches, hair loss, pain or numbness in extremities, local reactions at injection site, and temporary reduction in bone density. You may get a localized allergic response, in which case the drug is stopped.
e. Endometrial biopsy - uterine cramping, small risk of infection or uterine perforation. A local anesthesia may be required.

f.   Transfer of embryos - minimal discomfort, minimal risks of developing infection which, in some cases, requires hospitalization and intravenous antibiotic treatment.

g.   Psychological distress - sometimes associated with assisted reproductive technology procedures.

h.   Multiple births, miscarriages, ectopic pregnancies, congenital abnormalities - If a pregnancy is successfully established, multiple pregnancies (20–25% chance of twin pregnancy, 1–5% chance of triplet pregnancy, and a rare chance of a higher number of babies), miscarriage, ectopic pregnancy, stillbirth and/or congenital abnormalities may occur. The likelihood of multiple births, tubal pregnancies, and miscarriage is increased with ovum donation as compared to spontaneously occurring pregnancy. The risks of developing an abnormal fetus are no greater than the risk associated with a spontaneously occurring pregnancy (about 5%).

i.   Sexually Transmitted/Infectious Diseases - Although eggs donors are screened for sexually transmitted diseases there is a risk that HIV, hepatitis, gonorrhea, syphilis, cytomegalovirus, or other sexually transmitted diseases or infections may be transmitted. The long-term risks to an infant from such transmission can include mental retardation, developmental retardation, physical anomalies (abnormalities), and death. The woman and spouse are also at risk of contracting all such sexually transmitted diseases. This latter complication can include death as in the case of AIDS or hepatitis. A woman can require a hysterectomy if she develops a pelvic infection. It can cause such severe pain that intercourse is no longer possible. Daily life can also be affected.

V. Other Matters

a.   We accept this act as our own, and acknowledge our obligation to and agree to care for, support, and otherwise treat a child born as a result of this procedure in all respects as if it were our natural born child.

b.   We understand that during pregnancy, childbirth and delivery the same types of complications can arise as with a child conceived by sexual intercourse. It is also possible that the resulting child or children could be born abnormal, possess undesirable traits or hereditary tendencies, or be possessed of any of the other problems or disabilities of children conceived by sexual intercourse.

c.   We understand that insurance coverage for any or all of the above procedures may not be available and that we will be personally responsible for the expenses of this treatment. In particular, we understand that we are responsible for all costs related to the ovum donation and subsequent fertilization and transfer including medications, blood tests, medical evaluations, social services screenings, psychological evaluations, and surgical procedures. We hereby authorize The Brigham and Women's Hospital, Inc. to release such information from our medical records as may be necessary for the settlement of all claims for payment of these charges.

d.   We understand and agree that the IVF Team may conclude that our donor is not a suitable donor candidate based on her medical evaluation, social services screening, psychological evaluation and/or her screening for hereditary and sexually transmittable diseases. We further understand and agree that we will not be provided with the reasons for such conclusion unless the donor consents.

e.   We have been assured that all information about us and our treatment will, to the extent allowed and required by law, be kept confidential and that neither our identity nor specific medical details concerning us will be revealed without our consent. Specific medical details may be revealed in professional publications as long as our identity is concealed.

f.   Brigham and Women's is a teaching hospital. Residents, interns, nursing students, and medical students participate in patient care and performance of surgery and/or procedures under supervision of a senior physician or nurse. We consent to this participation. We consent to the observation of our surgery by Brigham and Women's medical and/or nursing, students/staff for educational purposes. At all times, our personal wishes control the extent of our participation in educational programs.

g. We consent to, authorize, and request the authorities of The Brigham and Women's Hospital, Inc., to dispose of bodily fluids or tissue, including, if any, unfertilized and abnormally fertilized eggs. Such tissue or bodily fluids may be photographed during surgery and/or be preserved for diagnostic, scientific, or teaching purposes. We understand that the disposition of fertilized eggs, if any, will be governed by a separate consent form, which is attached.

h. We have read this consent form and the information packet provided by Brigham and Women's Hospital, and have had the opportunity to discuss this decision with a physician and a social worker/psychologist. All of our questions have been answered to our satisfaction.

OUR SIGNATURE BELOW CONSTITUTES OUR ACKNOWLEDGEMENT (1) that we have read, understood and agreed to the foregoing, (2) that the proposed operation(s) or procedure(s) have been satisfactorily explained to us and that we have all the information that we desire, (3) that we received a copy of the form and (4) that we hereby request the procedures described above and give our authorization and consent.

Recipient's signature: _____
                                                                    Date

Recipient's Husband's signature: _____
                                                                    Date

Witness's signature: _____
                                                                    Date

PART TWO. DISPOSITION OF EGGS FOR OVUM DONATION RECIPIENTS

This form should be signed by ovum donation recipients.

Your ovum donor will undergo ultrasound-guided egg retrieval. An average of 7 eggs are obtained in any one retrieval. This number may vary widely however, from 0 to 40. Of the eggs retrieved, an average 60% will be able to be successfully fertilized. In any particular individual, however, the successful fertilization rate may vary from 0% to 100%. Generally it is not advisable to transfer more than 5 fertilized eggs to a patient in any one cycle. It is therefore possible that more eggs may be retrieved from your donor than may be utilized by you in a single cycle. If this occurs there are three options available to you. These three options are described below. Please read them carefully. **AFTER YOU HAVE READ THEM, YOU AND YOUR HUSBAND SHOULD SIGN YOUR NAMES UNDERNEATH THE ONE PREFERRED OPTION. BOTH OF YOU MUST SELECT AND SIGN THE SAME OPTION.** If you have any questions, please discuss them with your physician. **If it is necessary or advisable for us to deviate from the option you have selected, you will be informed.** In addition, in certain circumstances special arrangements concerning these options can be made by consultation with your physician.

Option One

We will inseminate all normally appearing eggs that are retrieved from your donor. This will maximize your chance of becoming pregnant. However, because of the unacceptable medical risk to both mother and babies resulting from high order multiple births, no more than 5 fertilized eggs will be transferred into your uterus. Any remaining fertilized eggs will be discarded in a manner according to hospital policies.

If you wish to elect this option you and your husband should sign here.

_____ _____   _____ _____
Wife's Signature   Date   Witness   Date

_____ _____
Husband's Signature   Date

Option Two

We will inseminate all normally appearing eggs that are retrieved from your donor. This will also maximize your chance of becoming pregnant. No more than 5 fertilized eggs, however, will be transferred into your uterus. Any remaining fertilized eggs which are developing normally will be cryopreserved (frozen). If you select this option you will be given further information about cryopreservation, and you will be required to sign a separate consent form.

If you wish to elect this option you and your husband should sign here.

_____ _____   _____ _____
Wife's Signature   Date   Witness   Date

_____ _____
Husband's Signature   Date

Option Three

If you do not wish to discard or cryopreserve any fertilized eggs not transferred into your uterus in the initial cycle, then we will inseminate no more than 5 eggs at the time of egg retrieval. All eggs which successfully fertilize will be transferred into your uterus. This could decrease your chance of becoming pregnant if fewer than 4 eggs successfully fertilize.

If you wish to elect this option you and your husband should sign here.

_____ _____   _____ _____
Wife's Signature   Date   Witness   Date

_____ _____
Husband's Signature   Date

Revised July 7, 1992

Appendix 10-D

Known Ovum Donor Consent

BRIGHAM AND WOMEN'S HOSPITAL
IVF-ET/GIFT PROGRAM

I.   I have been asked to donate eggs* to _____, ("recipient") who cannot have children because she has no ovaries, or has ovaries which do not produce viable eggs, or her eggs are genetically abnormal, or she has disease which causes her eggs to be unavailable even by surgical procedure such as is ordinarily used in a program of in vitro fertilization.

II. Procedure

I understand that the following is a summary of the procedures to be followed with regard to my participation as an ovum donor:

a.   In order to be approved as a donor, I understand that I will be screened (during an interview in which I agree to give full disclosure) for hereditary and genetic diseases and for sexually transmitted disease, including but not limited to gonorrhea, syphilis, chlamydia, hepatitis, and HIV (human immunodeficiency virus). This will require cultures of my cervix and blood tests. I also hereby verify that I have not, to my knowledge, contracted HIV or used intravenous drugs, nor have I or my sexual partner had sexual contact with a homosexual male, someone infected with HIV, or someone who used intravenous drugs. A thorough psychosocial assessment will be conducted on me as well as on the recipient couple.

b.   I will need to take medications which will cause my ovaries to produce one or more eggs. These fertility medications are taken by subcuticular and intramuscular injection, and include drugs such as Leuprolide acetate or related drugs, Metrodin, and Pergonal. I will also take antibiotics which may include but are not limited to Doxycycline and Ampicillin. I may be on medication for several weeks.

c.   For part of the time I am on these medications, I will require daily blood sampling, taken by a needle in the vein.

d.   Transvaginal ultrasound examinations will be performed at appropriate times (often daily for about one week) to determine the number and size of developing follicles in my ovaries.

e.   I understand that the eggs are gathered only after they have matured within the ovary for the proper length of time. In practical terms, the eggs are gathered at midcycle, approximately cycle day 10–15. I also understand that precise timing requires some personal flexibility in scheduling the exact day of the egg retrieval.

f.   When the monitoring reveals adequate follicular maturity, I will receive an injection of hCG, a natural hormone substance which initiates the final egg maturation process.

g.   Approximately 34 hours following the hCG injection, my eggs will be collected by an ultrasound-guided puncture of my ovaries with a needle placed in my vagina. In order to minimize the discomfort of the egg retrieval procedure, I will be given a spinal anesthesia or intravenous sedation.

---

*The terms "ovum" and "egg" are used interchangeably throughout this material.

h. I agree not to have unprotected sexual intercourse (without a condom) from the time the ovulation stimulating drugs are begun until after the egg retrieval is completed to guard against pregnancy and transmission of infectious diseases.

i. The eggs obtained in this manner will be inseminated in the laboratory by sperm from the husband of the intended recipient, or if necessary, a donor's sperm. If fertilization takes place, the fertilized egg(s) will then be transferred into the uterus of the recipient with the hope that a pregnancy will ensue.

j. If there are many eggs, the recipient couple may choose to inseminate all of them, or only some of them and discard the others. If following insemination, there are many fertilized eggs, the recipient couple may choose to cryopreserve some of the embryos for future use.

III. Potential Risks and Discomforts

I further understand that the following are some of the risks and discomforts associated with these procedures:

a. Blood drawing - mild discomfort and some risk of developing a bruise at the needle site.

b. Fertility Drugs - moderate weight gain, mood changes, stomach pressure, headaches, allergic reaction, and hyperstimulation of the ovaries (5% chance in any cycle). In very rare cases, hyperstimulation could lead to very enlarged ovaries and an increased susceptibility to develop blood clots necessitating hospitalization. In very rare cases, it may also lead to the development of fluid in the abdomen or lungs, kidney failure, or stroke. In extremely rare cases, an enlarged hyperstimulated ovary will rupture. This may necessitate general anaesthesia and major surgery, with all the inherent risks. Loss of one or both ovaries is possible. The risk of hyperstimulation is minimized if the follicles are aspirated as is planned to occur at my egg retrieval. The risk increases if, after taking the fertility medications to stimulate my ovaries, I choose not to undergo egg retrieval. There also exists an unlikely possibility of a lasting effect on my pelvic organs, including pain, irregular menstrual function, or impairment of my future fertility.

c. Antibiotics - possible allergic reaction which, in rare cases, may be severe.

d. Ultrasound egg retrieval - Many patients experience mild to moderate discomfort after the procedure. Potentially serious complications include bleeding, infection, and injury to the bowel or blood vessels. In extremely rare circumstances, surgery may be necessary to repair damage to internal organs or to control significant internal bleeding (i.e., hemorrhage). Anesthesia will be necessary for the egg retrieval. (The risks associated with anesthesia will be explained during an consultation with an anesthesiologist.) There may be additional risks of donating eggs, which at the present time have not been identified. Since it is theoretically possible that not all of the developed eggs will be recovered at the time of retrieval, there is a risk that I may become pregnant if I engage in unprotected intercourse during the egg donation cycle(s).

e. Ultrasound examinations - no known risks, minimal discomfort.

f. Psychological distress - sometimes associated with assisted reproductive technology procedures.

g. Inconvenience - monitoring procedures during the period of stimulation, and the time needed to perform the egg retrieval itself will result in a certain amount of inconvenience and lost time.

IV. Other Matters

a. I hereby waive any right and relinquish any claim for myself, my heirs, administrators, or executors, to the donated eggs or cryopreserved embryos or any pregnancy or offspring resulting from them.

The recipient couple may regard the eggs, embryos, and resultant offspring as their own once the donation has been completed.

b. All ordinary costs related to the ovum donation including medications, blood tests, medical and psychological evaluations, and surgical procedures will be the responsibility of the recipient. I understand, however, that complications might arise resulting in additional medical and hospital expenses. I represent to the hospital that I have medical insurance in effect to cover such additional expenses. I further understand that I am solely responsible to the Hospital for any such medical or hospital costs not covered by my insurance, although I am free to make separate arrangements with the recipient for reimbursement of such expenses.

c. I have been assured that all information about me and my treatment will, to the extent allowed and required by law, be kept confidential and that neither my identity nor specific medical details concerning me will be revealed without my consent. Specific medical details may be revealed in professional publications as long as my identity is concealed.

d. I understand that the results of my medical evaluations, and my screening for hereditary and sexually transmittable diseases will be reviewed with me. I further understand that I will be asked to permit the recipient couple to be provided with the results of my screening for hereditary and genetic diseases. In the event that I do not consent to this disclosure, the recipient couple will not be provided with this information, and under such circumstances, I will not be permitted to serve as a donor. I also understand that I may not be permitted to serve as a donor based on the results of my medical or psychological evaluation. In this event, the reasons for this determination will not be provided to the recipient couple without my consent.

e. Brigham and Women's is a teaching hospital. Residents, interns, nursing students, and medical students participate in patient care and performance of surgery and/or procedures under supervision of a senior physician or nurse. I consent to this participation. I consent to the observation of my surgery by Brigham and Women's medical and/or nursing, students/staff for educational purposes. At all times, my personal wishes control the extent of my participation in educational programs.

f. I consent to, authorize, and request the authorities of The Brigham and Women's Hospital, Inc., to dispose of bodily fluids or tissue, including, if any, unfertilized and abnormally fertilized eggs. Such tissue or bodily fluids may be photographed during surgery and/or be preserved for diagnostic, scientific, or teaching purposes.

g. I have read this consent form and the information packet provided by Brigham and Women's Hospital, and have had the opportunity to discuss this decision with a physician and a social worker/ psychologist. All of my questions have been answered to my satisfaction.

MY SIGNATURE BELOW CONSTITUTES MY ACKNOWLEDGMENT (1) that I have read, understood and agreed to the foregoing, (2) that the proposed operation(s) or procedure(s) have been satisfactorily explained to me and that I have all the information that I desire, (3) that I received a copy of the form and (4) that I hereby request the procedures described above and give my authorization and consent.

_____   _____
Witness   Date   Donor's Signature   Date

                                           _____
                                           Donor's Husband's Signature   Date

Revised July 7, 1992

Appendix 10-E

Recipient/Spouse Consent for Receiving Donated Eggs (Anonymous Donor)

FAULKNER CENTRE FOR REPRODUCTIVE MEDICINE
OVUM DONATION PROGRAM

Name_____ Date _____

You have requested that you receive donated eggs from another woman for the purpose of achieving a pregnancy. A donor is a person who undergoes ovarian stimulation for the purpose of providing eggs to another individual, or an IVF patient who produces eggs in excess of those which will be used for her own cycle.

Your decision whether or not to participate will not prejudice your future relations with the Faulkner Centre for Reproductive Medicine or the Faulkner Hospital. If you decide to participate, you are free to discontinue participation at any time.

FCRM Policy Regarding Numbers of Eggs Fertilized

The purpose of stimulating ovulation is to achieve pregnancy for the recipient of that cycle. However, occasionally more eggs are obtained than will be used for a recipient couple. It is the policy of the Faulkner Centre for Reproductive Medicine (FCRM) not to cryopreserve excessive numbers of embryos. To that end, a maximum of 15 eggs will be inseminated in any given cycle which we hope will allow for embryo transfer in the stimulated cycle and at least one additional embryo transfer following cryopreservation and thawing. For those recipients who do not elect to freeze embryos, no more than 7 eggs will be inseminated. Those eggs in excess of 15 (or 7 if freezing is not desired) are deemed to be excess tissue, and may be discarded or may be used at the discretion of the FCRM for appropriate purposes including, but not limited to, research in accordance with the Faulkner Hospital Institutional Review Board. You may choose to donate excess eggs to other persons for the purposes of achieving conception. However, this will not be done without your express permission. Please initial this option to indicate your decision.

I agree to have excess eggs donated to other people for the purpose of achieving conception.

_____   _____
   Yes   No

Screening of Participants

The egg recipient, her spouse, and the egg donor, must each provide a detailed history, including a comprehensive medical history looking for familial diseases before they are allowed to enter the donor egg program. Additional screening may include:

    a.   physical examination of the egg recipient and the donor, including pelvic examination.
    b.   detailed social histories of each person, including history of habits and substance ingestion. History

of sexual relationships outside that of the immediate couple will be privately discussed, and the conversation may be of a personal nature.

c. screening for inheritable diseases according to history and ethnic background is performed. Genetic karyotypes of egg donor and spouse of egg recipient may be arranged at the recipient's request.

d. psychological screening and preparation with a qualified mental health professional include standard questionnaires. Multiple visits are mandatory.

e. Screening generally includes but is not limited to the following:

1. Gonorrhea (Recipient, Donor)
2. Syphilis (Recipient, Donor)
3. Blood type and Rh (Recipient, Donor, Spouse)
4. Mycoplasma (Recipient)
5. Hepatitis B (Recipient, Donor, Spouse)
6. Toxoplasmosis (Recipient)
7. Rubella (Recipient)
8. Cytomegalovirus (Recipient, Spouse)
9. Hepatitis C (Recipient, Donor, Spouse)
10. Human immunodeficiency virus (HIV) (Recipient, Donor, Spouse)
11. Other as appropriate by history.

With respect to screening for contagious disease, it is understood that there are limitations to technology; despite strict adherence to protocol, contagious diseases may be transmitted from one individual to another, specifically from egg donors to egg recipients. The chances of this occurring are unlikely, but exist nonetheless.

Monitoring Cycles

Even if you have normal menstrual cycles, it may be necessary to prepare your uterus for receiving an embryo. In some instances, your cycle may be monitored before the actual donor cycle to be certain your uterine lining is favorable for embryo transfer. In either event, the following procedure will be utilized:

a. Several weeks of hormonal therapy must occur. This includes administration of the steroid hormones estradiol and progesterone. Estradiol is administered either by pills or in patches worn on the skin. Potential side effects of this medication include water retention, local skin irritation, bruising of the skin, and in cases of genetic tendency, blood clots in the legs, hypertension and stroke. You should not smoke cigarettes while taking this medication. If you have regular menstrual cycles, you may also need to take a medication called Lupron or Synarel, which permits manipulation of your cycle for timing. If these medications are necessary, you will be asked to sign a separate consent form.

The other medication, progesterone, is given by injection, suppository or a lozenge. Side effects of this medication include local swelling and infection at the site of injection, allergic reactions to the oil (peanut or sesame), or to the preservative in the solution. Additional side effects would be irritation, itching or pain secondary to the injection, and bleeding from the injection site. You will be advised how to administer this medication by a properly trained expert.

b. At least one endometrial biopsy must be performed if this is a monitoring cycle. An endometrial biopsy is not performed in the donor cycle. The biopsy entails passing a small instrument into the uterus and taking a very small tissue sample from the top of the uterine cavity. Although oral analgesics and a local anesthetic are administered before the procedure, it can be painful. Very rarely, it results in a small hole in the top of the uterus, which usually closes on its own within several days. Bleeding and infection are possible, but rare.

c.   Blood work must be drawn frequently during the monitoring cycle. Side effects include pain, bleeding at the site of venepuncture, swelling and bruising, and potentially, if repeated samples are drawn, iron deficiency anemia. It is suggested that you take an iron supplement while you are undergoing the monitoring process.

Cycle of Embryo Transfer

When a donor becomes identified, you may begin treatment with estradiol which may continue anywhere from two days to six weeks. The day after the oocyte donor receives human chorionic gonadotropin (hCG), one day before her egg retrieval, you will begin progesterone. On the day of the egg retrieval, your husband will produce a semen specimen unless, as previously agreed upon, a frozen anonymous semen specimen is to be placed with the donor eggs to initiate fertilization.

Embryo transfer is accomplished in the operating room a few days later. Four hours later you will be discharged home. We recommend very limited activity at home for several days and afterward light activity. During that time, progesterone should be continued.

During the entire egg recipient cycle, frequent blood sampling is necessary to assess your hormone levels and adjust hormone doses. Hormones may continue to be required for up to 100 days.

Because the psychological effects (if any) of receiving eggs are unknown, you may be contacted periodically after the procedure by a member of our team to inquire how you are feeling after your experience. Referral for counselling can be made if needed.

Chances of Success Following Embryo Transfer of Donated Eggs

If multiple embryos are transferred, there can be multiple pregnancies, up to and sometimes exceeding the number of embryos transferred. There are many obstetrical, physical and social side effects resulting from multiple pregnancy. A short list includes but is not limited to the following:

1.   Maternal
   a.   Exacerbation and new onset of gestational diseases such as gestational diabetes, hypertension and preeclampsia. By definition, the pregnancy is high risk, and a physician qualified to care for high risk pregnancy patients should be contacted early in the pregnancy.
   b.   Exacerbation of preexisting medical diseases, sometimes irreversibly.
   c.   Birth accidents, such as rupture of umbilical cord, separation of the placenta, low lying placenta, and uterine rupture.
   d.   Preterm labor, the incidence of which increases with the number of fetuses in the uterus.
   e.   Necessity for delivery by Caesarean section.
2.   Fetal
   a.   Prematurity, low birth weight, umbilical cord accidents, death of one fetus.
   b.   Lowered I.Q. scores resulting from maldevelopment, prematurity and crowding in the uterus.

Birth Defect and Familial Disorders

The incidence of major birth defects in singleton pregnancies is 4 to 6 percent in the general population.

Even with the most precise screening methods possible, there is a chance that a pregnancy resulting from reproductive technology, utilizing donated eggs or sperm, can result in a child with birth defects, medical problems, learning disabilities, handicaps, cerebral palsy or other unforeseen difficulties. Some of these problems can arise from genetic abnormalities that cannot be detected with modern screening tests. Some of them can result from birth accidents, and illness during pregnancy. By accepting a donated oocyte or sperm you should be taking a similar risk of having children who have serious problems as you would be if you were to conceive on your own. Unknown information may increase the risk somewhat.

Ownership of Embryos Resulting from Egg Donation

It is understood that once eggs are removed for donation, the donor relinquishes all control of those eggs to FCRM for the above purpose. The resulting embryos are the responsibility solely of the recipient couple in conjunction with FCRM. The recipient couple becomes legally responsible for the fate of the embryos, including decisions concerning them and storage costs of freezing excess embryos. The donor has no responsibilities or rights in relation to such embryos.

The potential recipient of an act of egg donation understands that the potential donor may change her mind about the donation until the time of egg retrieval.

Offspring Resulting from Egg Donation

Offspring resulting from egg donation are the children of the recipient couple. It is understood that the egg donor may not claim any responsibility or parenting rights for those children, even if the egg donor and embryo recipient are related.

The recipient couple is fully responsible for all offspring, regardless of the outcome of the pregnancy, until the child reaches the age of consent. Because of the newness of egg donation, this is an area with limited legal precedence and FCRM cannot assure recipients or donors of the enforceability of this situation.

Financial Responsibility

The cost of one ovum donation cycle may approach $_____. Insurance companies vary in the extent of coverage and methods of reimbursement. The Faulkner Centre for Reproductive Medicine will work with you to ensure that you receive maximum benefits, but you are responsible for all charges. Depending on your insurance coverage, you will be asked to give partial payment before the cycle begins. In addition, recipients who choose to use the New England Gamete Repository are responsible for payment to that agency in the sum of $_____ to $_____ depending on the protocol used to cover compensation to the donor for time, risk and inconvenience and administrative costs. In most cases donor compensation is not reimbursed by any insurance company. In the event that the donor has a complication directly related to the egg donation stimulation or procedure which manifests itself within 60 days of the egg donation stimulation or procedure that is not covered in full by any insurance, any and all costs incurred by the donor will be the responsibility of the recipient. If the donor cycle is cancelled for reasons beyond the donor's control, a pro-rated expense for her time, risk and inconvenience is the recipient's responsibility.

Confidentiality

FCRM will make every reasonable effort to keep information about your participation in the egg donation program confidential and will only disclose information with your permission.

It is understood and agreed that the donation of eggs will be on an anonymous basis. It is also understood and agreed that no entry will be made on the donor's medical record as to the disposition of any eggs that may be obtained. Furthermore, there will be no entry on the personal record of any recipient as to the source of the donated eggs. However, because of the necessity and desire of the physicians to keep certain medical records, a separate record may be made and retained by your physicians in which entries may be made concerning the source and disposition of donated eggs.

It is understood that there is a possibility that insurance claims or other records may inadvertently reveal the identity of one or both parties. While the Faulkner Centre will avoid this disclosure to the extent possible, the recipient and donor assume the risk of identification.

We are obliged to inform you about the Centre's policy in the unlikely event that physical injury occurs. If, as a result of your participation, you experience physical injury from known or unknown risks of the procedures as described, immediate medical care and treatment, including hospitalization if necessary, will be made available. No monetary compensation, however, is available, and you will be responsible for the costs of such medical treatment.

I have read the above consent and all questions have been answered to my satisfaction. I have read and initialed the appropriate choice on page one. I understand and agree to the consent.

_____   _____
Egg Recipient   Date

_____   _____
Witness   Date

_____   _____
Husband   Date

_____   _____
Witness   Date

Appendix 10-F

Known Egg Donor Consent

FAULKNER CENTRE FOR REPRODUCTIVE MEDICINE
OVUM DONATION PROGRAM

Name_____   Date _____

You have agreed to donate eggs for the purpose of producing a pregnancy in another woman. A donor is a person who undergoes ovarian stimulation for the purpose of providing eggs to another individual, or an IVF patient who produces eggs in excess of those which will be used for her own cycle.

Your decision whether or not to participate will not prejudice your future relations with the Faulkner Centre for Reproductive Medicine or the Faulkner Hospital. If you decide to participate, you are free to discontinue participation at any time.

FCRM Policy Regarding Numbers of Eggs Fertilized

The purpose of stimulating ovulation is to achieve pregnancy for the recipient of that cycle. However, occasionally more eggs are obtained than will be used for a recipient couple. It is the policy of the Faulkner Centre for Reproductive Medicine (FCRM) not to cryopreserve excessive numbers of embryos. To that end, a maximum of 15 eggs will be inseminated in any given cycle which we hope will allow for embryo transfer in the stimulated cycle and at least one additional embryo transfer following cryopreservation and thawing. For those recipients who do not elect to freeze embryos, no more than 7 eggs will be inseminated. Those eggs in excess of 15 (or 7 if freezing is not desired) are deemed to be excess tissue, and may be discarded or may be used at the discretion of the FCRM for appropriate purposes including, but not limited to, research in accordance with the Faulkner Hospital Institutional Review Board. You may choose to donate excess eggs to other persons for the purposes of achieving conception. However, this will not be done without your express permission. Please initial this option to indicate your decision.

I agree to have excess eggs donated to other people for the purpose of achieving conception.

_____   _____
Yes   No

Screening of Participants

The egg donor, the egg recipient, and her spouse must each provide a detailed history, including a comprehensive medical history looking for familial diseases before they are allowed to enter the donor egg program. Additional screening may include:

a. physical examination of the egg recipient and the donor, including pelvic examination.
b. detailed social histories of each person, including history of habits and substance ingestion. History of sexual relationships outside that of the immediate couple will be privately discussed, and the conversation may be of a personal nature.

c. screening for inheritable diseases according to history and ethnic background is performed. Genetic karyotypes of egg donor and spouse of egg recipient may be arranged at the recipient's request.

d. psychological screening and preparation with a qualified mental health professional including standard questionnaires. Multiple visits are mandatory.

e. Screening generally includes but is not limited to the following:
   1. Gonorrhea (Recipient, Donor)
   2. Syphilis (Recipient, Donor)
   3. Blood type and Rh (Recipient, Donor, Spouse)
   4. Mycoplasma (Recipient)
   5. Hepatitis B (Recipient, Donor, Spouse)
   6. Toxoplasmosis (Recipient)
   7. Rubella (Recipient)
   8. Cytomegalovirus (Recipient, Spouse)
   9. Hepatitis C (Recipient, Donor, Spouse)
   10. Human immunodeficiency virus (HIV) (Recipient, Donor, Spouse)
   11. Other as appropriate by history.

With respect to screening for contagious disease, it is understood that there are limitations to technology; despite strict adherence to protocol, contagious disease may be transmitted from one individual to another, specifically from egg donors to egg recipients. The chances of this occurring are unlikely, but exist nonetheless.

Ovulation Induction for the Purpose of Egg Retrieval

Medications:

Once screening of all parties has been accomplished and the egg recipient has been properly prepared to receive donated egg(s) to the satisfaction of the IVF team, the egg donor will enter into the treatment phase of the process. The medications will be given to you by daily intramuscular injection, for perhaps as long as ten to fourteen days depending upon your clinical and laboratory findings. During this time, daily blood specimens, not greater than two teaspoons, are taken. At an appropriate time, you will begin to have daily ultrasounds, a technique used to determine the size of the follicles (a fluid filled sac which contains the egg) in your ovaries. This employs sound waves which are not thought to be harmful to your body. The egg donor will receive individual instruction about the use and risks of these medications. Medication protocols will be individualized based on donor's medical history and physical status.

Most medications will be administered to you by daily intramuscular injection, for perhaps as long as ten to fourteen days, depending upon the clinical and laboratory findings. The medications that may be administered—clomiphene citrate, FSH (Metrodin), human menopausal gonadotropin (Pergonal), and human chorionic gonadotropin—might cause the ovaries to become enlarged and overstimulated in 5% of cases or less. This condition is reversible. A possible risk of ovarian cancer associated with the use of fertility medication has been raised but not proven.

Ovarian overstimulation syndrome is characterized by mild lower abdominal discomfort and swelling due to the accumulation of fluid in the abdomen. The treatment for this syndrome is bed rest, usually at home but rarely requiring hospitalization. In extremely rare instances, serious complications could occur such as blood clots and strokes. Ovarian hyperstimulation usually lasts from one to four weeks following administration of human chorionic gonadotropin (which is given two days before oocyte retrieval). If you are receiving medication and it appears that you could develop a severe form of ovarian hyperstimulation syndrome, your cycle might be cancelled and you will not receive human chorionic gonadotropin, and will not go to the operating room for oocyte retrieval. A donor's cycle may also be cancelled if hormone levels are not optimal or egg follicles fail to grow appropriately.

Other possible side effects of the medications include swelling, redness and slight pain at sites of injection. Occasionally, patients have an allergic reaction to the medications. Patients receiving ovulation induction medications generally have higher than usual estrogen levels and may experience tiredness, mood swings or nausea because of the increased estrogen.

Egg Retrieval:

When ultrasound and blood work indicate that the eggs are ready for collection, the egg donor receives an injection of human chorionic gonadotropin (HCG) that causes the eggs to mature. Egg retrieval is performed approximately 34 hours later.

Egg retrieval is performed under sterile conditions in the operating room using sufficient intravenous sedation and local anesthesia for comfort. If at any time you feel uncomfortable during the procedure you can ask for additional medication.

Briefly, an egg retrieval is performed as follows:

1. The patient is taken to the operating room and an IV is inserted. Blood is drawn.
2. IV sedation is administered by a member of the anesthesia team and local anesthesia is administered by the gynecologist.
3. Vaginal ultrasound is used to guide a small sterile needle through the vagina into the egg chambers. The upper portion of the vagina is only approximately one-half inch away from the ovaries. The eggs are removed in their fluid and taken to the laboratory. It is possible that eggs may not be present or may not be retrieved.

    The eggs that we obtain in this manner will be mixed with sperm in the laboratory. If fertilization takes place, the fertilized egg(s) will then be transferred into the uterus of the infertile recipient in the hope that a pregnancy will ensue.
4. The egg donor is taken to the recovery room where she must stay for approximately four hours. She can then be discharged from the hospital.
5. A follow up visit one week after the egg retrieval is mandatory to be certain there is no evidence of severe ovarian hyperstimulation. A few brief questionnaires will be given to you at that time to be filled out. A follow up visit with a member of our mental health team is also required.
6. Because the psychological effects (if any) of donating eggs are unknown, you may be contacted periodically after the procedure by a member of our team to inquire how you are feeling after your experience. Referral for counseling can be made if needed.

The risks involved in egg retrieval are those of any minor procedure, including: infection and injury to the bowel, blood vessels, or other structures. There is also a possible risk that the needle stick used to obtain the eggs from the ovaries might cause bleeding. Ovarian bleeding or rupture may rarely occur but could lead to open abdominal surgery for control of bleeding or repair or removal of the ovary. Every measure will be taken to prevent these occurrences, and the possibility of occurrence is very small. Theoretically there could be a potential loss of fertility resulting from having a transvaginal ultrasound guided egg retrieval, but to our knowledge no such loss has ever been reported.

It is understood and agreed that the donation of eggs will be on a nonanonymous basis, which means that you and your recipient know one another and have agreed to this donation with each other. It is also understood and agreed that no entry will be made on your personal medical record as to the disposition of any eggs that may be obtained. Furthermore, there will be no entry on the personal record of any recipient as to the source of the donated eggs. However, because of the necessity and desire of the physicians to keep certain medical records, a separate record may be made and retained by your physicians in which entries may be made concerning the source and disposition of donated eggs.

Ownership of Embryos Resulting from Egg Donation

It is understood that the donor may change her mind about the donation at any time until the egg retrieval. Withdrawal will not prejudice further relations with the Faulkner Centre for Reproductive Medicine or the Faulkner Hospital.

It is understood that once eggs are removed from a donor, or excess eggs are removed from an IVF donor, the donor relinquishes all control of those eggs to FCRM for the above agreed to purposes. The eggs and resulting embryos belong to the recipient couple and/or the FCRM and the donor has no responsibilities or rights of any kind in relation to such embryos.

If the recipient couple in conjunction with FCRM decides to freeze excess embryos, it is under their jurisdiction to do so, without knowledge or consent from either the donor or her spouse.

Offspring Resulting from Egg Donation

Offspring resulting from egg donation are the children of the recipient couple. It is understood that the egg donor may not claim any responsibility or parenting rights for or obligations to those children, even if the egg donor and embryo recipient are related. The recipient couple is fully responsible for all offspring, regardless of the outcome of the pregnancy, until the child reaches the age of consent. Because of the newness of egg donation, this is an area with limited legal precedence and FCRM cannot assure recipients or donors of the enforceability of this situation.

Pregnancy Incidental to Egg Donation

Most egg donors are young fertile women. It is understood that they will be more fertile during the month that they undergo treatment and egg retrieval. Some eggs may be incidentally released into the donor's reproductive system around the time of an egg retrieval. Therefore, there is a possibility that the egg donor may conceive during the treatment cycle. Unless the egg donor desires conception, she should seek the advice of the physicians on the IVF team or her private gynecologist about the use of contraceptive methods or abstinence during the treatment cycle.

Confidentiality

FCRM will make its best effort to keep information about your participation in the egg donation program confidential and will only disclose information with your permission.

Benefit

I understand that there is no direct benefit to me from oocyte donation.

Financial Responsibility

The recipient couple has been informed that they are responsible for all charges incurred as part of the egg donation procedure. This includes but is not limited to physician, laboratory and hospital charges. The recipient's insurance company may cover all or part of these charges, but the recipient couple is solely responsible for any unpaid monies.

We are obliged to inform you about the Centre's policy in the unlikely event that physical injury occurs. If, as a result of your participation, you experience physical injury from known or unknown risks of the procedures as described, immediate medical care and treatment, including hospitalization if necessary, will be available. No monetary compensation, however, is available. The Faulkner Centre for Reproductive Medicine will help to bill the appropriate insurance company for any additional expenses but the Faulkner Centre will not be responsible for the costs of such care. In the event that the donor has a complication directly related to the egg donation stimulation or procedure which manifests itself within 60 days of the egg donation stimulation or procedure that is not covered in full by any insurance, any and all costs incurred by the donor will be the responsibility of the recipient who has been advised of this fact.

I have read the above consent and all questions have been answered to my satisfaction. I have read and initialed the appropriate choice on page one. I understand and agree to the consent for the donation of oocytes and procedures necessary to it.

_____   _____
Egg Donor   Date

_____   _____
Witness   Date

_____   _____
Husband (if married)   Date

_____   _____
Witness   Date

Appendix 10-G

Anonymous Egg Donor Consent

**FAULKNER CENTRE FOR REPRODUCTIVE MEDICINE
OVUM DONATION PROGRAM**

Name_____ Date _____

You have agreed to donate eggs for the purpose of producing a pregnancy in another woman. A donor is a person who undergoes ovarian stimulation for the purpose of providing eggs to another individual, or an IVF patient who produces eggs in excess of those which will be used for her own cycle.

It is understood that the donor may change her mind about the donation at any time until the egg retrieval. Withdrawal will not prejudice further relations with the Faulkner Centre for Reproductive Medicine or the Faulkner Hospital.

FCRM Policy Regarding Numbers of Eggs Fertilized

The purpose of stimulating ovulation is to achieve pregnancy for the recipient of that cycle. However, occasionally more eggs are obtained than will be used for a recipient couple. It is the policy of the Faulkner Centre for Reproductive Medicine (FCRM) not to cryopreserve excessive numbers of embryos. To that end, a maximum of 15 eggs will be inseminated in any given cycle which we hope will allow for embryo transfer in the stimulated cycle and at least one additional embryo transfer following cryopreservation and thawing. For those recipients who do not elect to freeze embryos, no more than 7 eggs will be inseminated. Those eggs in excess of 15 (or 7 if freezing is not desired) are deemed to be excess tissue, and may be discarded or may be used at the discretion of the FCRM for appropriate purposes including, but not limited to, research in accordance with the Faulkner Hospital Institutional Review Board. You may choose to donate excess eggs to other persons for the purposes of achieving conception. However, this will not be done without your express permission. Please initial this option to indicate your decision.

I agree to have excess eggs donated to other people for the purpose of achieving conception.

_____   _____
   Yes   No

Screening of Participants

The egg donor, the egg recipient, and her spouse must each provide a detailed history, including a comprehensive medical history looking for familial diseases before they are allowed to enter the donor egg program. Additional screening may include:

a.   physical examination of the egg recipient and the donor, including pelvic examination.
b.   detailed social histories of each person, including history of habits and substance ingestion. History of sexual relationships outside that of the immediate couple will be privately discussed, and the conversation may be of a personal nature.

c. screening for inheritable diseases according to history and ethnic background is performed. Genetic karyotypes of egg donor and spouse of egg recipient may be arranged at the recipient's request.
d. psychological screening and preparation with a qualified mental health professional including standard questionnaires. Multiple visits are mandatory.
e. Screening generally includes but is not limited to the following:
    1. Gonorrhea (Recipient, Donor)
    2. Syphilis (Recipient, Donor)
    3. Blood type and Rh (Recipient, Donor, Spouse)
    4. Mycoplasma (Recipient)
    5. Hepatitis B (Recipient, Donor, Spouse)
    6. Toxoplasmosis (Recipient)
    7. Rubella (Recipient)
    8. Cytomegalovirus (Recipient, Spouse)
    9. Hepatitis C (Recipient, Donor, Spouse)
    10. Human immunodeficiency virus (HIV) (Recipient, Donor, Spouse)
    11. Other as appropriate by history.

With respect to screening for contagious disease, it is understood that there are limitations to technology; despite strict adherence to protocol, contagious disease may be transmitted from one individual to another, specifically from egg donors to egg recipients. The chances of this occurring are unlikely, but exist nonetheless.

Ovulation Induction for the Purpose of Egg Retrieval

Medications:

Once screening of all parties has been accomplished and the egg recipient has been properly prepared to receive donated egg(s) to the satisfaction of the IVF team, the egg donor will enter into the treatment phase of the process. The medications will be given to you by daily intramuscular injection, for perhaps as long as ten to fourteen days depending upon your clinical and laboratory findings. During this time, daily blood specimens, not greater than two teaspoons, are taken. At an appropriate time, you will begin to have daily ultrasounds, a technique used to determine the size of the follicles (a fluid filled sac which contains the egg) in your ovaries. This uses sound waves which are believed not harmful to your body. The egg donor (and her spouse) will receive individual instruction about the use and risks of these medications. Medication protocols will be individualized based on donor's medical history and physical status.

Most medications will be administered to you by daily intramuscular injection, for perhaps as long as ten to fourteen days, depending upon the clinical and laboratory findings. The medications that may be administered—clomiphene citrate, FSH (Metrodin), human menopausal gonadotropin (Pergonal), and human chorionic gonadotropin—might cause the ovaries to become enlarged and overstimulated in 5% of cases or less. This condition is reversible. A possible risk of ovarian cancer associated with the use of fertility medication has been raised but not proven.

Ovarian overstimulation syndrome is characterized by mild lower abdominal discomfort and swelling due to the accumulation of fluid in the abdomen. The treatment for this syndrome is bed rest, usually at home but rarely requiring hospitalization. In extremely rare instances, serious complications could occur, including blood clots and strokes. Ovarian hyperstimulation usually lasts from one to four weeks following administration of human chorionic gonadotropin (which is given two days before oocyte retrieval). If you are receiving medication and it appears that you could develop a severe form of ovarian hyperstimulation syndrome, your cycle might be cancelled and you will not receive human chorionic gonadotropin, and will not go to the operating room for oocyte retrieval. A donor's cycle may also be cancelled if hormone levels are not optimal or egg follicles fail to grow appropriately.

Other possible side effects of the medications include swelling, redness and slight pain at sites of injection. Occasionally, patients have an allergic reaction to the medications. Patients receiving ovulation induction medications generally have higher than usual estrogen levels and may experience tiredness, mood swings or nausea because of the increased estrogen.

Egg Retrieval:

When ultrasound and blood work indicate that the eggs are ready for collection, the egg donor receives an injection of human chorionic gonadotropin (HCG) that causes the eggs to mature. Egg retrieval is performed approximately 34 hours later.

Egg retrieval is performed under sterile conditions in the operating room using sufficient intravenous sedation and local anesthesia for comfort. If at any time you feel uncomfortable during the procedure you can ask for additional medication.

Briefly, an egg retrieval is performed as follows:

1. The patient is taken to the operating room and an IV is inserted. Blood is drawn.
2. IV sedation is administered by a member of the anesthesia team and local anesthesia is adminis-tered by the gynecologist.
3. Vaginal ultrasound is used to guide a small sterile needle through the vagina into the egg chambers. The upper portion of the vagina is only approximately one-half inch away from the ovaries. The eggs are removed in their fluid and taken to the laboratory. It is possible that eggs may not be present or may not be retrieved.
4. The egg donor is taken to the recovery room where she must stay for approximately four hours. She can then be discharged from the hospital. Donated ova are inseminated with sperm and resulting embryos are transferred to the recipient in two to three days.
5. A follow-up visit one week after the egg retrieval is mandatory to be certain there is no evidence of severe ovarian hyperstimulation. A few brief questionnaires will be given to you at that time to be filled out. A follow-up visit with a member of our mental health team is also required.
6. Because the psychological effects (if any) of donating eggs are unknown, you may be contacted periodically after the procedure by a member of our team to inquire how you are feeling after your experience. Referral for counseling can be made if needed.

The risks involved in egg retrieval are those of any minor procedure, including: infection and injury to the bowel, blood vessels, or other structures. There is also a possible risk that the needle stick used to obtain the eggs from the ovaries might cause bleeding. Ovarian bleeding or rupture may rarely occur but could lead to open abdominal surgery for control of bleeding or repair or removal of the ovary. Every measure will be taken to prevent these occurrences, and the possibility of occurrence is very small. Theoretically there could be a potential loss of fertility resulting from having a transvaginal ultrasound guided egg retrieval, but to our knowl-edge no such loss has ever been reported.

It is understood and agreed that the donation of eggs will be on an anonymous basis, which means that you have agreed to donate your eggs but you and your recipient do not know one another. It is understood and agreed that no entry will be made on your personal medical record as to the disposition of any eggs that may be obtained. Furthermore, there will be no entry on the personal record of any recipient as to the source of the donated eggs. However, because of the necessity and desire of the physicians to keep certain medical records, a separate record may be made and retained by your physicians in which entries may be made concerning the source and disposition of donated eggs.

Ownership of Embryos Resulting from Egg Donation

It is understood that once eggs are removed from a donor, or excess eggs are removed from an IVF donor the donor relinquishes all control of those eggs to FCRM for the above agreed to purposes. The eggs and resulting embryos belong to the recipient couple and/or the FCRM and the donor has no responsibilities or rights of any kind in relation to such embryos.

If the recipient couple in conjunction with FCRM decides to freeze excess embryos, it is under their jurisdiction to do so, without knowledge or consent from either the donor or her spouse.

Offspring Resulting from Egg Donation

Offspring resulting from egg donation are the children of the recipients. It is understood that the egg donor may not claim any responsibility or parenting rights for or obligations to those children, even if the egg donor and embryo recipient are related.

The recipient couple is fully responsible for all offspring, regardless of the outcome of the pregnancy, until the child reaches the age of consent. Because of the newness of egg donation, this is an area with limited legal precedence and FCRM cannot assure recipients or donors of the enforceability of this situation.

Pregnancy Incidental to Egg Donation

Most egg donors are young fertile women. It is understood that they will be more fertile during the month that they undergo treatment and egg retrieval. Some eggs may be incidentally released into the donor's reproductive system around the time of an egg retrieval. Therefore, there is a possibility that the egg donor could conceive during the treatment cycle. Unless the egg donor desires conception, she should seek the advice of the physicians on the IVF team or her private gynecologist about the use of contraceptive methods or abstinence during the treatment cycle.

Anonymity

The anonymity of all parties will be strictly maintained to the best of our ability. General physical characteristics of the egg donor and medical information about her will be available to the egg recipient as will additional biographical information provided by the donor for the purpose of being given to the recipient. Neither the name nor identifying information of the donor will be given to the recipient under any circumstances, or entered in the hospital record of the recipient. A separate confidential record will be kept by the Faulkner Centre. The donor will receive no other information about the recipient, the outcome of the donation procedure, or the resulting pregnancy, should one occur. Any information obtained about any of the individuals involved (donor, donor's spouse, recipient, recipient's spouse) will remain confidential and will only be disclosed with the consent of that individual.

However, there is the possibility that insurance claims or other records may reveal the identity of one or both parties. While the Faulkner Centre for Reproductive Medicine will avoid this disclosure to the extent possible, the recipient and donor assume the risk of identification.

Benefit

It is understood by all parties that there will be no medical benefit to the donor from egg donation.

Financial Responsibility

The recipient couple understands that they are responsible for all charges incurred as part of the egg donation procedure. This includes but is not limited to physician, laboratory and hospital charges. The recipient's insurance company may cover all or part of these charges, but the recipient couple is solely responsible for any unpaid monies.

We are obliged to inform you about the Centre's policy in the unlikely event that physical injury occurs. If, as a result of your participation, you experience physical injury from known or unknown risks of the donation procedures as described, immediate medical care and treatment, including hospitalization, if necessary, will be available. No monetary compensation, however, is available. The Faulkner Centre for Reproductive Medicine will help to bill the appropriate insurance company for any additional expenses but the Faulkner Centre will not be responsible for the costs of such care. In the event that the donor has a complication directly related to the egg donation stimulation or procedure which manifests itself within 60 days of the egg donation stimulation or procedure that is not covered in full by any insurance, any and all costs incurred by the donor will be the responsibility of the recipient who has been advised of this fact.

In addition, the anonymous donor identified by the New England Gamete Repository will be compensated for her time, risk and inconvenience the sum of $_____ for a fully medicated cycle or $_____ for a clomiphene stimulated cycle. This amount will be pro-rated should cancellation occur for reasons beyond your control. This will be paid to the donor by the New England Gamete Repository within ten working days of her post egg retrieval follow-up visits. IVF patients who donate excess eggs do not receive any compensation from the Faulkner Centre for Reproductive Medicine or any other source for time, risk and inconvenience associated with the egg donation.

I have read the above consent and all questions have been answered to my satisfaction. I have read and initialed the appropriate choice on page one. I understand and agree to the consent for the donation of oocytes and procedures necessary to do it.

_____	_____
Donor	Date
_____	_____
Witness	Date
_____	_____
Husband (if married)	Date
_____	_____
Witness	Date

Appendix 10-H

Informed Consent for Anonymous Egg Donor[1]

PENNSYLVANIA REPRODUCTIVE ASSOCIATES
PENNSYLVANIA HOSPITAL ANONYMOUS OOCYTE DONOR PROGRAM

1. I hereby authorize and direct Pennsylvania Reproductive Associates ("PRA") including physicians, nurses, reproductive laboratory biologists, mental health professionals, and such assistants as may be selected by them ("IVF team"), to treat me in accordance with the laboratory protocols for in vitro fertilization and embryo transfer ("IVF-ET"), and I hereby consent to such treatment as outlined in this consent statement.

2. I understand that the consenting participants in this procedure include me as the egg donor, the recipient's husband ("husband") who will provide the sperm and the recipient wife ("wife") who will carry the fertilized egg(s) (embryo(s)) if they should result in fertilization and/or embryo development.

3. I understand that the purpose of my participation in the IVF program is to provide fertilizable eggs for the recipient wife and husband in their attempt to achieve a viable pregnancy.

4. I understand that the eggs donated by me and sperm collected from the husband will be mixed under the process of in vitro fertilization. If the donated egg(s) are fertilized, and divide appropriately, the resulting embryo(s) will be transferred to the wife. Embryo(s) from the treatment cycle may be cryopreserved (frozen) if consented to by the recipient couple for replacement at a later date. The disposition of any cryopreserved embryo(s) will be determined solely by the recipient couple as outlined in the PRA cryopreservation consent form.

5. I have also had the opportunity to attend an individual and/or group egg donation information seminar given by the IVF team to educate me as to the policies, procedures and risks associated with my participation as an egg donor. I have discussed the process of egg donation and related procedures with members of the IVF team and have reviewed explanatory literature of the procedures which was made available to me by the IVF team. All questions related to my participation as an egg donor have been answered to my satisfaction.

6. The oocyte donor and the recipient husband and wife, must provide a detailed history including a comprehensive medical history to explore for familial (inherited) diseases before being approved as a participant in the egg donor program and/or an egg donor in a specific case.
The steps for application and acceptance into the egg donor program include the following:

a) a physical examination of the egg donor including a pelvic exam and a PAP smear if appropriate;
b) a detailed social history of each participant, including history of habits, substance use, and previous sexual relationships. Previous sexual relationships outside that of the immediate couple may be privately discussed with members of the IVF medical and psychological team;
c) screening for inheritable diseases according to history and ethnic background of egg donor and spouse of oocyte recipient when appropriate;
d) psychological screening, testing, consultation and an interview with a psychologist or other mental health professional. I understand that the psychological impact of being an egg donor is unknown and that I have had an opportunity to explore all relevant issues with a psychologist. I also understand that psychological records, results of tests, and interview notes will be kept confidential and

---

[1] Note: This consent form was being revised at the time this book went to press. For updated forms, please contact Mary English, RN, Director of Clinical Services, Pennsylvania Reproductive Associates, Eighth and Spruce Streets, Spruce Building, Suite 786, Philadelphia, PA 19107 (215) 829-5095.

will only be used to determine whether to proceed with my participation as an egg donor. I further understand that PRA and the IVF team members cannot be held responsible for any negative psychological consequences for participating as an egg donor in the program.

e) infectious disease screening will include at a minimum the guidelines set forth by the American Fertility Society titled "Minimal Screen for Gamete Donations" as follows:

1. gonorrhea culture;
2. chlamydia culture;
3. mycoplasma culture;
4. Hepatitis B surface antigen;
5. Hepatitis C;
6. RPR (test for exposure to syphilis);
7. cytomegalic virus;
8. Human Immunodeficiency Virus;
9. RH factor;
10. other disease screening as appropriate by history, or as indicated in future evaluation.

I represent that all requests for medical and family history will be answered truthfully and to the best of my knowledge. I further agree to follow all medical instructions given to me by the IVF team. During the time I am involved in this program, I agree not to smoke cigarettes, marijuana or other substances, drink alcoholic beverages or use any illegal drugs or prescription or non-prescription medications without the consent of one of the IVF team physicians.

Prior to and during the time of my participation in the program, I agree to immediately inform the IVF team, in writing of any material change in my circumstances which may reasonably impact my health, including, but not limited to any illnesses or exposure to communicable diseases.

Once screening of all participants is completed and the egg recipient has been properly prepared to receive donated egg(s) to the satisfaction of the IVF team, the egg donor will be permitted to begin the treatment phase of the process.

OVULATION INDUCTION IN PREPARATION FOR EGG RETRIEVAL

I understand that in order to produce several oocytes (eggs) for donation, I will need to take medication on a specified schedule to stimulate my ovaries. I also understand that although I may have a normal menstrual cycle, it will be necessary for me to take medication that will suppress my normal menstrual cycle (Lupron) so that my ovaries can be stimulated with natural hormones (Pergonal, Metrodin) and ovulation controlled to optimize the timing of ovulation and the quality of eggs retrieved.

I understand that Lupron is given by subcutaneous injection for approximately two weeks prior to the stimulation of my ovaries with fertility medications. Once my cycle is suppressed, as documented by pelvic ultrasound and serum hormonal studies and the recipient has begun hormonal replacement to prepare her uterus for embryo transfer, intramuscular hormonal injections (Pergonal, Metrodin) will begin. The medications administered are concentrated forms of natural hormones produced by the body and will be given by intramuscular injection for approximately 9 to 12 days. At various times during this period, I will be asked to have blood and/or ultrasound tests to evaluate the ovarian response and hormonal levels. When results from blood and ultrasound monitoring reveal that mature follicles and adequate hormonal values exist, I will receive another injection (hCG) (another concentrated form of natural hormones) to mature the eggs and control ovulation for the timing of egg retrieval. Finally, I understand that the medication protocols used to induce ovulation are based on my past medical history and physical status.

I understand that despite adequate suppression of my ovarian cycle and appropriate stimulation with fertility medications, that I may not achieve an adequate hormonal and ovarian response. In such circumstances, my cycle will be cancelled, and egg retrieval will not be performed. Before attempting another cycle, if agreed to by me and deemed appropriate by the IVF team, I will have to wait at least one cycle for the effects of ovarian stimulation to subside.

Risks of Ovulation Induction

I understand that there are associated risks and consequences with the use of ovulation induction medications as outlined below:

1) Ovulation induction drugs will cause the ovaries to become temporarily enlarged and may result in the development of benign ovarian cysts. Rarely would such changes produce severe complications, i.e. twisting of the ovary, rupture of the ovary or fluid and electrolyte imbalances. However, if any of these symptoms occur, it may be necessary to require hospitalization and may in rare cases result in the removal of one or both ovaries.

In less than 5% of the cases, the ovaries may become severely stimulated, which is a condition that is reversible and referred to as severe ovarian hyperstimulation syndrome.

Ovarian hyperstimulation is characterized by mild lower abdominal discomfort, fluid retention with subsequent weight gain due to the accumulation of fluid in the abdomen. The treatment for this syndrome is bedrest, usually at home but may require, in some cases, hospitalization. In extremely rare circumstances, serious complications may occur. These conditions usually last from one to four weeks following administration of hCG (given to trigger ovulation). If you are receiving medication and it appears that you could develop a severe form of ovarian hyperstimulation, your cycle may be cancelled, and you will not receive hCG or have an egg retrieval. Again, your cycle may also be cancelled if normal levels are not optimal or ovarian follicles fail to grow appropriately.

Other side effects from the medications include, but are not limited to:

1) swelling, redness and slight pain at injection sites;
2) allergic reactions to the medications;
3) fatigue, mood swings and nausea, which may be attributed to higher estrogen levels;
4) temporarily impaired vision.

Finally, as part of the ovulation induction process, I am aware that I will be asked to abstain from strenuous exercise or sexual activity during a specific time period of the treatment cycle.

Pregnancy incidental to egg donation is also a potential risk. Eggs may be incidentally released into the reproductive system around the time of an egg retrieval. Therefore, it is possible that I may conceive during a treatment cycle. Unless I wish to become pregnant, I am advised that I should seek advice about use of contraceptive methods or abstain from intercourse.

EGG RETRIEVAL

I understand that when daily ultrasound and blood hormonal assays reveal that my eggs are ready for collection, I will receive an injection of human chorionic gonadotropin (hCG) in order to induce final maturation of the eggs and time my ovulation for retrieval within approximately 33 to 36 hours.

I recognize that egg retrieval utilizes a vaginal ultrasound probe to guide a needle through the vaginal wall into the ovary. This procedure is performed under sterile conditions in the IVF laboratory and will require the use of local anesthesia in the cervix and intravenous analgesia. The procedure generally lasts approximately 45 minutes and is outlined as follows:

1) upon arrival to the IVF laboratory, an intravenous line will be started by one of the IVF nurses;
2) at the appropriate time for the retrieval, IV sedation will be administered;
3) a speculum will be inserted into my vagina, the vagina will be cleansed with saline and a local anesthesia will be administered to the cervix. The speculum will be removed, and the vaginal probe, a cylindrical device with an ultrasound transducer on the tip, will be introduced into the vagina. The needle guide attached to the probe guides the needle through the vaginal wall into the follicle. The needle is connected to a closed aspiration system. Often many follicles can be aspirated in the ovary with only one puncture. As the follicles and fluid are aspirated, they are given to the laboratory biologist for microscopic examination, in order to identify the eggs. After the follicles are aspirated from one ovary, the probe is directed to the opposite ovary, and again, an attempt will be made to puncture all follicles. It is possible that eggs may not be present in every follicle or that no eggs may be retrieved.

Following the retrieval, I am advised that I must stay in the recovery area for at least one hour before getting dressed and being discharged. I understand that one of the consequences of the procedure may be light to moderate amounts of vaginal bleeding. I understand that the medications may make me feel drowsy. I further understand that I will be observed by IVF personnel following the procedure to ensure that there are no observable abnormal effects from the medication. I also understand that I must stay home the remainder of the day following the retrieval and have someone near or closely available, should I develop any untoward effects. Finally, I am aware that because of the effects of the medication, I should not drive on the day of my egg retrieval.

Risks of Egg Retrieval

The risks involved in egg retrieval are those associated with any minor surgical procedure—primarily bleeding and infection. There is the potential for intra-abdominal bleeding, damage to ovaries and/or infection, but available clinical experience and evidence suggests that the risks are low. Every measure will be taken to prevent these occurrences, and to minimize the associated risks. Theoretically, if a pelvic infection should result from an ultrasound retrieval, there is the potential for loss of fertility resulting from this infection, but no such fertility loss for an egg donor has been reported to date. There is also the remote possibility that surgery may be necessary to control the infection which could result in the loss of one or both ovaries.

OWNERSHIP RIGHTS FOR EMBRYOS
RESULTING FROM EGG DONATION

Once I have given up my eggs for donation at retrieval, my participation in the egg donor process is completed although I am aware that I will be asked to return to PRA for a follow-up exam within 7 to 10 days. My donated oocytes are inseminated with the sperm of the recipient's husband and any resulting embryos are transferred to the recipient within 2 to 3 days, or cryopreserved if optimal synchronization has not been attained. It is my understanding that once the eggs are removed from me and have been inseminated by the sperm of the recipient spouse, the resulting embryos are the sole responsibility of the recipient couple, and I have no further responsibilities, rights, or obligations in relation to such embryos or their disposition and any remaining eggs whether or not fertilized.

RESULTANT OFFSPRING

Any offspring resulting from egg donation and IVF are the children of the recipient couple.

It is understood that the egg donor has no rights, claims or responsibilities for any offspring or any rights or claims against the recipient couple, even if the egg donor and embryo recipient are related unless there are separate contractual agreements between the parties.

The recipient couple is fully responsible for any and all offspring, regardless of the outcome of the pregnancy.

ANONYMITY

I understand that the identity of the recipient couple(s) will not be revealed to me (unless I am a "known" egg donor, i.e., sister, relative, or volunteer friend) and that my identity will not be revealed to the recipient couple(s). In addition, I understand that I may not be given any information concerning oocyte, fertilization, pregnancy establishment or pregnancy outcome, if donation is anonymous. I understand that the IVF team will exercise their best efforts to ensure that the anonymity of all parties will be strictly maintained. I am aware, however, that should the egg recipient achieve pregnancy as a result of my donated eggs, the Ovum Donor Personal History Form, including my medical, social and psychological history, will be available to the recipient, excluding all identifying information. A separate confidential record will be kept by Pennsylvania Reproductive Associates and the IVF team. In addition, I am aware that I will receive no information about the recipient, and that any information obtained concerning any of the individuals involved (donor, donor spouse, recipient spouse) shall remain confidential and will only be disclosed with the written consent of that individual. I understand that PRA will exercise every effort to ensure the confidentiality of identifying information but cannot guarantee that an inadvertent disclosure of information might not occur and compromise the confidentiality of the participants.

POTENTIAL RESEARCH STUDIES

I understand that this procedure will be performed as part of the In Vitro Fertilization Program of Pennsylvania Reproductive Associates, Inc., ("PRA"), at Pennsylvania Hospital or at the Plymouth Meeting facility, and that the results of all such procedures performed as part of the program will be subject to extensive study. I understand that all information obtained will be handled confidentially and that neither my identity nor specific medical details will be revealed by the doctors or staff without any consent, or court order, except that specific medical details may be revealed in professional publications if my identity is concealed. I agree to refrain from granting interviews or having any contact with the news media, unless said contact is approved in advance by the IVF team.

FINANCIAL RESPONSIBILITY

I understand that the recipient couple is responsible for all charges incurred as part of the egg donation procedure. This includes, but is not limited to, physician, laboratory, and hospital charges as well as charges incurred by Pennsylvania Reproductive Associates. The recipient's insurance may or may not cover all of these charges, but I, as the egg donor, will not be responsible for any unpaid monies. If, as a result of my participation, I experience physical injury from known or unknown risks directly related to any medical procedures performed or medications received, immediate medical attention and treatment, including hospitalization, if necessary, will be available and the responsibility for these charges will be borne by Pennsylvania Reproductive Associates.

I hereby specifically waive any right to pursue any claims, demands or actions for damages or monies against Pennsylvania Reproductive Associates including but not limited to claims for medical malpractice, pain and suffering, loss of consortium and loss of time from work other than for the costs of hospitalization and medical treatment specifically set forth above which charges will be borne by Pennsylvania Reproductive Associates.

COMPENSATION

As a participant in the anonymous egg donor program of Pennsylvania Reproductive Associates, I understand that I will be compensated for my time, inconvenience, and effort for screening, ovulation induction, and egg retrieval. My compensation, depending on the length of my participation, may vary and will be reviewed and agreed to with me prior to my treatment cycle.

My request and authorization for treatment in your program is purely voluntary. I understand that I may revoke this consent at any time and that my present or future care at Pennsylvania Reproductive Associates will not in any way be affected by that decision. I agree that this consent may only be revoked in a signed written submission delivered to a member of the IVF team. This consent extends to Pennsylvania Reproductive Associates and the IVF team to whom I have entrusted my care and any others assisting, associated with, or designated by those parties.

I certify that I have read and fully understand this consent statement which has been preceded by an explanation by a member(s) of the IVF team, as well as a written explanation, and that the explanations referred to are fully understood by me. I have had the opportunity to ask the IVF team additional questions, and if asked, am satisfied with the answers provided. I have no further questions and fully intend to be legally bound by my consent to the procedures outlined in this consent statement as evidenced by my signature below.

_____   _____

Donor   Date

_____   _____

Witness   Date

Appendix 10-I

Informed Consent for Egg Donor Recipient and Husband—In Vitro Fertilization and Embryo Replacement Utilizing Donor Oocytes

PENNSYLVANIA REPRODUCTIVE ASSOCIATES
IN VITRO FERTILIZATION PROGRAM

1.   We hereby authorize and direct Pennsylvania Reproductive Associates ("PRA") including physicians, nurses, reproductive laboratory biologists, mental health professionals, and such assistants as may be selected by them ("IVF Team") to treat us in accordance with the laboratory protocols for in vitro fertilization and embryo replacement (IVF-ER) protocols, and we hereby consent to such treatment as outlined in this consent statement.

2.   We understand that the consenting participants in this procedure include the egg donor, and us as a couple consisting of the wife as the egg recipient ("Wife") who will carry the fertilized egg(s) (embryos) if they should result in fertilization and/or embryo development and the husband ("Husband") who will provide the sperm which will be used to attempt to fertilize the egg(s).

3.   We understand that the purpose of our participation in the IVF program is to achieve a viable pregnancy resulting from the fertilization of the donors egg(s) with the Husband's sperm for replacement in the Wife's uterus.

4.   We understand that an egg(s) taken from the egg donor and sperm collected from the Husband will be mixed under the process of in vitro fertilization. If the donated egg(s) are fertilized, and divide appropriately, the resulting embryo(s) will then be replaced in the Wife, either by a standard intrauterine embryo replacement, or by laparoscopy with a tubal embryo transfer. We are aware that if the Wife's cycle is unable to be adequately synchronized with that of the donor, the option of cryopreservation of the embryo(s) will be made available to us with appropriate signed informed consents.

5.   We have also had the opportunity to attend an IVF information seminar given by the IVF team during which time the policies, procedures and risks associated with our participation in the egg donor program were explained to us. This included our participation and responsibilities as the egg recipient and sperm donor, as well as those of the egg donor. We have discussed the process of egg donation and related procedures with members of the IVF team and have reviewed explanatory literature of the procedures which was made available to us by the IVF team. All questions related to our participation as egg recipient and sperm donor have been answered to our satisfaction.

6.   The egg donor, the recipient Wife and sperm donor Husband must each provide a detailed history including a comprehensive medical history to attempt to ascertain the presence or absence of familial (inherited) diseases before being approved as a participant in the egg donor program.

The steps for application and acceptance into the egg donor program include the following:

    a.   screening of all participating parties, i.e., egg donor, egg recipient and egg recipient's Husband.

    b.   a physical examination, including a pelvic exam and a PAP smear if appropriate of both the egg donor and egg recipient.

    c.   a detailed social history of each person, including history of habits, substance use and previous sexual relationships.

    d.   screening for inheritable diseases according to history and ethnic background of egg donor and Husband (sperm donor) when appropriate; (genetic karyotype chromosomal analysis may also be done on the egg donor if requested by the Husband and Wife at their expense).

    e.   psychological screening, testing, consultation and interviews with a psychologist or other qualified mental health professional.

    f.   infectious disease screening will include at a minimum the guidelines set forth by the American Society for Reproductive Medicine titled ("Minimal Screen for Gamete Donations"), and may in addition include screening for both the recipient couple and the donor as follows:

       1.   gonorrhea culture;

       2.   chlamydia culture;

       3.   chlamydia antibody;

       4.   mycoplasma culture;

       5.   Hepatitis B surface antigen;

       6.   Hepatitis C;

       7.   RPR (test for exposure to syphilis);

       8.   cytomegalic virus;

       9.   Human Immunodeficiency Virus;

     10.   drug and alcohol screen;

     11.   RH factor;

     12.   other disease screening as appropriate by history, or as indicated in future evaluation.

With respect to screening for contagious diseases, we understand that there are limitations to technology and that despite strict adherence to protocol, contagious diseases may be transmitted from one individual to another, specifically from egg donors to egg recipients. The chances of this occurring are unlikely, but exist nonetheless. Once screening of all parties has been accomplished and the Wife has been properly prepared to begin treatment to the satisfaction of the IVF team, the Wife will begin the treatment phase of the process.

PSYCHOLOGICAL COUNSELING/INTERVIEW

Psychological screening of the donor will only assess the donor's motivation for participation and the presence of any current major psychiatric issues such as psychosis, bipolar disorder or major depression will screen out the donor. All medical and psychological information is provided by the donor and the accuracy of that information cannot be guaranteed. In cases where the donor is a known relative or friend, psychological counseling and evaluation may be limited to that in a clinical interview.

We understand as the recipients of the donor's eggs, regardless of whether the donor is known or anonymous that we as a couple will be asked to have a counseling interview to discuss relevant issues as to the use of donor eggs. Such issues include but are not limited to anonymity, secrecy and any other issues that might be specific to our circumstances or concerns. We further understand that PRA and the IVF team members cannot be held responsible for any negative consequences for participating as an egg recipient in the program.

TEST TREATMENT CYCLE—SYNCHRONIZATION

We understand that even if the Wife has normal menstrual cycles, it will be necessary for her to receive medication to prepare her uterus for receiving an embryo. In addition, it will be necessary for her to be on replacement therapy with estrogen and progesterone so that her cycle can be synchronized with that of the egg donor to increase the chances of pregnancy. If the Wife does not have ovulatory function, she will receive a combination of estrogen and progesterone, in the form of oral and injection preparations. If the Wife has ovulatory function, she may need to take a medication called Lupron, which will allow her ovulatory function to be suppressed, and permit manipulation of her cycle for synchronization purposes. The following procedure(s) may be utilized:

1.   Several weeks of hormonal therapy may have to occur. This includes sequential administration of the hormones estrogen and progesterone. Estrogen is administered either by pills or in patches worn on the abdomen. Potential side effects of this medication include water retention, local skin irritation and bruising of the skin. More serious but rarer complications include blood clots in the legs or lung, hypertension and stroke. Smoking cigarettes while taking this medication is forbidden. Again, if the Wife has ovulatory function, she may be taking her estrogen and progesterone after suppression has been achieved with Lupron. The Wife will be given estrogen therapy in a step-like fashion to mimic those levels of estrogen achieved in a normal menstrual cycle.

At the appropriate time, a progesterone therapy will be added to the estrogen. This may include progesterone therapy including progesterone vaginal suppositories, oral micronized preparations of progesterone, or progesterone in oil administered by injection which will be given in varying doses to again mimic the normal secretion of progesterone in a normal cycle. Potential side effects of this medication may include local swelling and infection at the site of injection, allergic reactions to the oil (peanut or sesame), or preservative in the solution and/or allergy to the preparation used to make progesterone suppositories. Additional side effects could be irritation, itching or pain secondary to the injection and bleeding from the injection site. We understand that we will be advised how to have this medication administered by a properly trained expert.

2.   The Wife may have to undergo a test cycle before her treatment cycle which will include taking a cycle of estrogen and progesterone as described above, possibly in conjunction with one or more endometrial biopsies to assess endometrial development, and appropriateness for transfer of embryos. This may also include one or more ultrasounds to assess endometrial thickness and serial serum hormone levels to evaluate effectiveness of hormone replacement. If a biopsy should have to be performed, we are aware that this entails passing a small instrument into the uterus and taking a very small tissue sample from the top of the uterine cavity.

During the test cycle, as well as the treatment cycle, we understand that the Wife may have to have bloodwork drawn frequently during the monitoring phase. Side effects of blood drawing may include pain, bleeding at the site of the venepuncture, swelling and bruising, and potentially, if repeated samples are drawn, iron deficiency anemia.

Finally, one or more monitoring (test) cycles may be required to establish favorable conditions for embryo transfer. This will, of course, depend on individual circumstances and responses to the first cycle. On rare occasions, more than one test cycle may be required.

EMBRYO TRANSFER CYCLE DONOR PARTICIPATION

We understand that after a thorough evaluation and screening, both medically and psychologically, an egg donor will be matched with the Wife. We understand that frequent blood tests and ultrasound studies of the egg donor, as well as the Wife, will be done to determine impending ovulation and optimal synchronization of cycles. The egg donor will be admitted to the IVF suite for egg retrieval, in most cases by ultrasound retrieval, when her ovulatory process is at the appropriate stage as determined by the IVF treatment team, in order to obtain as many eggs as possible from her ovaries. At that point, the mixture of the egg donor's eggs with the Husband's sperm will be performed in an attempt to allow fertilization to occur. Any resulting embryos will be transferred into a different medium which will permit early growth and cleavage outside the uterus. Following several cell divisions, any viable embryo(s) will be placed in the Wife's uterus by means of a small plastic catheter inserted through the vagina and cervix.

Alternatively, the IVF treatment team may suggest replacement of the embryos directly into the fallopian tube by means of laparoscopy (tubal embryo transfer - TET). Another alternative procedure is placement of donor eggs and the Husband's sperm directly into the Wife's fallopian tube (gamete intra fallopian tubal transfer - GIFT). This is done prior to fertilization. We may exercise the option of cryopreservation for any embryos in excess of four (4) for replacement in subsequent cycles, after appropriate consultation and execution of informed consent forms.

POTENTIAL CONSEQUENCES RESULTING FROM TRANSFER OF MULTIPLE EMBRYOS

If multiple embryos are transferred, multiple pregnancy can occur up to and sometimes exceeding the number of embryos transferred. There are many potential obstetrical, physical and psychological consequences that may result from multiple pregnancy. The list includes but is not limited to the following:

1. Maternal
   a. Possible increased risk of gestational diseases such as gestational diabetes, hypertension and preeclampsia.
   b. Possible increased risk of exacerbating preexisting medical diseases, sometimes irreversibly.
   c. Increased risk of birthing accidents, such as rupture of umbilical cord, separation of the placenta, low lying placenta, and uterine rupture.
   d. Increased risk of preterm labor, which increases with the number of fetuses in the uterus.
   e. Increased risk of the necessity for delivery by Caesarean Section.
2. Fetal
   a. Increased risk of prematurity, low birth weight, umbilical cord accidents, death of one or more fetuses.
   b. Increased risk of lower I.Q. scores resulting from maldevelopment, prematurity and crowding in the uterus.
3. Selective Reduction Option

We understand that the statistical chances of achieving pregnancy are increased when 3–4 embryos are transferred, and that the transfer of more than 4 embryos increases the chances of multiple gestation.

In the event that a multiple pregnancy results, placing the mother and/or fetuses at risk, the option of selective embryo reduction may be exercised. This entails the aspiration of one or more gestational sacs from the mother's uterus.

We have been advised of the risk of multiple gestation and its potential medical impact, and understand that selective reduction may be recommended to us in order to preserve the health of both mother and fetus(es).

If selective reduction is an unacceptable option to us, we have discussed the maximum number of embryos to be transferred in order to meet the goals of a) optimizing the achievement of pregnancy, and b) avoiding a potentially harmful multiple gestation.

BIRTH DEFECTS

The incidence of major birth defects in singleton pregnancies is approximately 2 percent in the general population.

Even with the most precise screening methods possible, there is a chance that a pregnancy resulting from reproductive technology, utilizing donated eggs as in any pregnancy can result in a child with birth defects, medical problems, learning disabilities, handicaps, cerebral palsy and other unforeseen difficulties. Some of these problems can arise from genetic abnormalities that cannot be detected with modern screening tests. Some of them can result from birth accidents, and illness during pregnancy. We recognize that we will be taking a similar risk in accepting a donated oocyte as we would if we were to conceive on our own. Results to date of IVF, GIFT and other assisted reproductive technologies (ART) have shown no increased risk of abnormal infants when compared to a spontaneous pregnancy.

OWNERSHIP OF EMBRYOS RESULTING FROM EGG DONATION

We understand that once the egg(s) are removed from a donor and have been inseminated by the sperm of the Husband, the resulting embryo(s) are our sole responsibility. We understand and agree that we are legally responsible for the resulting embryos. The donor has no responsibilities, rights or obligations in relation to such embryo(s).

We understand that the potential donor may change her mind about the donation until the time that the Husband's sperm inseminates the egg(s). Once the Husband's sperm have been added to the egg(s), the egg(s) and resulting embryos become our sole responsibility and the egg donor's rights are terminated as of that time.

OFFSPRING RESULTING FROM EGG DONATION

Any offspring resulting from egg donation and IVF are our children and we specifically assume all legal rights and obligations normally associated with having offspring. We understand that the egg donor may not claim any responsibility or parenting rights for the resultant offspring, even if the egg donor is related to us, except where there is a separate written contractual agreement between the parties.

We understand and agree that we are fully responsible for any and all offspring regardless of the outcome of the pregnancy.

ANONYMITY

We understand that the identity of the egg donor will not be revealed to us (unless the egg donor is already known to us, i.e., sister, relative, or volunteer friend) and that our identity will not be revealed to the egg donor.

We understand that the IVF team will exercise their best efforts to ensure that the anonymity of all parties will be strictly maintained. We further understand that should I achieve pregnancy as a result of the donated eggs, the Ovum Donor Personal History Form (ODPH), which includes the egg donor's medical and social history, will be made available to us, excluding all identifying information. We also understand that a separate confidential record will be kept by Pennsylvania Reproductive Associates and the IVF team. In addition, we are aware that we will receive no information other than the ODPH form about the egg donor. Any information obtained concerning any of the individuals involved shall remain confidential and will only be disclosed with the express written consent of that individual. We understand that PRA will exercise every effort to ensure the confidentiality of identifying information but cannot guarantee that an inadvertent disclosure of information might not occur and compromise the confidentiality of the participants.

POTENTIAL RESEARCH STUDIES

We understand that this procedure will be performed as part of the In Vitro Fertilization Program of Pennsylvania Reproductive Associates, Inc., ("PRA"), at Pennsylvania Hospital or at the Plymouth Meeting facility, and that the results of all such procedures performed as part of the program may be subject to extensive study. We understand that all information obtained will be handled confidentially and that neither our identity nor specific medical details will be revealed by the doctors or staff without specific consent, or a court order, except that medical details may be revealed in professional publications if our identity is concealed. We agree to refrain from granting interviews or having any contact with the news media, unless said contact is approved in advance by the IVF team.

FINANCIAL RESPONSIBILITY

We understand that we are responsible for all charges incurred as part of the egg donation procedure whether or not there is a successful procedure. This includes, but is not limited to, physician, laboratory, and hospital charges as well as charges incurred by Pennsylvania Reproductive Associates. Our insurance may or may not cover all of these charges, but we, as the egg recipient and sperm donor, will be responsible for any unpaid monies.

PROGRAM PARTICIPATION

We understand that our participation in the Pennsylvania Reproductive Associates-IVF program is purely voluntary. We further understand that we may revoke this consent and that our present and future care at Pennsylvania Reproductive Associates will not in any way be affected by that decision. We agree that this consent may only be revoked in a signed written submission delivered to a member of the IVF team. This consent extends to Pennsylvania Reproductive Associates and the IVF team to whom we have entrusted our care and any others assisting, associated with, or designated by those parties.

We certify that we have read and fully understand this consent statement which has been preceded by an explanation by a member(s) of the IVF team, as well as a written explanation, and that the explanations referred to were fully understood. We have had the opportunity to ask the IVF team additional questions, and if asked, are satisfied with the answers provided. We have no further questions and fully intend to be legally bound by our consent to the procedures outlined in this consent statement as evidenced by our signatures below.

_____   _____
Witness   Wife (Egg Recipient)

_____   _____
Witness   Husband (Sperm Donor)

                                   _____
                                   Signature of Physician
                                   Obtaining Consent from Husband and Wife

                                   Date: _____

Physician Certification

I hereby certify that I am a member of the IVF team and that I or one of my colleagues have discussed, and explained, all aspects of In Vitro Fertilization and Embryo Replacement Utilizing Donor Oocytes with _____ and _____, and in my opinion, each fully understands what I said, as well as the matters set forth in the foregoing consent form which has been executed prior to this certification.

_____

Signature of Physician

_____

Date

PART III

SOCIAL/ETHICAL ISSUES

Prior to 1993, gamete donation received little public attention. Sperm donation was performed quietly for a select group of patients. Egg donation was primarily performed for a limited number of prematurely menopausal women. However, an article published that year on egg donation performed on naturally menopausal women over the age of 50 created a wave of excitement, shock, and fear. Society could no longer bury its collective head and ignore the fact that the reproductive life span of a woman was neither finite nor defined by menopause. Just as contraception a generation ago gave women more control over timing reproduction, egg donation freed women to delay childbearing indefinitely.

This section explores the social/ethical issues of gamete donation. Chapter 11 provides insight into establishing an ethics advisory board in conjunction with a gamete donation program. Chapter 12 explores the issues associated with providing egg donation for women over 50. Chapter 13 reviews the religious issues associated with gamete donation. In Chapter 14, patient perspectives on gamete donation are provided. Chapter 15 discusses the ethical considerations associated with gamete donation. Chapters 16 and 17 provide two perspectives on explaining gamete donation to children, the former that of an experienced pediatrician who deals with the children and families who result from gamete donation and the latter that of an experienced psychologist whose primary counseling exposure is prior to and during the conception. The last chapter in this section, Chapter 18, attempts to enlighten the reader regarding some of the potential gamete donation issues that can be anticipated as a result of the genome project.

Because advances in assisted reproductive technologies evolve at such a rapid pace, what can be done will have to be balanced continuously with what should be done and how best to do it.

Machelle M. Seibel, M.D.

11

Charting Uncharted Waters: The Role of the Ethics Advisory Committee

PAULA A. HINDLE, R.N.

Several decades ago, reproductive medicine focused on preventing pregnancy. Now technology is directed toward creating life. The techniques include artificial insemination, in vitro fertilization, surrogacy, gamete intra-fallopian transfer procedures, and gamete donation. Although the clinical procedures have been well-defined and have become common practice, the ethical, moral, and legal issues are not as clearly defined or prescribed. So how do clinicians navigate through the uncharted waters of the ethical, moral, and legal issues associated with gamete donations?

Two resources are available to clinicians to provide a forum to review, direct, and discuss the issues associated with reproductive medicine. These two resources are the institutional review board and a hospital ethics committee. This chapter will look at the history, roles, and usefulness of each of these resources. Finally, one organization's experience will be described to highlight the usefulness of these structures.

INSTITUTIONAL REVIEW BOARDS

Institutional review boards were developed in the 1960s as a result of the Helsinki Declaration. The purpose of these boards was to review the ethical issues of proposals for biomedical research. The Helsinki Declaration defined a code of ethics to direct human experimentation and differentiated between experimentation on patients and healthy subjects. This declaration was later amended to include a justification of the need to do biomedical research but was also expanded to require an explicit assessment of the risks and benefits of the research and mandated informed consent. Institutional review boards are regulated by both federal and state government regulations that define the composition of the committee and direct the boards' activities.

The function of the institutional review board is to review biomedical research to ensure the rights of the human subjects and to ensure compliance with the principles of the Helsinki II declaration (Table 11.1) (Gutteridge F, et al., 1982, p. 1796). The Helsinki II accord also states that the research procedure be spelled out in a written proposal. These proposals should include the information shown in Table 11.2 (Gutteridge F, et al., 1982, pp. 1798–1799).

Such a review board is designed to deal with ethical issues associated with biomedical research. It is primarily useful in directing the clinician when the practice or procedure is experimental. Therefore an institutional review board deals only with the ethical issues involved in developing technology. It does not deal with application of the technology once it has become a standard practice. George Annas,

TABLE 11.1. Principles of the Helsinki II Declaration

The investigators must be scientifically qualified and competent to carry out the proposed research.

The proposed research must be properly designed.

There must be an assessment of the benefit in relation to risk.

There must be an equitable section of the subjects.

Adequate informed consent must be obtained from the subjects.

The subjects' privacy must be respected.

The extent to which subjects are protected against the possible untoward effects of interventions must be considered.

TABLE 11.2. Content of Research Proposals

The identity of the institution responsible for the technical and administrative support of the proposal.

The identity and qualification of, and facilities available to the investigator(s) responsible for conducting the research.

The objectives of a justification for the proposed research, including a discussion of the risks and benefits to individual subjects.

A description of (i) the experimental design and statistical analysis of the study and the criteria for discontinuation; (ii) evidence establishing the safety and quality of any drugs or other chemicals used.

A summary of the experimental protocol.

A precise description of the procedures used to select and recruit subjects, to obtain informed consent, and to assure confidentiality of personal information referable to individual subjects. Any special incentives or treatment offered to subjects for their participation should be indicated.

Arrangements for providing medical care and/or financial compensation for subjects injured as a result of the research.

the Director of the Law, Medicine, and Ethics Program at Boston University Schools of Medicine and Public Health, wrote, "The success of Institutional Review Boards can be traced to their very specific mandate, their standards of decision-making (spelled out in federal regulation), and their support by the medical and research funding communities" (Annas GJ, 1991). Where does the clinician turn when ethical issues arise from a proven technology? Another resource that is available for guidance is a hospital bioethics committee.

ETHICS COMMITTEE

Bioethics committees were created to deal with the moral and ethical dilemmas arising from the use of established technology. The birth of bioethics can be traced to 1962 and the development of the arteriovenous shunt and cannula, which made chronic hemodialysis possible. Unfortunately, the demand for dialysis severely exceeded the availability of the technology. To remedy that problem, a small group was established to determine which patients would have access to hemodialysis.

A number of other events have caused bioethics to flourish. For example, the first cardiac transplant evoked questions concerning the source of organ donations. These questions led to the development of the brain death criteria that are now accepted by most states. The Quinlan and Baby Doe cases brought forward discussions concerning the issues of quality of life and the right to refuse treatment. These, as well as subsequent similar cases, led to the implementation of the Patient's Self Determination Act in 1989.

Unlike institutional review boards, bioethics committees are not regulated by the state or federal government. They are established to have a forum for discussing the moral and ethical impact of medical technology. In the Karen Ann Quinlan case, for example, the

New Jersey Supreme Court suggested that an ethics or bioethics committee was the more suitable arena in which to discuss the issues of quality of life and the right to refuse treatment. This premise is supported by the Joint Commission for the Accreditation of Hospital Organizations, which requires each of its accredited organizations to have a mechanism to discuss ethical issues.

In hospitals the role of the bioethics committee is typically threefold and includes case review, education, and policy development (Jonsen AR, 1993). Ethics committees are typically composed of physicians, nurses, social workers, clergy, and administration representatives. Some hospitals may also include hospital board members, community representatives, and/or legal counsel. Members of the committee should be well-versed in the issues concerning the technology of patient care.

In its case review function, the ethics committee serves in a consultative role to assist clinicians, nurses, physicians, and social workers when difficult case-specific treatment decisions must be made. To date, most of these issues are related to the end of life such as withdrawing treatment and whether or not to resuscitate. However, with the recent developments in reproductive medicine and genetics, the focus of ethics committees should be broadened to address issues related to creating life.

Besides case review, an ethics committee assumes educational responsibilities for its members, clinicians, patients, families, and the community in general. The content of education includes ethical conceptual frameworks, medical technology and its application, and ethical/legal implications such as brain death criteria and the right to refuse treatment legislation. The committee must also be aware of cultural and religious values that may affect both the physician's and the patient's decision making.

The third function of the ethics committee is related to policy development. Historically, the ethics committee is the group to formulate the policies for whether or not to resuscitate, refusal of treatment, and/or brain death policies.

Besides hospital ethics committees, many professional groups are now establishing their own ethics committees, for example, the American College of Obstetrics and Gynecology (ACOG) and the American Society for Reproductive Medicine (ASRM). The major focus of these groups is policy development. Recently, the ASRM developed a definition of pre-embryos and embryos. These definitions gave direction to the specialists: "Currently, the responsibility for establishing policies on the transfer or non-transfer of pre-embryos lies with the programs that offer medical assistance in reproduction" (Annas GJ, 1991).

Ethics committees have many advantages, but they also have some disadvantages. "As argued by Marsha D. Fowler, it is a serious mistake to perceive them (ethics committees) as the right hand of God working vengeance on the morally errant practitioner" (Hipps RS, 1992), but "the situation is one of health care professionals, as persons of good will, who are caught in the snare of complex moral dilemmas, resulting from technologic-scientific capability, a plurality of sociocultural and professional values and obligations, and the milieu of uncertainty that always attends health care and moral decision making" (Hipps RS, 1992).

In case reviews, an ethics committee can determine whether all relevant information is available, facilitate communication, clarify the ethical issues, assist in conflict resolution, provide staff support, and recommend other recourses as needed such as legal recourse. Richard S. Hipps identified additional advantages of an ethics committee (Table 11.3) (Hipps RS, 1992, pp. 165–166).

Some disadvantages of hospital ethics committees are associated with a concern about interfering in the physician-patient relationship, impingement on the physician's decision making, threats to confidentiality, and legal

TABLE 11.3. Ethics Committee Advantages

A core group of health care professionals is identified within an institution who are knowledgeable about medicolegal/ethical issues.

A forum for interdisciplinary dialogue related to ethical issues of patient care is established, which supports the concept of holistic care.

The patient becomes the focus of ethical dilemmas.

An objective body is established to consult on ethical issues and provide assistance to those in need during difficult decision-making times.

The gap is filled between societal values and the reality at the bedside.

The committee can act in a preventative capacity against litigation and crisis.

Hospital ethics committees project a good public image by communicating that all relevant factors related to patient care are taken into consideration.

Some third payers and governmental bodies are recommending the formation of hospital ethics committees for the above reasons and in an attempt to curtail runaway health care costs.

concerns. Pitfalls to which ethics committees can succumb include protecting the organization and/or becoming a rubber stamp review board. Also, the greater the decision-making responsibility, the greater the potential legal liability for the committee members and the institution. With careful attention to avoid these potential pitfalls, an ethics committee can be a wonderful resource for clinicians.

Historically, hospital ethics committees have focused on end-of-life issues. However, there is now a significant need to look at the moral and ethical issues associated with reproductive medicine. In this area of specialty the legal, moral, and ethical issues are just beginning to be discussed. There are few, if any, clear directives. Thus it is not surprising that

ACOG and ASRM were compelled to institute ethics committees to address the issues and to establish guidelines for the use of reproductive technology.

Case Example. One hospital in Boston has used an ethics committee as a forum to discuss issues surrounding the use of reproductive technology. Faulkner Hospital is a 250-bed community teaching hospital. Its ethics committee was a Board Committee as designated by the hospital bylaws. The committee was made up of its chairperson, two nurses, several physicians from the Department of Medicine, a surgeon, an emergency room physician, pastoral care representatives, two board members, and a representative from hospital administration. The committee's role and responsibility were as previously described: case review, education, and policy development.

When Faulkner established the Centre for Reproductive Medicine, its medical director suggested that hospital administration establish an ethics committee specifically to address issues associated with in vitro fertilization (IVF). The committee supported the request to create a subcommittee to specifically address the issues in reproductive medicine with the recommendation that a committee member from the hospital ethics committee be on the IVF subcommittee. This member would then periodically report to the hospital committee the issues discussed and any guidelines developed by the IVF ethics committee.

The IVF ethics committee consists of its chairman, the Medical Director of Reproductive Medicine, staff nurses, physiologists, several clergy, psychiatric staff, a social worker, an attorney, a hospital administration representative (also the representative from the hospital's ethics committee), a pediatrician, ethicists, and support staff within the Centre for Reproductive Medicine. The committee meets quarterly to address and discuss issues facing the staff. Issues related to gamete donation and preimplantation genetics have been the primary focus most recently. The IVF committee also continues the threefold function of case review, education, and policy development.

The committee discusses issues to determine criteria for appropriateness of donors and recipients and discussions about genetic history of potential donors. For example, should an individual with a family history of substance abuse, cardiac disease, or diabetes be eligible for gamete donation? Through these discussions, guidelines for gamete donation were developed.

Examples of other issues discussed included policies and procedures that were developed to protect confidentiality of donors. The committee has also considered what background information should be collected on the donor for future disclosure to the resulting donor offspring. All of these issues deal with the impact of reproductive technology versus the development of new or experimental technology. An institutional review board could not, and would not, appropriately address the issues facing the clinicians. However, a focused ethics subcommittee provides an appropriate forum to assess the impact of new medical technology on the patient and society and to suggest guidelines for its application.

The effectiveness of ethics committees, in general, has yet to be assessed. No one has been able to determine appropriate measures of effectiveness. However, in the case of this particular hospital, the depth of discussion in dealing with difficult questions concerning gamete donation, clinicians would describe the ethics committee as being extremely helpful in identifying relevant information for the discussion, differing points of view, the patient's perspective, and the potential legal issues.

As I stated earlier, there are still few legal or societal guidelines in reproductive medicine. However, the use of an ethics committee can be an excellent vehicle for identifying the issues and establishing guidelines surrounding this technology.

REFERENCES

1. Annas GJ. (1991) Ethics committees: From ethical comfort to ethical cover. Hastings Center Report 21(3):19, 20.
2. Gutteridge F, Bankowaski Z, Curran W, Dunne J. (1982) The structure and functioning of ethical review committees. Social Science Medicine 6:1796, 1798–1799.
3. Hipps RS. (1992) Are hospital ethics committees really necessary? J Medical Humanities 13(3):164, 165–166.
4. Jonsen AR. (1993) The birth of bioethics. Special Supplement, Hastings Center Report 23(6):51–54.

12

Egg Donation in Women Over the Age of Fifty

MARK V. SAUER, M.D.
RICHARD J. PAULSON, M.D.

INTRODUCTION

The practice of donating oocytes obtained from young women to treat infertile women with or without functioning ovaries has become a well-established method (Morris RA, Sauer MV, 1993; Sauer MV, Paulson RJ, 1992a). Similar to other assisted reproductive techniques, this treatment was originally intended for women under the age of 35. Early clinical trials of oocyte donation principally involved women with premature ovarian failure. However, over the past decade the age of recipients has progressively increased, and pregnancies have been established in women older than 40 (Pantos K, et al., 1993; Sauer MV, et al., 1993a) and, more recently, in women older than 50 (Sauer MV, et al., 1993a; Antinori S, et al., 1993). These reports substantiate the clinical observation that the uterus retains its receptivity for embryo implantation and development well beyond the age of natural menopause. In fact, it appears that as long as adequate doses of exogenously administered estrogen and progesterone are administered, the patient's chronologic age is unimportant in establishing pregnancy. Thus oocyte donation makes childbearing possible in virtually any woman with a normal functioning uterus (Seibel MM, Richards C, 1990). Considerable controversy has surrounded the application of assisted reproduction to older women. There is an ongoing debate as to whether a maximum age should be established beyond which women would be excluded from care. Since no definite physiologic limit exists to preclude pregnancies in recipients, restrictions would need to be imposed on the basis of the wisdom or ethics of extending care to the older population.

This chapter focuses on the evolution of oocyte donation as a method to treat age-related infertility and how it may be safely applied to women of advanced reproductive age. Attention is directed toward the actual screening of recipients. The obstetric outcomes following therapy are also profiled. Additionally discussed are the ethical issues surrounding the application of this method to older couples.

FACTORS RESPONSIBLE FOR INTRODUCING OOCYTE DONATION TO OLDER WOMEN

There are many reasons behind the increasing interest in fertility expressed by older patients. First, a shift in the population toward older individuals has occurred. The proportion of women between the age of 35 and 50 has significantly increased over the past decade

(Spencer G, 1984). Individuals whom the media have tagged "baby boomers" are starting to enter their fifties. Second, women often defer childbearing to fulfill educational and vocational pursuits. The availability of modern and effective measures of contraception has allowed women to plan their families through gaining control over reproduction. Divorce, which is more prevalent today than in the past, also influences the age of women attempting to conceive. Following the dissolution of a marriage and subsequent remarriage, many women are faced with beginning new families. However, since fecundity decreases with age, these individuals may be unpleasantly surprised as they encounter difficulties in conceiving with their new spouse. Finally, oocyte donation has received tremendous media attention. Older individuals are now well-educated about assisted reproductive methods. In our experience, most women presenting for fertility care over the age of 40 are self-referred. Thus a combination of changing demographics and a newly developed successful method of treatment is responsible for producing increasing numbers of patients.

NATURAL FERTILITY IN THE PERIMENOPAUSE

Fertility rates in natural populations begin to fail after age 30 and demonstrate a steep decline in live births after 35 (Maroulis GB, 1991). By 50 years of age, fertility potential is reduced to less than 0.5% of that noted for women during the third decade of life. However, despite low fecundity rates, spontaneous conceptions still occur. Approximately one in 10,000 live births are to mothers over 50 (Office of Population Censuses and Surveys, 1991a, 1991b). Unfortunately, a high degree of pregnancy wastage also occurs during this period of reproductive life. Spontaneous abortions are expected in 30–50% of all clinical

pregnancies in older mothers following assisted reproduction procedures, most of these losses being attributed to aneuploidy (Lauritsen JG, 1976). Anomalies in live births are also increased. For example, whereas the incidence of Down syndrome is less than one per 1,000 live births in mothers aged 25, the risk rises to as high as 150 per 1,000 live births by the age of 50 (Hook EB, 1981).

It appears that a state of "reproductive menopause" exists approximately ten years before the actual cessation of menses. This transition has been termed the "perimenopause," and during this time, traditional therapies designed to enhance fertility potential have a substantially decreased likelihood of success. This is evident in the clinical and ongoing pregnancy rates of women over the age of 40 undergoing in vitro fertilization (Table 12.1) (Medical Research International and the American Fertility Society Special Interest Group, 1990, 1991, 1992; Society for Assisted Reproductive Technology, 1993). Live birth rates following assisted reproduction in this group are generally less than 10%. Furthermore, the majority of these pregnancies occur in the relatively younger women whose age is nearer to 40. Essentially no data exists for

TABLE 12.1. Performance of Women 40 Years and Older Undergoing In Vitro Fertilization in the United States as Reported Annually to the National Registry of the American Fertility Society

Year	No. ET	Clinical Pregnancies*	Deliveries
1988	198	20 (10%)	8 (4%)
1989	287	34 (12%)	16 (6%)
1990	350	38 (11%)	23 (7%)
1991	1970	270 (14%)	181 (9%)

ET = embryo transfer.

*Percentage of pregnancies per actual transfer attempt.

pregnancy success following assisted reproduction in women beyond 45, and few if any patients would be candidates for therapy using their own oocytes by the age of 50.

It appears that evolution has precluded most women from reproducing after age 40 and certainly by the age of 50. Unlike the ovaries of other mammals, the human ovary has essentially exhausted its supply of oocytes by the time menopause occurs. Fewer than 0.001% of the original ovarian complement of oocytes are ever ovulated. The majority of oocytes and their follicles are destined to be lost to atresia (Gosden RG, 1987). Histologic studies indicate that by the time one reaches menopause, most individuals have only a few thousand oocytes remaining (Block E, 1952). In general, these gametes are not recruited and follicular development is not observed, regardless of the level of gonadotropin used to induce ovulation. There is also a sharp decline in follicular mass with advancing age, suggesting that an accelerated rate of follicular atresia occurs during the final decade before menopause (Richardson SJ, et al., 1987). Furthermore, the declining pool of available primordial follicles from which to recruit eggs for ovulation is also accompanied by a decreasing absolute number of growing follicles (Gosden RG, 1987).

Animal studies suggest that the mammalian uterus undergoes age-related changes that are detrimental to reproduction. Both implantation and pregnancy rates are decreased in older animals (Werner MA, et al., 1991), even if transferred embryos are obtained from younger animals and placed into older females (Holinka CF, et al., 1979). Older females are essentially unable to achieve pregnancy. In addition, the number of implantation sites per animal and the proportion of animals noted to have any implantation decline significantly with age (Harman SM, Talbert GB, 1970).

Other factors may also influence the relationship between the early conceptus and the endometrial environment. These include the rate and normal pattern of development of ova in the older female reproductive tract, the delayed uterine sensitivity to blastocysts and implantation secondary to decreased capacity of older uterine tissue to take up steroids, and the less efficient uterine response to a decidualizing stimulus as seen in the mouse, rat, and hamster (Werner MA, et al., 1991). Thus an age-related decline in fertility as the result of a uterine factor appears to exist in rodents as evidenced by infertility, implantation failure, and prenatal mortality (Thorneycroft IH, Soderwall AL, 1969; Talbert GB, Krohn PL, 1966; Maibenco HC, Krehbiel RH, 1973).

Similar arguments for an age-related decline in human fertility due to a "uterine factor" have been proffered (Levran D, et al., 1991; Meldrum DR, 1993). The best measure of uterine receptivity results from comparing individual embryo implantation rates in humans of various ages undergoing in vitro fertilization and embryo transfer. Women under 30 can experience implantation rates as high as 20% per embryo transferred, whereas implantation rates in women aged 36 and older are typically closer to 9%. After the age of 40, individual embryo implantation rates are usually less that 5% (Wood C, et al., 1992). It is known that uterine blood flow decreases in association with declining levels of estradiol (deZiegler D, et al., 1991; Goswamy RK, et al., 1988). This naturally occurs during the menopause and may therefore adversely affect the local uterine environment. The identification of estrogen receptors in the wall of the uterine artery further supports this hypothesis (Perrot-Applanat M, et al., 1988). Fibrotic changes are visible in the walls of the uterine arterial musculature (Sauer MV, et al., 1993b) that may further accentuate these physiologic changes by interfering with local blood flow.

Finally, approximately half of spontaneously aborted pregnancies are chromosomally normal, suggesting that local endomyometrial factors are responsible for the losses. Whether this is a primary target organ effect or secondary to the aging corpus luteum's inability to support a pregnancy remains unknown (Blaha GC, 1970).

Oocyte and embryo donation to older women using gametes obtained from younger individuals provides an ideal opportunity to study the contribution of each of these two variables independent of the other. Formerly, it was not possible to dissociate the impact of the gamete from the influence of the local endometrial environment on the normal development of the early embryo. When adequate hormone replacement is provided, endometria developing in menopausal women between 40 and 60 years of age demonstrate a normal histologic, ultrasonographic, and steroid receptor response (Sauer MV, et al., 1993b). Endometrial samples taken from younger women with ovarian failure receiving a hormone replacement regimen are indistinguishable from those of older women using the same hormone replacement. Thus it appears that if adequate amounts of exogenous estrogen and progesterone are provided, most uteri respond with normal endometrial morphology, regardless of age. Further testimony to the adequacy of this newly generated environment is the high rate of implantation and delivery observed in women of advanced reproductive age undergoing oocyte donation (Sauer MV, et al., 1992; Flamigni C, et al., 1993). Implantation, clinical pregnancy, and delivery rates have been four to five times higher than those experienced by patients of the same age using their own gametes (Table 12.2). More important, women over the age of 50 are highly unlikely to successfully conceive using assisted reproductive techniques and autologous oocytes.

DEVELOPMENT OF OOCYTE AND EMBRYO DONATION AND ITS APPLICATION TO MENOPAUSAL WOMEN

The transfer of preimplantation embryos conceived either in vitro or in vivo from one female to another has been successfully performed in over a dozen different mammals (Sauer MV, 1993). The method was first demonstrated in the rabbit 100 years ago and subsequently perfected by the animal husbandry business to revolutionize cattle breeding (Seidel GE, 1981). Modifications of the uterine lavage technique practiced in animals led to the establishment of the first embryo donation pregnancy in humans in 1983 (Bustillo JE, et al., 1984). Simultaneous attempts at embryo donation using in vitro fertilized oocytes donated by women undergoing controlled ovarian hyperstimulation resulted in a live birth in 1984 (Lutjen P, et al., 1989). Table 12.3 highlights the early results of several centers using a variety of transfer techniques (Sauer MV, et al., 1988; Sauer MV, Paulson RJ, 1990; Borrero C, et al., 1989; Abdulla HI, et al., 1989; Rotsztejn DA, et al., 1990).

As more and more pregnancies became established in hypergonadotropic-hypogonadal women receiving sex steroid replacement, the demand for oocyte donation services increased. By 1989, reports of successful pregnancies in menopausal women beyond the age normally attributed to "premature" had been published (Sauer MV, et al., 1990; Serhal PF, Craft IL, 1989). There was an initial reluctance to transfer embryos to women over the age of 40 based on the belief that the aforementioned "uterine factor" existed in aging animals and that embryo donation to "older" women would result in markedly decreased implantation rates. Delivery rates were ex-

TABLE 12.2.   Results of the Transfer of Fertilized Donor Ova in Women 40 Years of Age and Older with Ovarian Failure Compared with Women under 40 Years of Age with Ovarian Failure and Women 40 Years of Age and Older Undergoing Standard In Vitro Fertilization and Embryo Transfer

	≥40 Years Old with Donor IVF	<40 Years Old with Donor IVF	≥40 Years Old with Standard IVF
Recipients	65	35	57
Cycles	93	46	79
Oocytes per recipient (mean±SD)	15.2±9.0	15.3±6.8	6.7±4.1*
Fertilized oocytes/oocyte retrieved (fertilization rate %)	48.2	62.0	39.2
Transfer cycles	86	43	70
Embryos transferred per cycle, (mean±SD)	4.4±1.0	4.7±0.7	2.9±1.2**
Implantation rate per transferred embryo (%)	19.7	15.9	4.8*
95% confidence interval	16.1, 24.5	11.1, 21.7	2.3, 8.7
Ratio of clinical pregnancies per transfer attempt, n (%)	34/86 (39.5)	14/43 (32.6)	8/70 (11.4)
95% confidence limits	29.2, 50.7	19.1, 48.5	5.1, 21.3
Ratio of ongoing pregnancies per transfer, n (%)	29/86 (33.7)	13/43 (30.2)	6/70 (8.6)
95% confidence limits	23.9, 44.7	17.2, 46.1	3.2, 17.7

IVF = in vitro fertilization.

*$P < 0.05$ comparing women 40 years of age and older undergoing standard IVF with either group undergoing oocyte donation.

**$P < 0.05$ comparing women under 40 years of age undergoing oocyte donation and either group of women 40 years of age and older. Confidence limits determined by binomial distribution.

TABLE 12.3.   Early Attempts at Oocyte and Embryo Donation for Treatment of Premature Menopause

Investigator	Method	No. Cycles	No. Clinical Pregnancies
Sauer/Buster	Uterine lavage	90	4
Sauer	IVF	26	16
Borrero	GIFT	19	11
Abdulla	ZIFT	10	4
Rotsztejn	TET	11	9

TABLE 12.4. Egg Donation in Women Over Age 40

Investigator	Age Range (years)	Replacement Protocol*	Clinical Preg Rate (%)
Serhal and Craft	42–47	E2 Valerate/P-IM or oral P	36.5
Abdulla	40–44	E2 Valerate/P-Supp or P-IM	18.2
	45–49		9.1
Pantos	40–54	E2 Valerate/P-Supp	31.7
Navot	40–45	E2 transdermal/P-IM	14.7
Sauer	40–55	Micronized E2/P-IM	34.5

*E2 = estradiol; P = progesterone; IM = intramuscular; Supp = vaginal suppository.

pected to be further compromised by an anticipated high rate of miscarriage. Remarkably, trials of oocyte donation among women in their forties exhibited similar implantation and pregnancy rates, favorable obstetrical results, and reduced miscarriage rates compared to younger recipients (Table 12.4) (Abdulla HI, et al., 1990; Navot D, et al., 1991).

Following the reported successes of women in their forties, an increasing number of women over 50 began requesting oocyte donation. At the University of Southern California a protocol similar to that used for women in their forties demonstrated that a functional endometrium could be induced in patients in their fifties (Sauer MV, et al., 1993b). This was followed by an attempt at oocyte donation (Sauer MV, et al., 1993a). Of fourteen couples who passed the original screening, nine achieved pregnancy. Only one

pregnancy was lost, resulting in a clinical pregnancy rate of 38%. Since publication of this preliminary series, more women have been enrolled for study. Current published results of oocyte donation to women over the age of fifty are listed in Table 12.5. This experience suggests that embryo implantation and pregnancy rates parallel those seen in younger women. Thus uterine receptivity is retained well beyond natural menopause.

DEMOGRAPHICS OF WOMEN SEEKING OOCYTE DONATION

Demographic differences exist between older aged recipients and women with premature ovarian failure (Table 12.6) (Sauer MV,

TABLE 12.5. Published Pregnancies in Women Over the Age of 50

Investigator	No. Patients	No. ET	Implantation Rate	Clinical Pregnancy Rate	Delivery Rate
Sauer	14	21	19%	8/21 (38%)	7/21 (33%)
Antinori	11	11	11%	4/11 (36%)	3/11 (27%)
Flamigni	10	14	10%	4/14 (29%)	4/14 (29%)

TABLE 12.6. **Comparing Demographics of Recipients with Respect to Age**

	<30 Years Old	30–39 Years Old	40–49 Years Old	50–60 Years Old
Age of patient (mean years)	27.7	35.2	43.9	52.4
Age of spouse (mean years)	30.4	36.9	43.8	45.6
Years married	4.8	5.2	5.7	8.3
Remarried (%)	0.0	10.1	54.2*	66.6*
Parity	0.1	0.1	0.6	2.2*
Anonymous (%)	47.2	63.7	80.0*	80.8*
Foreign national (%)	0.0	6.8	1.8	11.1*
Elective abortions (%)	12.5	15.3	28.0*	5.6
Cosmetic surgery (%)	0.0	3.4	37.4*	33.3*
Infertility surgery (%)	0.0	16.9	34.6*	16.7
History ART[†] (%)	0.0	33.9*	38.3*	5.5

*$p < 0.05$.

[†]ART = assisted reproductive technologies.

Paulson RJ, 1992b). In general, older recipients are more likely to be divorced and remarried, to have been pregnant previously, and to have undergone an elective termination of pregnancy. Older individuals are more prone to choose the anonymous form of oocyte donation and usually have had little if any exposure to assisted reproductive care. Both husband and wife are usually employed in a full-time vocation and are often professionally educated. A large minority have undergone cosmetic surgery, usually in an attempt to maintain a youthful appearance.

WHY ARE WOMEN IN THEIR FIFTIES SEEKING OOCYTE DONATION?

There are as many reasons for women to seek treatment as there are individuals. In many instances, oocyte donation represents the first real opportunity to benefit from any assisted reproductive technique. For example, individuals who were 35 years of age in 1978 and were found to have irreparable tubal disease were considered sterile. These same individuals would have been 40 years of age in 1983 and rejected by many IVF programs on the basis of poor success rates among women of advanced reproductive age. Finally, by 1993, when these individuals were 50 years old, it became possible for them to attempt oocyte donation. Ironically, these patients' chances for successfully conceiving now are better than they were at either of the earlier times.

In other cases the woman has remarried and wishes to provide her new (and frequently younger) spouse with a child. Fifty percent of the women who were initially screened were grandmothers, having had children with a previous husband. In each of these cases the new spouse had never fathered a child. It is obvious that women who have raised children to adulthood during a previous marriage are well aware of the rigors of child rearing.

In other cases, individuals married late in life and never had an opportunity to conceive because of age-related infertility. Our oldest pregnant patient, a woman delivering at the age of 56, fits this description. She was married at 48 to a man who had never fathered a child.

She experienced menopause at age 52. Nine months after her first attempt at oocyte donation, she delivered a healthy baby boy.

STEPS INVOLVED IN THE SCREENING AND PREPARATION OF RECIPIENTS

Screening of candidates for oocyte donation has focused on evaluating their overall health. Of concern are the obstetrical risks of older mothers (Cunningham FG, Leveno KJ, 1989). Tests characterizing cardiovascular health are important, since the stress of pregnancy on the heart is known to be significant. Baseline assessments include tests for diabetes, hyperlipidemia, and exercise tolerance. A generalized search for occult malignancies is undertaken. A number of cancers, including those of the breast, uterus, and cervix, have been discovered. Table 12.7 lists the surveillance screens that are employed at the University of Southern California.

The reproductive potentials of men and women who are interested in oocyte donation are also ascertained. In the male this includes a routine semen analysis and semen culture. Tests of sperm function utilizing the hamster penetration assay are performed for men who have not previously proven fertility. Women must undertake an evaluation of the uterine cavity that includes a hysterosalpingogram, transvaginal ultrasound examination, and an endometrial biopsy.

Several different hormone replacement regimens have been used with success in establishing pregnancy (Sauer MV, 1991). Most commonly, oral estradiol, in either micronized or valerate form, is prescribed. Delivery may be provided in sequential step-up fashion to mimic the natural fluctuations that occur in serum estradiol or as a fixed continuous dose (Leeton J, et al., 1991). Pregnancy rates are not different for the two methods. Synchronization with the donor is typically undertaken, the recipient beginning medications four to five days in advance of the donor's injecting gonadotropin (Figure 12.1). Estrogen may also be delivered transdermally with good results (Steingold KA, et al., 1991). Progesterone is needed to induce secretory changes and to decidualize the endometrium in preparation for embryo implantation. Most commonly, intramuscular progesterone has been used. Al-

TABLE 12.7. Prescreening Examination of Patients Over Age 50 Before Embryo Donation

Medical	Infectious Disease (Both Partners)
Stress treadmill electrocardiography	HIV
Mammography	Syphilis
Chest Radiography	Hepatitis screen
Oral glucose tolerance test	
Fasting insulin	**Reproductive Factors**
Fasting cholesterol and blood lipoproteins	Transvaginal ultrasonography of pelvis
Chemistry panel	Endometrial biopsy on hormone replacement
Prothrombin time/partial thromboplastin time	Semen culture
Thyroid-stimulating hormone	Semen analysis
Blood count with platelets	Hamster egg penetration test (HEPT)
Cervical smear (Pap)	

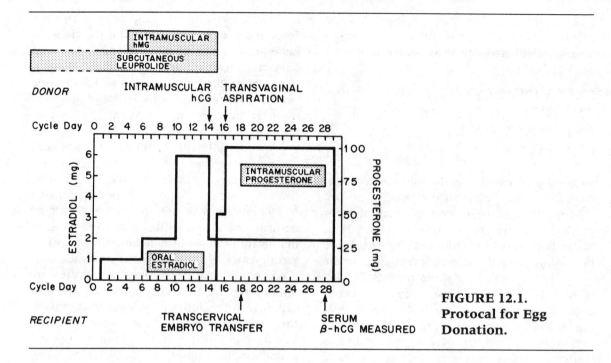

**FIGURE 12.1.
Protocal for Egg
Donation.**

ternative regimens using suppositories or encapsulated micronized progesterone have also resulted in pregnancies.

Morphologic analysis of endometrial biopsies taken from women using these formulations have defined certain unique characteristics (Sauer MV, et al., 1991). Biopsies obtained on the twenty-first day of the artificial cycle (midluteal) typically demonstrate a slight delay in maturation in the glandular compartment. This occurs in 15–25% of samples. If the endometria of these same patients are resampled later (day 26–28), biopsies are most commonly in phase. This implies a "catch-up" phenomenon. Transvaginal ultrasound images on the twenty-first day of the cycle usually denote a full thickness lining of approximately 10 mm. Receptors for progesterone and estrogen are likewise characteristic of luteal endometria. A "practice transfer" using embryo transfer catheters is performed at the time of

the biopsy to ascertain the length and contour of the endometrial cavity. This ensures that a transcervical embryo transfer can be easily accomplished at a later date.

OBSTETRICAL MANAGEMENT AND DELIVERY

It is likely that 25–50% of women undertaking embryo donation will experience pregnancy. Since women over the age of 35 are generally considered to be high-risk obstetrical patients, it is reasonable to assume that all women beyond the natural menopause are at equally high risk. Further complicating care is the fact that 20–35% of established pregnancies are multiple gestations.

It is important to visualize the early pregnancy using transvaginal ultrasound. Supernumerary implantation sites commonly occur and may or may not develop normally. Often, abnormal implantations occur adjacent to a normally developing embryo. These abnormal sacs eventually collapse and occasionally bleed, causing tremendous anxiety, but rarely result in a miscarriage. Patients are maintained on hormone replacement through the first fourteen weeks of gestation, following which time it appears safe to discontinue medications (Devroey P, et al., 1990; Schneider MA, et al., 1993). We have arbitrarily assigned a serum through level of 30 ng/mL for progesterone as the criterion for discontinuing medications at that time. Serial measurements of estradiol and progesterone are not useful, since the prescribed regimen results in pharmacologic levels of these steroids.

Delayed childbearing is associated with adverse perinatal outcomes, as was recently reported by the Swedish Medical Birth Registry (Cnattingius S, et al., 1992). A summary of the obstetrical experience of 173,715 nulliparous Nordic women aged twenty years and older revealed that mothers over the age of 40 experience a 1.5–2-fold increased risk for growth retardation, preterm labor, and late fetal and early neonatal deaths. Stillbirth rates also rose sharply after the age of 40. Women older than 35 are also known to be at high risk for developing gestational diabetes, hypertension, preterm labor, and growth retardation (Naeye RL, 1983; Kirz DS, et al., 1985).

Table 12.8 reports the obstetrical outcomes of women 50 years of age or older who successfully conceived in our program. Although antenatal complications were commonly experienced, most developed secondary to multiple gestations. A tendency toward gestational hypertension may exist, although results are too preliminary to know whether this phenomenon will persist. Once pregnancy is es-

TABLE 12.8. Obstetrical Outcome of 15 Consecutive Pregnancies to Women Age 50 Years or Older

	No. (%)	Mean + SD*	Range
Age (years)		52.3±2.1	50–56
Nulliparous	8/15 (53%)		
Gestational age at delivery (weeks)	37.2±2.7		32–41
Birth weight (grams)†	2912.7±908		1800–4680
Multiple gestations	7/15 (47%) (6 twins, 1 triplet)		
Cesarean section	10/15 (67%)		
Complications	8/15 patients		
Gestational hypertension	7		
Gestational diabetes	2		
Pre-eclampsia	1		
Premature labor	3		

*SD = standard deviation.
†Not adjusted for multiple gestations.

tablished, referral to fetal maternal medicine specialists is important for monitoring both diabetes and early signs of hypertension. Serial ultrasound assessments provide evidence of fetal growth retardation. Late occurring complications, particularly stillbirth, may best be avoided by an aggressive approach to delivery. With full knowledge of the gestational age of these patients, attempts at inducing labor near term (38+ weeks) should be considered judicious. A stillbirth has been reported in one 43-year-old woman who was allowed to carry her pregnancy beyond term (Sauer MV, Paulson RJ, 1991).

A QUESTION OF REPRODUCTIVE CHOICE: WHEN IS TOO OLD TOO OLD?

Therapy for infertility joins a growing group of medical interventions that are now offered to older individuals on a limited basis. In considering each case, risks are assessed and weighed against the potential benefits in making a final decision. Controversy has surrounded whether the decision to proceed with oocyte donation poses unacceptable risks. In weighing the arguments for and against treatment the potential benefit of therapy should be viewed from the perspective of the recipient. Women whose ovaries do not produce viable oocytes, regardless of their chronologic age, have no option for achieving pregnancy without the use of donated oocytes. Most women over the age of 50 technically fall into this group. A restriction of oocyte donation inherently means a restriction of reproductive choice (Seibel MM, 1992; Seibel MM, et al., 1994).

It is undeniable that on an actuarial basis, life expectancy at the age of 50 is less than that at 35. However, the life expectancy of a healthy woman at 50 is certainly of adequate duration to allow her time to raise a child to adulthood. Throughout history, men have been able to father children essentially without any age barriers. No societal taboos or reproaches await fathers even in their seventies. The fact that such arguments have now arisen regarding women who want to become mothers in their fifties underscores the gender bias of our society toward parenting.

It has been suggested that the relationship between a child and parents who are over the age of 50 may be associated with an increased "generation gap." This implies that older parents are less capable of coping with the physical and psychological stress of parenting. However, such arguments are pure speculation and simply indicate the need for consideration of this issue by the prospective parents before undergoing oocyte donation. It is not uncommon for children who lose parents as a result of injury or illness to be raised by grandparents whose chronologic age would in most instances approximate that of these older individuals. In fact, in many cultures, grandparents traditionally assume the bulk of the responsibility for raising their children's children. The wisdom and maturity of these older individuals may be quite advantageous to the offspring. As our demographic analysis indicates, older couples certainly have the financial resources and in general more time to spend with their families during this time of their life.

Individuals should be able to seek help and have available to them the full spectrum of medical treatment that is available to society at large. As with any new form of therapy, the exact risks and long-term consequences of oocyte donation to women of advanced reproductive age remain unknown. Accordingly, this method should be applied under carefully controlled protocols, preferably approved by institutional review boards. Establishment of reasonable guidelines (The American Society for Reproductive Medicine, 1994), rather than absolute rules, regarding any form of medical therapy should be based on scientific knowledge and governed by peer review.

FUTURE CONSIDERATIONS

The widespread application of oocyte donation to increasing numbers of women of advanced reproductive age is inevitable. Despite attempts in several countries to limit or even prohibit oocyte donation, it is unlikely that legislative bodies in the United States will restrict such therapy. Increasing numbers of women in their forties and now in their fifties are seeking fertility care in this country. For many of these biologically older women, oocyte donation represents the only true hope for motherhood as use of their own gametes is essentially doomed to failure and adoption is rarely permitted.

Vigilant surveillance is imperative in the screening of all these individuals. To maximize success, a thorough health assessment is mandatory. It should be expected that occasional abnormalities will be discovered. Some problems may preclude an attempt at oocyte donation. In other cases, discovered ailments should be defined but will remain relative contraindications. Medical screening necessitates a primary care approach by the fertility specialist and the development of discriminatory criteria from which to practice.

Concerns that have been raised regarding the potential harm to "the fabric of society" by allowing older individuals the opportunity to become parents seems unfounded. The demand for oocyte donation in women over the age of 50 has recently increased. However, when the number of these pregnancies is compared to those occurring in the population at large, the numerical contribution is minimal. Typically, in countries where oocyte donation is restricted, no similar laws exist placing age limits on males or regulating the use of donated sperm to procreate. Precluding healthy women from availing themselves of a successful alternative for reproduction while allowing men access to fertility care should be considered sexist and prejudicial. We believe that, as is true in most cases of social evolution, with increasing numbers of accumulated cases it is likely that acceptance will follow.

REFERENCES

1. Abdulla HI, Baber RJ, Kirkland A, Leonard T, Studd JWW. (1989) Pregnancy in women with premature ovarian failure using tubal and intrauterine transfer of cryopreserved zygotes. Br J Obstet Gynecol 96:1071–1075.
2. Abdulla HI, Baber R, Kirkland A, Leonard T, Power M, Studd JWW. (1990) A report on 100 cycles of oocyte donation: Factors affecting the outcome. Hum Reprod 5:1018–1022.
3. Antinori S, Versaci C, Gholami GH, Panci C, Caffa B. (1993) Oocyte donation in menopausal women. Hum Reprod 8:1487–1489.
4. Blaha GC. (1970) The influence of ovarian grafts upon young donors on the development of transferred ova in aged golden hamsters. Fertil Steril 21:268–273.
5. Block E. (1952) Quantitative morphological investigation of the follicular system in women: Variations at different ages. Acta Anat (Basel) 14:108.
6. Borrero C, Remohi J, Ord T, Balmaceda JS, Rojas F, Asch RH. (1989) A program of oocyte donation and gamete intra-fallopian transfer. Hum Reprod 4:275–279
7. Bustillo JE, Buster JE, Cohen S, Thorneycroft IH, Simon JA, Boyers SP, Marshall JR, Seed RW, Louw JA, Seed RG. (1984) Nonsurgical ovum transfer as a treatment of infertile women: Preliminary experience. JAMA 251:1171–1173.
8. Cnattingius S, Forman MR, Heinz WB, Isotalo L. (1992) Delayed childbearing and risk of adverse perinatal outcome. JAMA 268:886–890.
9. Cunningham FG, Leveno KJ. (1989) Pregnancy after 35. In: Cunningham FG, MacDonald PC, Gant NF, eds. Williams Obstetrics, 18th edition, Suppl 2, pp. 1–12.
10. Devroey P, Camus M, Palermo G, Smitz J, Van

Waesberghe L, Wisanto A, Wijbo I, Van Steirteghem AC. (1990) Placental production of estradiol and progesterone after oocyte donation in patients with primary ovarian failure. Am J Obstet Gynecol 162:66–70.

11. deZiegler D, Bessis R, Frydman R. (1991) Vascular resistance of uterine arteries: Physiological effects of estradiol and progesterone. Fertil Steril 55:755–779.

12. Flamigni C, Borini A, Violini F, Bianchi L, Serrao L. (1993) Oocyte donation: Comparison between recipients from different age groups. Hum Reprod 8:2088–2092.

13. Gosden RG. (1987) Follicular status at the menopause. Hum Reprod 2:617–721.

14. Goswamy RK, Williams G, Steptoe PC. (1988) Decreased uterine perfusion: A cause of infertility. Hum Reprod 3:955–959.

15. Harman SM, Talbert GB. (1970) The effect of maternal age on ovulation, corpora lutea of pregnancy and implantation failure in mice. J Reprod Fertil 23:33–39.

16. Holinka CF, Yueh-Chu T, Caleb EF. (1979) Reproductive aging in C57B2/6J mice: Plasma progesterone, viable embryos and resorption frequency throughout pregnancy. Biol Reprod 20:1201–1211.

17. Hook EB. (1981) Rates of chromosomal abnormalities at different maternal ages. Obstet Gynecol 58:282–285.

18. Kirz DS, Dorchester W, Freeman RK. (1985) Advanced maternal age: The mature gravida. Am J Obstet Gynecol 152:7–12.

19. Lauritsen JG. (1976) Aetiology of spontaneous abortions: A cytogenetic and epidemiologic study of 288 abortuses and their parents. Acta Obstet Gynecol Scand 52:282–285.

20. Leeton J, Rogers P, King C, Healy D. (1991) A comparison of pregnancy rates for 131 donor oocyte transfers using either a sequential or fixed regime of steroid replacement therapy. Hum Reprod 6:299–301.

21. Levran D, Ben-Shlomo I, Dor J, Ben-Rafael Z, Nebel L, Mashiach S. (1991) Aging of endometrium and oocytes: Observations on conception and abortion rates in an egg donation model. Fertil Steril 56:1091–1094.

22. Lutjen P, Trounson A, Leeton J, Findlay J, Wood C, Renou P. (1989) The establishment and maintenance of pregnancy using in vitro fertilization and embryo donation in a patient with primary ovarian failure. Nature 307:174–175.

23. Maibenco HC, Krehbiel RH. (1973) Reproduc-

tive decline in aged female rats. J Reprod Fertil 32:121–123.

24. Maroulis GB. (1991) Effect of aging on fertility and pregnancy. Semin Reprod Endocrinol 9:165–175.

25. Medical Research International and the American Fertility Society Special Interest Group. (1990) In vitro fertilization/embryo transfer in the United States: 1988 results from the National IVF/ET Registry. Fertil Steril 53:13–20.

26. Medical Research International and the American Fertility Society Special Interest Group. (1991) In vitro fertilization/embryo transfer in the United States: 1989 results from the National IVF/ET Registry. Fertil Steril 55:14–23.

27. Medical Research International and the American Fertility Society Special Interest Group. (1992) In vitro fertilization/embryo transfer in the United States: 1990 results from the National IVF/ET Registry. Fertil Steril 57:14–23.

28. Meldrum DR. (1993) Female reproductive aging: Ovarian and uterine factors. Fertil Steril 59:1–5.

29. Morris RA, Sauer MV. (1993) Oocyte donation in the 1990s and beyond. Asst Reprod Rev 3:211–217.

30. Naeye RL. (1983) Maternal age, obstetric complications, and the outcome of pregnancy. Obstet Gynecol 61:210–216.

31. Navot D, Bergh PA, Williams MA, Garrisi GJ, Guzman I, Sandler B, Grunfeld L. (1991) Poor oocyte quality rather than implantation failure as a cause of age related decline in female fertility. Lancet 337:1375–1377.

32. Office of Population Censuses and Surveys: (1991a) Abortion Statistics 1990, Series AB No. 17. London: HM Stationery Office.

33. Office of Population Censuses and Surveys: (1991b) Birth Statistics 1990, Series Fm 1 No. 19. London: HM Stationery Office.

34. Pantos K, Meimeti-Damianaki T, Vaxevanoglou T, Kapetanakis E. (1993) Oocyte donation in menopausal women aged over 40 years. Hum Reprod 8:488–491.

35. Perrot-Applanat M, Groyer-Picart MT, Garcia E, Lorenzo F, Milgram E. (1988) Immunocytochemical demonstration of estrogen and progesterone receptors in muscle cells of uterine arteries in rabbits and humans. Endocrinology 123:1511–1519.

36. Richardson SJ, Senikas V, Nelson JF. (1987) Follicular-accelerated loss and ultimate exhaustion. J Clin Endocrinol Metab 65:1231–1237.

37. Rotsztejn DA, Remohi J, Weckstein LN, Ord T,

Moyer DL, Balmaceda JP, Asch RJ. (1990) Results of tubal embryo transfer in premature ovarian failure. Fertil Steril 54:348–350.

38. Sauer MV. (1991) Hormone replacement prior to embryo donation to women with ovarian failure. Female Patient 16:51–60.

39. Sauer MV. (1993) Current status of oocyte donation. Contemp Obstet Gynecol 38:49–60.

40. Sauer MV, Paulson RJ. (1990) Human oocyte and preembryo donation: An evolving method for the treatment of infertility. Am J Obstet Gynecol 163:1421–1424.

41. Sauer MV, Paulson RJ. (1991) Consecutive pregnancies in a menopausal woman following oocyte donation. Gynecol Obstet Invest 32:118–120.

42. Sauer MV, Paulson RJ. (1992a) Understanding the current status of oocyte donation in the United States. Fertil Steril 58:16–18.

43. Sauer MV, Paulson RJ. (1992b) Demographic differences between younger and older recipients seeking oocyte donation. J Assist Reprod Genet 9:400–402.

44. Sauer MV, Bustillo M, Gorrill MJ, Louw J, Marshall JR, Buster JE. (1988) An instrument for the recovery of preimplantation uterine ova. Obstet Gynecol 71:804–806.

45. Sauer MV, Paulson RJ, Lobo RA. (1990) A preliminary report on oocyte donation extending reproductive potential to women over 40. N Engl J Med 323:1157.

46. Sauer MV, Stein A, Paulson RJ, Moyer D. (1991) Endometrial responses to various hormone replacement regimens in ovarian failure patients preparing for embryo donation. Int J Gynecol Obstet 35:61–68.

47. Sauer MV, Paulson RJ, Lobo RA. (1992) Reversing the natural decline in human fertility. JAMA 268:1275–1279.

48. Sauer MV, Paulson RJ, Lobo RA. (1993a) Pregnancy after age 50: Application of oocyte donation to women after natural menopause. Lancet 341:321–323.

49. Sauer MV, Miles RA, Paulson RJ, Press M, Moyer D. (1993b) Evaluating the effect of age on endometrial responsiveness to hormone replacement therapy: A histologic, ultrasonographic and tissue receptor analysis. J Asst Reprod Genet 10:47–52.

50. Schneider MA, Davies MC, Honour JW. (1993) The timing of placental competence in pregnancy after oocyte donation. Fertil Steril 59:1059–1064.

51. Seibel MM. (1992) To everything there is a season. Contemp OBGYN 37:153.

52. Seibel MM, Richards C. (1990) Hysterectomy in benign conditions: A procedure of the past? Lancet 335:600–601.

53. Seibel MM, Zilberstein M, Seibel S. (1994) Becoming parents after 100? Lancet 43:603.

54. Seidel GE, Jr. (1981) Superovulation and embryo transfer in cattle. Science 211:351–356.

55. Serhal PF, Craft IL. (1989) Oocyte donation in 61 patients. Lancet 1:1185–97.

56. Society for Assisted Reproductive Technology. (1993) Assisted reproductive technology in the United States: 1991 results for assisted reproductive technology generated from the American Fertility Society registry. Fertil Steril 59:956–962.

57. Spencer G. (1984) Projections of the population of the United States by age, sex, race: 1983–2080. Current Population Reports: Population Estimates and Projections. Washington D.C.: U.S. Department of Commerce, May 1984 (series p 25, no. 952).

58. Steingold KA, Matt DW, deZiegler D, Sealey JE, Fratkin M, Rexnikov F. (1991) Comparison of transdermal to oral estradiol administration on hormonal and hepatic parameters in women with premature ovarian failure. J Clin Endocrin Metab 73:275–280.

59. Talbert GB, Krohn PL. (1966) Effect of maternal age on viability of ova and uterine support of pregnancy in mice. J Reprod Fert 11:399–406.

60. The American Fertility Society (Sauer MV, Schmidt-Sarosi CL, Quigley MM). (1994) Guidelines for oocyte donation. Fertil Steril 59:5s–9s.

61. Thorneycroft IH, Soderwall AL. (1969) The nature of the litter size loss in senescent hamster. Anat Rec 165:343.

62. Werner MA, Barnhard J, Gordon JW. (1991) The effects of aging on sperm and oocytes. Semin Reprod Endocrinol 9:231–240.

63. Wood C, Calderon I, Crombie A. (1992) Age and fertility: Results of assisted reproductive technology in women over 40 years. J Asst Reprod Genet 9:482–484.

13

Religious Views Regarding Gamete Donation

JOSEPH G. SCHENKER, M.D.

Advances in reproductive technology now make it possible not only to assist couples achieve pregnancy, but also to alter the process of procreation per se. These advances in biological and medical sciences have created therapeutic resources possessing new powers with unforeseeable consequences for human life at its very beginning. Because these techniques could enable humans to go beyond the limits of reasonable dominion over nature, they are capable of constituting progress in the service of humanity while at the same time they could also involve serious risk (Pope John Paul, 1980).

Gamete donation has become an integral part of infertility treatment. Sperm, oocyte, and pre-embryo donation are highly successful procedures, undertaken to deliberately procure the creation of a child. Therapeutic donor insemination (TDI) is indicated for the treatment of male sterility. There are several accepted medical protocols for this treatment, and the overall success rate is 70–75% (Schenker JG, 1993). The majority of women will conceive within six cycles of treatment. Ovum donation provides a solution for women who were previously considered permanently infertile. The indications have expanded beyond patients with premature ovarian failure to include patients who are carriers of genetic disorders, patients with repeated in vitro fertilization (IVF) failures

(Schenker JG, 1992), and patients who are menopausal because of surgical castration, X-ray therapy, or chemotherapy. Oocyte donation is more standardized than IVF and results in better pregnancy and delivery rates per pre-embryo transfer (Schenker JG, 1991; Schenker JG, 1992). Yet these modalities of treatment raise serious legal, social, ethical, and religious problems. The religious aspects of the major religions toward gamete donation will be discussed in this chapter.

JEWISH LAW

Background

The Jewish religion is characterized by a strict association between faith and practical religious rulings. In principal, Jewish law is composed of two divisions: a written law and an oral law. The foundation of the written law is the Torah, the first five books of the Scripture, which are the origin of authority. The Torah is an expression of God's revelation, teaching, and guidance of mankind. The attitude toward the Torah is therefore one of reverence toward a holy divine text that includes moral values as well as practical laws. The oral laws interpret and elucidate the written Torah and regulate the new rules and customs. Its authority is derived from the written Torah.

The dominant parts of the oral law are Mishnah, Talmud, Post-Talmudic codes, and Responsa. Each of these four parts is discussed below.

Mishnah

The Mishnah is an early textbook of the Jewish oral law that was compiled systematically by numerous scholars over a period of several centuries. Its final form was established early in the third century of the common era. The Mishnah includes early traditional interpretation of the written Torah, original interpretation of the written Torah, ancient regulations that are not written in the Torah, and post-Bible regulations.

Talmud

During approximately three centuries following the final compilation of the Mishnah, the great interpreters (Amoraim) studied the six orders of the Mishnah and wrote a monumental composition called the Talmud. The Talmud includes commentaries and interpretative studies of Mishnah and Midrashim and established regulations and new customs.

Post-Talmudic Codes

After the compilation of the Talmud, an enormous amount of Talmudic knowledge was necessary for efficient ruling. The Post-Talmudic codes were intended to provide access to the laws, regulations, and customs of the Talmudic Halacha. Different scholars until the sixteenth century summarized and reviewed the Halachic conclusions of the Talmud in the Post-Talmudic codes. Among the scholars are Rashi (1040–1105), Rabbi Moshe Ben Nachman (1195–1270), and Rabbi Menachem Ben Shlomo Hameiri (1249–1316). The most prominent Post-Talmudic codes are listed in Table 13.1.

Responsa

The various attitudes of rabbinical scholars to the application of religion in a changing world are contained in Responsa. They provide analysis and discussion of the legal codes as the written opinion of qualified authorities to questions concerning all aspects of Jewish law from the time of the later Geonim to the present day. About 1,000 volumes containing more than half a million separate Responsa have appeared in print. Rabbinical scholars in recent times have dealt with the new problems that have arisen with the investigation and treatment of infertility such as artificial insemination and in vitro fertilization. Moreover, the Responsa of later Rabbinical authorities are often short monographs in which every text that is even remotely relevant to the point at issue is quoted and discussed.

The Jewish attitude to infertility can be

TABLE 13.1. Prominent Post-Talmudic Codes

1. She'iltot: Rav Akhai Ga'on Babylonia	A.D. 680–753
2. Halakhot: Rabbi Yitzhak Alfasi North Africa, Spain	A.D. 1013–1103
3. Maimonides: Rabbi Moshe Ben-Maimon Spain, Egypt	A.D. 1138–1205
4. Piskey Harosh: Rabbi Asher Ashkenazi Germany, Spain	A.D. 1250–1300
5. Shulkhan Arukh: Rabbi Yosef Karo Israel	A.D. 1488–1575

learned from the fact that the first Commandment from God to Adam was "Be fruitful and multiply." This is expressed in a Talmudic saying from the second century that says, "Any man who had no children is considered as a dead man." This attitude arises from the Bible itself and refers to the words of Rachel, who was barren and who stated, "Give me children or else I die."

According to the Hebrew law, the infertile couple should be diagnosed and treated as a single unit. One should first evaluate the female partner, and if pathology is not found, one may proceed to investigate the male. The male factors that should be evaluated are inadequate or abnormal production, ejaculation, or deposition of spermatozoa.

Jewish law has a positive attitude toward IVF and embryo transfer (ET) with the stipulation that the oocyte and the sperm are from the married couple. The various aspects of the "test tube baby" are discussed in the Responsa. Children born following IVF-ET are accepted according to Jewish Halachic Law.

Therapeutic Donor Insemination

The practice of TDI is not morally accepted by all infertile couples or their physicians, and is not accepted by most rabbinical authorities. For many centuries, rabbis have been discussing the principles involved in TDI. The discussions are based on ancient sources in the Talmud and the Codes of Jewish law. Talmudic passages from the fifth century recognized that procreation without intercourse was possible as exemplified by the Midrashic legend of Ben Sira's birth.

The legend is that the prophet Jermiah went to the bath house, where his semen entered the bath water. Soon after, Jermiah's daughter came and had a bath and became pregnant by her father, resulting in the birth of Ben Sira, who was recognized as a legitimate child. The legend has since been quoted many times in medical literature and in rabbinical Responsa dealing with TDI. Some rabbinical scholars deny the legend of Ben Sira's birth as having followed a conception "sine concubito."

Another ancient source indicating the possibility of conception without sexual intercourse is mentioned by Rabbi Elisah of Corbell in his work Haggahot Semak in the thirteenth century: "A woman may lie on her husband's sheets but should be careful not to lie on sheets upon which another man has slept lest she becomes impregnated by his semen."

In the modern era, rabbinical authorities have devoted much discussion to the practice of TDI. The discussions have focused on two issues:

1. Is it permissible according to Jewish law to perform TDI, or is the very act a transgression equivalent to adultery?
2. What is the status of the TDI offspring?

All Jewish legal experts agree that TDI using the semen of a Jewish donor is forbidden. It is the severity of the prohibition that is debatable. The question is whether TDI constitutes adultery, which is strictly forbidden by the Torah (the Pentateuch), or whether the injunction stems from the sources—mainly the legal complications of the birth of TDI offspring—as most of the experts hold. Some rabbinical authorities permit TDI when the donor is a non-Jew. This eliminates some of the legal complications related to the personal status of the offspring. However, if the semen donor is a gentile, the child is considered pagan (blemished); if the child is a female, she is forbidden to marry a Cohen (priest).

TDI according to Jewish law is prohibited for a variety of reasons: incest, lack of genealogy, and problems of inheritance. Semen donors for TDI as well as the physicians who use their semen are violating the severe prohibition against masturbation.

Some Halachic authorities prohibited a married woman who underwent the procedure of TDI to continue living with her husband. However, most rabbis state that without intercourse being involved, the woman is not guilty of adultery and is not prohibited from cohabiting with her husband. If the woman undergoes TDI without her husband's knowledge and consent, she must accept a divorce and forfeit any rights to financial support including her Ketubah (dowry) and alimony. TDI may not be used to fulfill the requirement of levirate (the obligation a man has to marry his deceased brother's wife). The child conceived through TDI is considered by many rabbinical scholars as having the status of a mamzer (bastard). The mark of bastardy severely limits the offspring's prospects for marriage in keeping with Jewish law, and this implies a severe functional handicap from a social point of view. Some rabbis consider the offspring to be legitimate, as Ben Sira was considered, while others consider the offspring to be "safek mamzer."

There are various views regarding the legal relationship that exists between the semen donor and the child born as a result of TDI. Some rule that no relationship exists; others hold that the child is considered the donor's child with all the associated legal complications such as incest, inheritance, levirate marriage, and custody. The majority opinion is that the donor has not fulfilled the mitzvah (obligation) of procreation by fathering a TDI child. The practice of TDI is accepted by part of the Jewish population in Israel, and according to the regulations of the Ministry of Health this practice is allowed under special regulations.

It is difficult to view fertilization with donor sperm as an act of adultery, but there may still be a legal prohibition against using donor sperm for IVF. This prohibition does not affect an unmarried woman as long as the possibility of bastardy is excluded. Scholars who oppose the IVF procedure claim that there is no pa-rental relationship in the IVF and ET procedures that may give an advantage to the offspring resulting from the use of donor sperm and the IVF technique. If there is no kinship, the offspring cannot be regarded as the product of an unacceptable genetic union and is thus at least as good for society as the offspring of a non-Jew and can marry a Jewess. In this case the paternity of the non-Jewish genetic father is not recognized, while the status of the offspring is that of an ordinary Jew almost without exception.

Oocyte Donation

Egg donation or embryo donation creates the problem of whom to consider as the mother: the oocyte donor or the women who carries and delivers the baby. If one of the women is Jewish and the other is not, the question about whether or not the child is Jewish will arise because according to Jewish law, the religious status of the child is determined by the mother. This interesting subject has an apparent precedent in the literature. According to ancient tradition found in the Talmud and Midrashim, Dinah, the daughter of Leah and Jacob, was first conceived in Rachel's womb, and Joseph, the son of Jacob and Rachel, was conceived in Leah's womb. Subsequently, they were exchanged; the male embryo that was in Leah's womb was removed and implanted within Rachel, and the female embryo was removed from Rachel's womb and implanted within Leah's. The result was that Leah gave birth to a daughter named Dinah and Rachel gave birth to a son called Joseph. This description is based on a Talmudic writing, and the Bible considers Dinah the daughter of Leah and Joseph the son of Rachel.

Contrary to the above Talmudic interpretation, Jewish law considers the sperm donor the father of the child resulting from TDI. Motherhood resulting from ovum donation or embryo donation is a divisible partnership—

between the donor who provided the egg and the recipient who provided the environment where the embryo was developed. Jewish law states that the child is related to the one who finished its formation, that is, the one who gave birth. A judgment is found in the Mishnah that states that if one person starts an action but does not complete it and another person continues and completes the action, the one who completed the action is considered to have done all of it. But the sources mentioned above do not reliably provide a final determination on the maternity and Jewishness of the child.

ISLAMIC LAW

Background

Islamic law—Sharia—is the heart of Islamic religion. It defines the pathway in which God wishes men and women to walk. Not only does it deal with matters of religious ritual, but it also regulates every aspect of political, social, and private life. It is derived primarily from the Quran and the Hadith, the traditions of the Prophet Mohamed. The Sharia is binding primarily for Muslim individuals, who are directly responsible to God, and it is not enforced by the state. According to orthodox Muslims, the law was founded through divine revelations that ended with the death of Mohamed. Therefore the Sharia is immortal.

There are two sources of Sharia in Islam: the primary sources (see Table 13.2) and the secondary sources (see Table 13.3). A good Muslim resorts to secondary sources of Sharia for matters that are not dealt with in the primary sources.

The Sharia classifies every human action without exception into one of five categories: (1) obligatory, (2) recommended, (3) permitted, (4) disapproved but not forbidden, and (5) absolutely forbidden. Even if the action is for-

TABLE 13.2. The Primary Source of Sharia in Chronological Order

1. The Holy Quran: the actual word of God.
2. The Sunna: the authentic traditions and sayings of the prophet Mohamed, as collected by specialists in Hadith.
3. Igmaah: the anonymous opinion of Islamic scholars of Aimma.
4. Analogy (Kias): the intelligent reasoning by which to rule on events that the Quran and Sunna did not mention through comparisons with rulings on similar or equivalent events.

bidden, it may be undertaken if the alternative would cause harm. The Sharia is not rigid. It provides latitude for adaptation to emerging situations in different eras and places. It also accommodates honest differences of opinion if they do not conflict with the spirit of its primary sources and are directed to the benefit of humanity. Muslim modernists have proclaimed the right of every qualified person to examine the sources of the Sharia law. The result is that in most Muslim countries today the Sharia laws are restricted and dominate only personal affairs.

Even in personal matters, much attention is currently given to ways of adapting Islamic law to modern times. The Muftis and Kadis adapt laws of personal status to the requirements of contemporary society. Progressive attitudes of

TABLE 13.3. The Secondary Sources of Sharia

1. Istihsan: the choice of one of several lawful options
2. Views of the Prophet's companions
3. Current local custom if lawful
4. Public welfare
5. Rulings of previous divine religions if not contraindicated by the primary sources of Sharia.

some religious leaders are revealed not only in family law but also with respect to other matters, especially those that relate to medical development in the field of reproduction.

Islam regulates the sexual relation and outlines its guidelines in the Quran. Sexual practice is allowed only between husband and wife within the framework of marriage. Having sexual relations outside the framework of marriage is forbidden. The Quran also outlines a system of punishment for both men and women who commit adultery. Over the centuries the method of punishment for adultery has increased from detention at home, blame, and oral humiliation at the beginning of Islam to whipping and even throwing stones at offenders later in Islam. This gradual increase in the severity of punishment reflects the smooth system of Islam in implementing its rules and instructions, as adultery was prevalent in the pre-Islamic era.

Islam has linked marital sex to procreation and family formation. The Hadith has also stressed the link between marital sex, procreation, and the establishment of the family. Though childbirth and child rearing are regarded as family commitments and not just biological and social functions, Islam states that not all marital sex leads to pregnancy and childbirth and some marriages will be childless. As Islam links sexual intercourse to procreation, only vaginal intercourse is permitted by the Quran. In addition, guidelines for sexual relation of the married couple are included such as privacy and avoidance of sexual intercourse during menstruation, puerperium, sickness, and disability.

Artificial Reproduction

Artificial reproduction is not mentioned in the primary sources of Sharia. However, because the importance of marriage, family formation, and procreation is affirmed when one of the marital functions such as procreation fails, Is-

lam encourages treatment of the situation. This is particularly true because adoption is not acceptable in Islam as a solution to the problem of infertility. According to Islam, attempts to cure infertility are not only permissible, but considered a duty. The Quran, as well as the Old Testament, gives a record of Abraham and Zakariya and proclaims having progeny as a great blessing from God. Therefore pursuing a remedy for infertility is legitimate and should not be considered rebellion against a fate decreed by God.

The duty of the physician is to help the barren couple achieve successful fertilization, conception, and delivery of a baby. The procedure of IVF/ET is accepted by Islam. However, it can be practiced only if it solely involves the husband and wife and is performed during the span of their marriage. According to Islam, the fusion of sperm and egg is a further step of the sexual act if it occurs within the time span of the legal marriage contract. Therefore no third party is permitted into the marital functions of sex and procreation whether providing eggs, sperm, embryos, or a uterus.

Therapeutic Donor Insemination (TDI)

The practice of TDI is strictly condemned by Islamic law and is considered adulterous. If the husband's infertility is beyond cure, the infertility should be accepted. TDI enhances the chances of inadvertent brother-sister marriages in a community, and it violates the legal system of inheritance. The procedure also entails registering the offspring of a man who is not the real father, which confuses lines of genealogy, the purity of which is of prime importance to Islam.

Ovum and Embryo Donation

Ovum donation is similar to sperm donation in that it involves intervention of a third party other than the husband and wife, and it is not permitted in Islam. Donation of embryos is also prohibited by Islamic law, as is adoption of a child.

CHRISTIAN VIEW

Background

Christianity is a religion that is centered on Jesus Christ as the supreme revelation of God and as Lord of his followers and is based on his teachings. Christianity comprises three principal divisions: the Roman Catholic Church, the Protestant churches, and the Orthodox Catholic churches. Christianity is particularly characterized by its universality and its attempts to extend its doctrine to all humankind through missionary activity.

The most striking development in the evolution of Christianity from its Jewish origin was the transition from a national religion (of the Jewish nation) to a universal religion. The Bible and the New Testament form the Scriptures that are sacred to Christians. The Old Testament emphasizes the idea of an agreement between God and his people and contains a record of Jewish history to show how faithfully they observed this agreement.

The New Testament contains promises made by God to humanity, as shown in the teaching and experiences of Christ and His followers. It consists of 27 books that make up the Canon, or all the books that Christians consider to be authoritative Scripture. The first four books are the Gospels according to Matthew, Mark, Luke, and John. They represent a collection of the acts and words of Jesus. The authors wrote them for teaching purposes. The Acts of the Apostles, a continuation of the Gospel of Luke, is a volume of history. Twenty-one documents called Epistles, or letters, follow. The New Testament ends with the Book of Revelation, or Apocalypse.

At the heart of Christianity are the issues of sexuality, marriage, and parenthood. The Church's intervention in the field of reproduction is inspired by the love that it owes to humanity, helping men and women to recognize and respect their rights and duties. Advances in technology have now made it possible to procreate apart from sexual relations through in vitro fertilization technique. In the early times of Christianity the Latin Fathers of the Church articulated the principles of a perspective on sexual intercourse. The central concern of their discussion was the liberation of the spirit from the flesh and not the problems of reproduction and the formation of the family. This attitude was mainly supported by Jerome and Augustine. Thus although there was some room in early Christian thought for the dignity of the human body and the propriety of reproduction, sexual intercourse was more often treated as a problem or a danger than as a positive opportunity or a part of the divine plan.

Roman Catholic Church

Background

The tradition of the Church recognizes in marriage and its indissoluble unity the only setting worthy of truly responsible procreation. The right to live is a fundamental one. In the Roman Catholic Church there are principles that are very important and guide the believers. The first principle is related to protecting human beings from the very beginning, which in the eyes of the Church means from conception. The second is that procreation is inseparable from the psychoemotional relation of the parents. However, from a moral point of view, a truly responsible procreation (vis-a-vis the unborn child) must be the fruit of the marriage. The fidelity of the spouses in the unity of marriage involves reciprocal respect of the right to become a father and a mother only through each other. "The child is a living image of the parents' love, the permanent sign of their conjugal union" (Pope John Paul II, 1982). The procreation may not be performed by the physician, and the physician's position must be limited to helping patients conceive and not causing the conception. The third principle is related to the personal norm of human integrity and dignity, and it should be taken into consideration in medical decisions, especially in the field of infertility.

The Vatican statement on assisted reproduction is very clear. It does not accept this treatment as a method of procreation. In 1956, Pope Pius XII declared that the attempts of artificial human fecundation in vitro must be rejected as immoral and absolutely unlawful (Pope Pius XII, 1956). The arguments of the Roman Catholic Church against the practice of IVF are that IVF involves disregard for human life and that IVF separates human procreation from sexual intercourse.

The Vatican instructions on respect for human life made a significant contribution to the discussions surrounding the new reproductive technologies. It was issued by the Congregation for the Doctrine of the Faith in February 1987, signed by Cardinal Joseph Ratzniger, and approved by Pope John Paul II. The document is a response to inquiries from episcopal conferences and individual bishops about the lawfulness of interventions into human reproduction. The key value in the instructions is respect for the dignity of the human person. The criteria for evaluating intervention in human reproduction are the respect, defense, and promotion of a human being; his or her primary and fundamental right to life; and his or her dignity as a person who is endowed with a spiritual soul and with moral responsibility.

Thus fertilization is licitly sought when it is the result of a conjugal act that is per se suitable for the generation of children to which marriage is ordered by its nature and by which the spouses become one flesh (Code of Canon Law, 1061). But from a moral point of view, procreation is deprived of its proper perfection when it is not desired as the fruit of a conjugal act specific to the love between spouses (Congregation for the Doctrine of the Faith, 1987).

Homologous Artificial Insemination (AIH)

The Church remains morally opposed to homologous or husband "in vitro" fertilization. Such fertilization is in itself illicit and in opposition to the dignity of procreation and of the conjugal union, even when everything is done to avoid the death of the human embryo.

Homologous artificial insemination within marriage cannot be accepted except in cases in which the technical means is not a substitute for the conjugal act but serves to facilitate and to help so that the act attains its natural purpose (Congregation for the Doctrine of the Faith, 1987). The exception is gamete intrafallopian transfer (GIFT), since sperm can be removed from the vagina after a normal sexual act and implanted into the fallopian tube, where fertilization will occur (Richards C, et al., 1993). Specifically, intercourse involves the use of a silastic condom that has a small perforation at the end so that neither masturbation nor contraception is employed.

Therapeutic Donor Insemination

Every pregnancy must occur within heterosexual marriage and must be the result of the conjugal act between the husband and wife. Thus therapeutic donor insemination is contrary to the unity of marriage, to the dignity of the spouses, to the vocation proper to parents, and to the child's right to be conceived and brought into the world in marriage and from marriage (Congregation for the Doctrine of the Faith, 1987). As was mentioned previously, such a method of conception also violates the rights of the child, compromises his or her paternal origins, and potentially interferes with the development of personal identity. This position eliminates any use of donor semen, whether for artificial insemination or for IVF. Furthermore, the artificial fertilization of a woman who is unmarried or a widow, whoever the donor may be, cannot be morally justified.

Ovum Donation

The practice of ovum donation is prohibited on the same basis as sperm donation.

Summary

The instruction is quite clear in its judgment on the reproductive technologies. The judgment is a rather clear and unambiguous "No." This analysis, though augmented by modern concepts of human dignity and moral rights, relies quite heavily on the traditional natural law analysis of the nature of intercourse having an inseparable procreative and unitive dimension. Therefore there can be absolutely no separation of any dimension of any aspect of reproduction. Consequently, the instruction prohibits in vitro fertilization, surrogate motherhood, cryopreservation of embryos, and most research on embryos and fetuses.

Eastern Orthodox Churches

Eastern Orthodox beliefs are based on the Bible and on Holy tradition (doctrines worked out mostly during early centuries of Christianity). The Eastern Orthodox Church was formally formed in A.D. 1054, when a split between the Eastern and Western Churches occurred.

The Eastern Orthodox Churches consist of several independent and self-governing Churches and some Churches that are not self-governing. The four governing Churches are Constantinople (Turkey), Alexandria (Egypt), Antioch (Damascus, Syria) and Jerusalem. Other major self-governing Churches, in order of size, are the Churches of Russia, Rumania, Serbia, Greece, Bulgaria, Georgia, and Cyprus. Eastern Orthodox Churches are also located in

Western Europe, North America, Central Africa, and the Far East, but they are not fully self-governing.

The three major orders of Orthodox clergy are bishops, priests, and deacons. The priesthood includes married and monastic clergy. Most married priests head parishes. Parochial clergy can marry only before ordination. Only unmarried priests can become bishops. According to the Eastern Orthodox Church marriage is one of the seven major sacraments. The Church permits divorce and allows divorced persons to remarry, but the first marriage is the greatest in the eyes of God.

In vitro fertilization and assisted reproduction are practiced in most countries in which Eastern Orthodox Church doctrine prevails. The Eastern Orthodox Church supports medical and surgical treatments of infertility. Nevertheless, in vitro fertilization and other assisted reproductive technologies are absolutely rejected by the Eastern Orthodox Church, which also opposes gamete donation, especially therapeutic donor insemination, on the basis that it is an adulterous act.

The Protestant Church

Protestantism resulted chiefly from the Reformation, a religious and political movement that began in Europe in 1517. The leaders protested an attempt by Roman Catholics to limit the practice of Lutheranism. Protestants disagree with other Christians about the relationship between humanity and God. As a result of this disagreement, certain Protestant beliefs differ from those of other Christians. These beliefs involve the nature of faith and grace and the authority of the Bible.

Most Protestants believe that the Bible should be the only authority of the religion, whereas the beliefs of Roman Catholics are based on both the Bible and the traditions of the Church. The traditions come from the declarations of Church Councils and Popes. They also come from short statements called creeds and from dogmas.

Most Protestants live in Europe and North America. A Protestant denomination is the state religion of a number of nations, including Denmark, Norway, and Sweden. Protestantism has strongly influenced the cultural, political, and social histories of those and other countries.

The Protestant Churches accept traditional treatment of infertility; assisted reproductive technologies are partly acceptable only when the gametes are from the married couple and when the procedure avoids damage to the pre-embryo. Sperm donation and oocyte donation are prohibited.

Anglican Church

During the Reformation of 1500 the Church of England separated from the Roman Catholic Church. Anglicanism spread as British colonists settled in North and South America, Africa, and Asia. Anglicans believe in the ancient faith of the Christian Church, as expressed in the Apostles' and Nicene creeds. Anglicans base their religion on Scripture, tradition, and reason and often view themselves as a bridge church between Roman Catholics and Protestants. They follow the Book of Common Prayer, which is the basis for doctrine and discipline as well as worship, but they acknowledge the right of national churches to revise the Book of Common Prayer according to their needs. The unity of Anglican Communion is symbolized by the Lambeth conference of bishops, which meets about every ten years in London. The conference can only advise the churches it represents. It serves mainly as a consulting and planning body. The Archbishop of Canterbury ranks as a senior bishop. The Anglican Church is the state religion of the United Kingdom.

Assisted reproductive technology was developed in the United Kingdom and Australia, where the Anglican Church prevails. As might be expected from that fact, the Anglican Church is more liberal toward the use of in vitro fertilization and allows semen collection by masturbation for artificial insemination by husband and for IVF but forbids the use of other semen and oocytes donated from a third party.

It should be mentioned that gamete donation is practiced in England and in some parts of Australia, Canada, and in other countries where the Anglican Church prevails by legislation.

HINDUISM

Background

The beliefs, practices, and socioreligious institutions of the people known as Hindus are found principally in India and parts of Pakistan, Bangladesh, Sri Lanka, Nepal, and Sikkim. Hinduism is also practiced in other parts of the world that have evolved from Vedism, the religion of the ancient Indo-European peoples who settled in India during the second millennium B.C.

Hinduism has no single book such as the Bible to serve as the source of its doctrine. Rather, it has many writings that contribute to its fundamental beliefs. The most important of these writings include the Vedas, the Puranas, the Ramayana, the Mahabharata, the Bhagavad-Gita, and the Manu Smiriti. The Manu Smiriti (Code of Manu) is a basic source of Hindu religious and social law. Part of it sets forth the basis of the caste system. Caste is India's strict system of social classes that began about 1500 B.C. The caste system includes thousands of subcastes, each of which has its own rules of behavior. Although the caste system has weakened through the years, it remains a strong influence on Indian life. Many Indians support the notion that social and religious duties are differently determined according to birth and inherent ability. This is the underlying principle of Dharma, the religious and moral law governing individual conduct.

Hinduism teaches that the soul never dies. When the body dies, the soul is reborn through a continuous process called reincarnation. The law of Karma is closely related to reincarnation. It states that every action of a person, no matter how small it is, influences how his or her soul will be born in the next reincarnation until he or she achieves spiritual perfection. The soul then enters a new level of existence, called Moksha, from which it never returns.

Hinduism exerts its influence from the power of its thought over society and not by formal institutional authority (see Table 13.4).

Indian society places such a high premium on fertility and procreation that Indian couples will sacrifice all they have to beget an offspring—especially a male offspring. Therefore assisted reproductive technologies are acceptable and practiced, including sperm donation. The Hindu view is that the sperm donor must be a close relative of the husband. The wife of a sterile male could be authorized to have intercourse with a brother-in-law or another member of the husband's family for the purpose of having a male offspring, but only after eight years of primary infertility or after eleven years if she delivers only female offspring. In practice, therapeutic donor insemination using anonymous donors is performed. Oocyte and embryo donations are acceptable.

BUDDHISM

Background

Buddhism, one of the major religions of the world, was founded in India about 500 B.C. by the Buddha. At various times, Buddhism has been a dominant religious, cultural, and social force in most of Asia, especially in India, China, Japan, Korea, Vietnam, and Tibet. In each area, Buddhism has combined with elements of other religions such as Hinduism and Shinto.

All Buddhists have faith in the Buddha, his teaching, called the Dharma, and the religious community he founded, called the Sangha. The basis of what Buddha preached in the Dharma is that existence is a continuing cycle of death and rebirth. Each person's position and well-being in life are determined by his or her behavior in previous lives. The word "Sangha" sometimes refers to the ideal Buddhist community, which consists of people who have reached the higher stages of spiritual development. In the strictest sense, Buddhism is an experience rather than a doctrine or system of beliefs; the Buddha's teaching was an attempt to communicate the experience of "awakening."

The ritual or worship of early Buddhism is very simple in character. There are no priests or clergy per se. The Sramanas or Bhikshus (mendicants) are simply a religious order, a class of monks who, to accomplish the speedier attainment of nirvana, have entered a course of greater sanctity and austerity than ordinary people. They have no sacraments to

---

TABLE 13.4. Hindu Concepts Related to Infertility

1. The soul is eternal and indestructible.
2. Regarding the concept of rebirth, the soul is viewed as not having a definite beginning and a definite end. It has a continuous process.
3. Marriage is sacred and permanent.
4. Male infertility is not a cause for divorce.
5. The emphasis on reproduction is not just on having children, but on having a male offspring.
6. It is religious duty to provide a male offspring. Therefore the wife of a sterile male could be authorized to have intercourse with a brother-in-law or another member of the husband's family for the purpose of having a male offspring (only after 8 years of infertility or 11 years when she delivers only female offspring).

administer or rites to perform for the people; every Buddhist is his or her own priest.

Buddhist councils are any of several assemblies convened in the centuries following the Buddha's death in 483 B.C. to recite approved texts of Scriptures and to settle doctrinal disputes. Little reliable evidence of the historical authenticity of the councils exists, and not all councils are recognized by all the traditions.

In the modern era a notable Buddhist council was the sixth, which convened in Rangoon from May 1954 to May 1956 to commemorate the 2500th anniversary of the Buddha's death. The entire text of the Pali Thervada canon was reviewed and recited by the assembly of monks.

Various Buddhist schools developed in India and in other Asian countries. The most influential schools include the Theravad, the Mahayana, the Mantrayana, and Zen. These schools have much in common, but they also differ in important ways.

The major centers of the Mantrayana school are in the Himalayan regions, Mongolia, and Japan. It stresses sexual symbolism and believes that sex should be used for holy purposes. The Zen school is practiced chiefly in Japan. The Buddhists in the different countries do not have an authorized view on new reproductive technologies. It should be mentioned that Buddhism has never been organized around a central authority. Therefore Buddhists of all types in various countries are individualistic, and even their Scriptures are not rigid.

According to Buddhism the three factors that are necessary for the rebirth of a human being are the female ovum, the male sperm, and the Karma. This Karma energy is sent forth by the dying individual at the moment of his or her death. Marriage within Buddhism does not have the high priority that it has in monotheistic religions. Marriage is considered to be the second best institution after monastic life. Traditionally, Buddhism has imposed strict ethics on priests while taking a relatively

lenient attitude toward laypeople. This means that Buddhist priests allow laypeople to do whatever they want to do as long as they do not harm others in concrete ways. According to Buddhism, any technology that is used to achieve conception is morally acceptable, and treatment should be given to unmarried as well as to married women. In vitro fertilization has been practiced in Japan since 1982 and is also practiced in other countries with Buddhist populations. The problem that arises is whether the oocyte and sperm have to be in their natural environment or not. If the crucial factor in the formation of human beings is the Karma energy, it is not necessary for the sperm and the ovum to be in their natural environment, and therefore in vitro fertilization should be accepted.

In Buddhism, donation of sperm is not prohibited, but this procedure should be used as little as possible because the parents in general may feel difficulties in taking care of a child who does not have their own genes, especially when a malformed child is born. There is also a danger that donation of sperm or an oocyte from a third party would involve commercialization and cause social problems, and donation of gametes could lead to eugenism.

In Japan, sperm donation is practiced, but ovum donation is prohibited. However, a child who is already born following TDI or ovum donation is accepted as the legitimate child of the social father who has given consent to therapeutic donor insemination and of the mother who delivered the child. The child also has a right to know his or her genetic father or mother when the child reaches maturity.

CONCLUSION

Since religious groups have been active in pressing their bioethical concepts on the public arena in different parts of the world, it is of importance to those who practice assisted reproduction to learn about the religious attitudes that relate to the problem of infertility and its therapeutic approach. Of primary importance is an awareness of the views of the main religions—Judaism, Christianity, Islam, Hinduism, and Buddhism—toward the practice of sperm and oocyte donation.

REFERENCES

1. Code of Canon Law, 1061.
2. Congregation for the Doctrine of the Faith. (1987) Instruction on respect for human life in its origin and on the dignity of procreation. Replies to certain questions of the day. Libreria Editrice Vaticanna.
3. Pope John Paul II. (1980) AAS 72:1126.
4. Pope John Paul II. (1982) AAS 74:96.
5. Pope Pius XII. (1956) AAS 48:471–473.
6. Richards C, Fallick M, Seibel MM. (1993) Gamete intrafallopian transfer and ultrasound-guided transcervical fallopian tube canalization. In Seibel MM, Kiessling AA, Bernstein J, Levin S (eds) Technology and Infertility: Clinical, Psychosocial, Legal and Ethical Aspects. Springer-Verlag. New York, New York.
7. Schenker JG. (1993) Genetic material donation: Sperm, oocyte, pre-embryo. Int J Obstet Gynecol 43.
8. Schenker JG. (1991) The therapeutic approach to infertility in cases of ovarian failure. Ann NY Acad Sci 626:414–430.
9. Schenker JG. (1992) Ovum donation: Ethical and legal aspects. J Assist Reprod and Genetics 9:411–418.

14

Consumer Perspectives on the Donor Egg Option

DIANE N. CLAPP, B.S.N., R.N.

Early in the 1940s, donor sperm programs were established for couples dealing with severe male factor infertility. In the 1990s, programs using eggs donated from fertile women became available to overcome infertility in women who could no longer use their own eggs or who had lost ovarian function. Many couples going through infertility view this as an exciting option that will fulfill their hope of carrying a pregnancy and allow them to have a genetically linked child together. Other couples view egg donation as just another carrot dangling in the medical pathway that prevents them from saying "enough is enough" and moving on with their lives. For some couples, the option of egg donation may come after they have stopped their efforts to achieve pregnancy. One 44-year-old woman said, "I feel both excited and upset about all the media press on donor eggs. After all those cycles of unsuccessful IVF, I was relieved to stop being an infertility patient. Now I am having to face all the big questions again. Can I put myself and my husband through the process? I thought we had made peace with our situation but now I am not sure." For others the donor egg option is presented to them immediately after a definitive diagnosis such as premature ovarian failure is made. "The doctor told me two things at once. First, that at age 36, I was in menopause and in the same breath he said that I was a great candidate for donor egg IVF. I need each piece of that news to sink in. First, I must realize that I'm never going to have my own child. Secondly, I must make decisions about my health and hormone replacement and what menopause means to me and my husband. Third, I have to think about the 'brave new world' of getting pregnant using another woman's eggs. I feel totally overwhelmed with it all."

Who are the couples who are considering egg donation as a treatment for their infertility? Most are battle-weary individuals who have been through months or years of infertility treatment. Many infertility patients describe their experience as an incredible roller coaster ride of monthly hopes and despair. Treatment fails, and they start again. Their self-esteem is shattered as they navigate the course of their infertility experience. Many women are left with a sense of no longer being in control of their body or their lives and struggling to maintain their self-image. As they approach a new treatment, they do so with a mixture of dread and hope; they hope that this will be "the cycle that works," but they dread the disappointment of a failed cycle. As the disappointments mount, a sense of hopelessness pervades all treatment.

All couples going through infertility experience a mourning and grieving process. Couples who are considering egg donation may be at the beginning or the end of this mourning process. In fact, the decision to proceed with egg donation may accentuate that process by ending one phase and shifting the couple into the next. The couple may be reluctant to express the usual concerns and sadness that often intensify after deciding to proceed with egg donation for fear of being rejected from the program. As one recipient said, "It was strange, I felt really good and excited about the donor we were working with, but I was surprised when a few days before the donor's eggs were collected, I wanted the cycle to stop and for the cycle to fall through. I wanted another chance to have a cycle *myself*. It was crazy, to have hope after all these years and to wish that someone would give me one more chance. I didn't tell anyone what I was feeling and it passed, but I guess I'll never stop wishing that it was me who could produce the eggs."

Couples considering egg donation face a series of difficult questions. The first is whether or not to use a donor. They must evaluate the impact of their decision on their partner and on the potential child and consider how being open or closed about their decision will affect the child, family, and friends. The question of whether to use an anonymous donor or a known donor must also be addressed. Finally, patients must decide which clinic they will use and when they will start the program.

The question of whether or not to consider egg donation requires both the man and the woman to take the time necessary for self-evaluation (Table 14.1). Accepting egg donation requires the couple to acknowledge the end of the genetic continuity they thought would one day occur. It is important that they discuss the biologic child they would have borne together. Thinking about how their child would have looked and even discussing the names they would have chosen can be helpful. Such discussions make the loss of their dreamed-of child more of a reality. Articulating what they like most in themselves and what they admire in their partner and

TABLE 14.1. Questions for Patients to Consider Before Proceeding to Egg Donation

- What does it mean to stop my own treatment and proceed with egg donation?
- Is there any coercion, either subtly or directly, on myself or my partner to proceed with this option?
- Have we acknowledged our worst fears and concerns about using a donated egg?
- Have we grieved for the loss of our biologic child?

wanted to pass on to their biologic child is important because a child born from a donated egg will have different qualities. Although the child will surely delight the parents in future years, he or she will be different nonetheless.

For some women the decision to move forward with egg donation may cause the woman to feel defective because another woman must provide the healthy egg that she could not provide. As one recipient recalls, "One of the hardest times for me was when the nurse called me at work to tell me that our donor had done an 'amazing job' and that she had produced ten good follicles. I called my husband at work and he was so excited. I hung up the phone and cried. I was so sad that I could never bring him that delight. If felt like I was celebrating another woman's victory." The decision to have children, the infertility workup and treatments, and ultimately the decision to pursue the donor egg option is usually a mutual struggle shared by the couple. But with the donor egg option there is the potential risk that one person, specifically the infertile woman, will feel left out of the process. If a pregnancy occurs, it will result from the husband's ability to produce good sperm and another woman's ability to produce viable eggs. Therefore any woman who is considering egg donation must think carefully about the treatment and ask herself whether using another woman's eggs will intensify smoldering feelings of low self-esteem.

The couple, too, must take careful inventory of how they feel. Neither must feel pressured to pursue this option before he or she is ready. To say "yes" just to make one's partner happy is not a good reason. To say "yes" because there is fear of the repercussions if one says "no" is also not a good reason for agreeing to use an egg donor. Meeting with a counselor to talk about all the issues is extremely important. "When we got my diagnosis, I felt that I was depriving Ralph, my husband, of his child. I want so much to let him have his own child. Donor egg seemed like the right option for us, but before we decided we met with a counselor to talk about adoption too. I would have been happy with either avenue, but Ralph really got in touch with how important it was to have a baby that was half of us."

Before making any decisions, the couple should look once again at their primary goals. Clearly, when they started the infertility process, their desire was to have a pregnancy and a child. At this junction they should reevaluate that goal by reconsidering why they initially wanted children and reframing that question in the context of their present life. Each partner should ask himself or herself how important being pregnant is and what it would mean for them if they never experienced a pregnancy. For some women, being pregnant is a major goal and a significant symbolic rite of passage into adulthood. Not being able to experience pregnancy, labor, and delivery and not being able to share that process with their partner and other women can be viewed only as a major loss. If neither pregnancy nor genetic continuity is as important as the desire to experience parenthood, then the couple may wish to consider adoption as an alternative.

During this stage, the couple may need time to consider and read about the option of child-free living. The couple is at a junction in their lives and their relationship and should look down both paths to know that they are making an informed decision based on consideration of all the options. For some couples, making the decision to stop treatment becomes difficult when they know that an option such as egg donation is available. They often feel that after investing all the time, money, and years of pain striving for a successful pregnancy, it is extremely difficult to turn away empty-handed, knowing that this option is available. Egg donation therefore places a subtle pressure on the couple to consider it. It is very important for the couple to assess what it would feel like if one of them said, "Enough is enough." In fact, it is helpful for each partner to ask the other that specific question.

When couples are in this decision-making mode, it is helpful for each of them to list the pros and cons of the donor egg option (Table 14.2). Having considered and processed the pros and cons, couples will need to determine their level of readiness to enter an egg donation program. Table 14.3 provides a useful checklist to assess couples' readiness to participate. One is most likely ready for egg donation if all of the questions can be answered "yes."

Once the couple has determined their readiness to participate in egg donation, they will want to anticipate their level of psychological preparedness. Table 14.4 lists some questions that couples find useful before moving forward with egg donation. Of central importance is the issue of secrecy versus openness. Not all couples have decided whether they will or will not tell the child. Couples who think they will not tell the child are advised to tell no one they are thinking of using a donor egg because anyone who knows may inadvertently betray a confidence. Couples who are considering being open about using egg donation should prepare and rehearse answers to questions they may be asked by family members and friends. It is advisable for partners to discuss ahead of time and agree on how much information they are comfortable sharing with the outside world.

TABLE 14.2. Pros and Cons of Egg Donation

Pros
- Depending on the donor egg program used, the couple may retain some control such as input into donor selection. The couple will certainly have control over the prenatal care and the nutritional status of the baby in utero.
- Couples will have the opportunity to experience the intimacy of sharing pregnancy, labor, and delivery together.
- The bonding process between the baby and its parents can start during the nine months of pregnancy.
- The fact that the baby will have half of the genetic properties of the couple is a major positive consideration for many couples considering this option.

Cons
- Egg donation does not guarantee a baby; each couple must look at the reality of the success rates for their donor's age group.
- Even donor egg pregnancies may miscarry.
- The donor may not stimulate well.
- Pregnancy achieved from a donor oocyte may take time to accept. Discussing ahead of time when in the pregnancy they think they will feel most anxious is helpful. (As with donor sperm insemination, many couples express high anxiety in the last trimester as they await the birth of the baby.)

For some people the concept of "third-party pregnancies" such as the use of a donated egg feels "bad" or shameful. If either partner experiences these feelings, the couple should try to understand why and who or where they came from. If there are moral or religious concerns, seeing a priest, minister, or rabbi can be helpful in sorting out these issues.

Donors, too, require evaluation for their level of preparedness. If a couple is using an anonymous donor, the clinic will have the total responsibility for this task. However, if the couple is using a known donor, they may wish to assist the clinic in this process or raise certain questions with family members or friends whom they are considering as potential do-

TABLE 14.3. Readiness Checklist for Egg Donation

- Have at least three months passed since you were told about this option, to allow enough time to absorb the fact that it appears you will not be able to have a genetic child together?
- Are you healthy enough to carry and deliver a pregnancy?
- Have you discussed the risks related to pregnancy, labor, and delivery for women in your age category with your doctor?
- Are you aware of the risks of multiple births with this procedure?
- Have you considered what you would do if you had a multiple pregnancy?
- Have you discussed the miscarriage rate for egg donation?
- Has the male been adequately evaluated recently, and is there a current semen analysis?
- Has the clinic explained the drug treatment used to prepare your uterine lining for the embryo transfer and any related side effects?
- Have you discussed any pre-existing medical condition with your physician to be certain that none of the medications, particularly estrogen, are contraindicated?

TABLE 14.4. Questions to Assess Psychological Preparedness of Recipient

- As a couple, have you seen a counselor or therapist to discuss the donor egg option, and in those sessions have you addressed the loss of not having your genetically related child?
- Have you discussed adoption and child-free living and feel that neither of these is appropriate for you at this time?
- Are you certain that neither of you is feeling pressured to choose the donor egg option?
- Have you discussed egg donation with at least one other couple who has done it?
- Have you discussed how you will feel when the donor stimulates well to determine whether the successful response of the donor will trigger feelings of being defective and being left out of the process?
- Have you discussed how you will feel if you invest your time, effort, and money into egg donation and the donor does not stimulate as well as you had hoped?
- Have you discussed whether or not to have genetic counseling to consider an amniocentesis, and what you would do if there were a problem with the fetus or if the baby were born with a birth defect?
- Have you discussed what you would do if you had a multiple pregnancy?
- Have you discussed the issues of secrecy and openness?

nors. Questions that help the couple evaluate the psychological preparation of the donor are listed in Table 14.5.

Once the decision is made to proceed with egg donation, the couple will have to choose a clinic to perform the procedure. Clinics vary greatly in donor screening and selection, as well as other important aspects of the procedure. Suggested questions to address to the clinic coordinator or the physician are listed in Table 14.6. Many of these questions reflect philosophical differences in the approach to egg donation and may have more or less weight for some couples. What is most important is mak-

TABLE 14.5. Questions to Assess Psychological Preparedness of Donor

- Has counseling been provided for the donor?
- Is counseling provided for her husband (if applicable) as well?
- When relevant, has the donor told her parents that she is donating eggs?
- If the donor has children, has she discussed the egg donation process with her children? If she has no children of her own, is she aware that she, like one in twelve couples in the United States, may encounter infertility when she tries to achieve a family of her own? How would she feel if this were the case and she had donated eggs in the past.
- What are the donor's expectations for future contact with the recipient and the child?
- Is the donor aware that she will need to take ovulation induction medications, and does she have adequate knowledge of the possible risks and complications from the medications?
- If you are using a known donor, what kind of relationship does the donor expect to have with you and your spouse?
- If you are using a known donor, what kind of a relationship does she expect to have with a child that is born through egg donation?
- Is the donor aware that you are considering the possibility of having chorionic villus testing or amniocentesis in the event of a pregnancy? Is she comfortable with the decision to have the test and, if necessary, to make decisions regarding terminating the pregnancy depending on the results of those tests?

TABLE 14.6. Questions to Help Evaluate Egg Donation Clinic's Policies

- Does the clinic recruit its own donors, and if so, how?
- Will the egg donor remain anonymous, or is there a protocol available that will allow some openness between recipient and donor?
- Are eggs taken from infertility patients?
- Has the donor proved her fertility, either by having children or by having participated in the egg donation program in the past? If she was a donor in the past, did she stimulate well, how many follicles did she produce, and was there good fertilization?
- How many times does the clinic use a particular donor, and is there a required waiting period before she can donate again?
- What are the ages of the youngest and the oldest donors?
- How does the clinic match the donor and the recipient, and who does the matching?
- Does the clinic provide pictures of the donor to the recipient?
- How much medical detail will the recipient couple receive about the donor?
- How long does the clinic keep medical records on the donor?
- Are the donor's eggs divided between two women, and, if so, how does the clinic determine who will be the primary and secondary recipient?
- Does the clinic use donors who have their own health insurance that will cover medical costs in the unlikely event of complications resulting from the ovulation induction or egg retrieval?
- If a patient brings a known donor, will she be able to use the eggs from that donor or will that donor's eggs be used anonymously for someone else and will she receive eggs from an anonymous donor?
- If a potential recipient recruits her own donor for a particular clinic, will the clinic use the same screening protocol that they would use for all donors, or will there be some changes in that protocol? If so, what would be eliminated?
- How long does the clinic maintain contact with the donor?
- Does the clinic have an ethical committee that evaluates ethical/legal issues regarding their egg donation program?
- Is the egg donation program a member of the American Society for Reproductive Medicine's Special Interest Group for Assisted Reproductive Technologies (SART)?
- Is the donor program open year round, or are there certain times of the year that it closes down?
- Is the donor program open during weekends and holidays should a retrieval or transfer be necessary?
- How many embryos does the clinic usually transfer per cycle?
- Does the clinic freeze extra embryos? How long will the clinic keep the embryos?
- Will the clinic release embryos to a different clinic should the recipient couple request it?
- How long will the clinic follow you if you get pregnant?
- What are the billing policies of the program?
- Is there a staff person at the IVF clinic who helps answer and deal with insurance-related issues?

ing sure that the issues that matter most to a particular couple are addressed openly.

To gain a sense of how successful the IVF clinic is, the consumer should consider how long the clinic has been doing egg donation IVF, the number of cycles that have been initiated, the number of embryos that have been transferred, the clinical pregnancy rate per embryo transfer, the ongoing pregnancy rate, the live birth rate, and the multiple pregnancy rate. It is also important to know what the clinic's miscarriage rate is. Consumers should ask these questions in the context of their age and diagnosis as recipients.

The potential recipient should also ask the clinic for information regarding survival rates for thawed embryos, pregnancy rates per frozen embryo transfer, and live birth rates per frozen embryo transfers for the past twelve months. It is also helpful to know what the required waiting period is after an unsuccessful frozen embryo transfer cycle before trying again.

Another important factor to consider is cost. Some of the expenses include the initial consultation, prescription drugs for the recipient and the donor, ultrasound and blood monitoring for the recipient and donor, and charges related to the egg retrieval, embryo transfer, and freezing and storing of embryos.

MOVING BEYOND THE DECISION

Once the couple has successfully gone through a donor oocyte program and found out that the woman is pregnant, the pregnancy will be precious and highly prized. Understandably, there is frequently heightened anxiety early in the pregnancy around the time of amniocentesis and later in the pregnancy just before delivery. But one can never expect the couple to forget how they achieved their pregnancy, and the presence of a third party will be a reality in their lives forever. Feelings about the use of donor eggs may surface at the birth of the child or when people comment on the child's close physical resemblances to either partner. Sometimes, old feelings associated with infertility surface during their child's adolescence and puberty. At that time, mothers see their daughters developing into young women. The daughter's transition into womanhood may trigger the mother's thoughts about her own infertility and the associated lack of control over her body. Separation issues are typical during both toddlerhood and adolescence. To gain autonomy, the toddler and adolescent have to assert themselves

and sometime reject parental influence. This can range from the adamant "no's" of toddlerhood to the blatant rejection of parental values that can occur during adolescence. Either of these can be very painful for the couple who strove so vigorously to become parents. During these stressful times, couples need to understand that these feelings have nothing to do with how good parents they have or have not been.

As with any life crisis, the trauma associated with infertility is never completely over. There are always some long-lasting effects from moving through a difficult time in one's life. It is important that the couple communicate and share their feelings as they go through these stressful times. As one mother of a baby achieved through egg donation said to me, "One of the most painful times for me was when my sister said, 'Oh, your daughter has our curly hair. It's just like mom's, and it's just like mine and yours.' I felt a knife in my heart because I knew the curls weren't from me. But, I took a deep breath and I thought about how it would have felt never to have held such a child in my arms. I thought about how I enjoyed combing those curls. Then I realized, it didn't matter where the curls came from, it just mattered that I have a baby who has curly hair in my life and that I am her mom."

GETTING SUPPORT

During the process of deciding to undergo donor egg treatment, couples and individuals benefit from having the support of a variety of people. Seeing a social worker or therapist to work through the decision-making part of this experience is, in my opinion, a crucial part of moving forward. This is particularly true if the couple have decided not to tell people about their decision to pursue this option. In addition, it is helpful to have a support network available to couples in the event that they would like to talk to other people going through the experience. There are several ways to achieve this. One is through the donor egg program itself. Many of these programs have developed a contact system or discussion groups in which couples can talk to other couples who have chosen this option. The national organization of RESOLVE, Inc. (1310 Broadway, Somerville, MA 02144-1731, 617/623-0744), which is based in Somerville, Massachusetts, has over 50 chapters throughout the country. RESOLVE's mission is to provide education, referral, and support to couples and individuals dealing with infertility. RESOLVE provides information on egg donation, and many RESOLVE chapters offer support groups for women or couples who are dealing with infertility. A copy of RESOLVE's "Ovum Donation: Questions to Consider Before Starting in a Program" appears at the end of this chapter (Appendix 14-A). Some chapters offer specialized groups for couples using egg donors as a way of achieving parenthood. By talking with others, couples become informed and empowered. Hearing what other people feel, they gain a perspective on how normal they are. They learn new ways of coping, and they gain knowledge about issues to consider in the future. Often these groups, which start at the time of decision making, evolve into parent support groups in which couples can share the joys, sorrows, and challenges of parenthood.

CONCLUSION

Egg donation is rapidly becoming a major form of treatment for certain types of infertility. However, because it introduces a third party into the reproductive process and is still a relatively new procedure, couples who are considering egg donation must consider the pros and cons of the procedure, determine their own readiness to move ahead, and ultimately select a clinic that is both successful and comfortable. This chapter was intended to provide guidance and perspective for patients who are possible candidates for egg donation.

SUGGESTED READINGS AND RESOURCES

1. Cooper S, Glazer E. (1994) Beyond Infertility: The New Paths to Parenthood. New York: Lexington Books.
2. Rubin P. (1993) How to Be a Successful Fertility Patient. New York: William Morrow and Co.
3. American Fertility Society (1209 Montgomery Highway, Birmingham, AL 35216, (205) 978-5000).
4. RESOLVE, Inc. (1310 Broadway, Somerville, MA 02144-1731) has a member-to-member contact system for people who are considering using a donor egg. RESOLVE also has their ART Workbook available.
5. Tan SL, Jacobs HS, Seibel MM. (1995) Infertility: Your Questions Answered. New York: Birch Lane.

Appendix 14-A

Ovum Donation: Questions to Consider Before Starting in a Program

DIANE N. CLAPP, B.S.N., R.N.

If you are considering using donor eggs, ask the following questions before starting in a program.

MEDICAL FACTORS

- How is your health in terms of getting pregnant (do you have cardiovascular problems, are you on medication, etc.)?
- Have you talked to your doctor about the risks relating to pregnancy, labor and delivery for women in your age category?
- Have you discussed the risks of multiple births?
- Have you asked about risk factors for having a miscarriage after embryo transfer?
- Is the male factor adequate? Has your husband been tested lately?
- Have you discussed the use of a natural or artificial cycle with estrogen and progesterone to prepare the endometrium lining of your uterus. Will the clinic require a mock cycle first? Which type of estrogen is used?

PSYCHOLOGICAL PREPARATION

- Have you as a couple gone for counseling to discuss the donor egg option?
- Is counseling provided for the donor?
- Is counseling provided for the donor's husband?
- Does the donor have children already? Has she discussed ovum donation with her children? If not, has she considered ramifications if later when she wants her own family, infertility is an issue?
- Is the donor aware of the need for ovulation induction and associated possible risks/complications?
- What legal contracts have been developed by the clinic?

RESOLVE
Infertility: Education Advocacy Support
1310 Broadway, Somerville, MA 02144-1731
HelpLine: 617/623-0744

Further information on this topic is available through RESOLVE factsheets. For a publications order form, please contact the local chapter or National RESOLVE Office at 1310 Broadway, Somerville, MA 02144-1731 or 617-623-0744.

- Has a written contract been negotiated? Specifics such as what to do with "extra" embryos, freezing embryos and paternal rights should all be clearly defined.
- Have you discussed what you will do if the child is born with any kind of birth related defect?
- Have you discussed the secrecy or openness issue relative to telling the child? Who, if anyone, will you tell that you are considering or trying this option?

Additional questions to consider if you are using a known or designated donor:

- Have you and the donor had *separate* legal counseling?
- Do recipients have any choice about donor selection?
- Clarify what type of screening and counseling is done for egg donors.
- What are costs? Do you have to pay the full amount if the donor doesn't stimulate well or if the eggs obtained are few or fertilization is poor?
- What is covered by insurance?
- What are the viable pregnancies or live birth rates from the donor egg program you are interested in?
- What kind of relationship do you and your spouse expect to have with the donor and have you discussed it with her?
- What kind of relationship do you expect the donor to have with the child and have you discussed that with her?
- Have you discussed your feelings about having an amniocentesis with the donor and have you discussed what to do if the test results indicate a problem with the fetus?

DONOR SELECTION AND EGG QUALITY, ETC.

- Who are the donors if anonymous?
- What is the age of the anonymous donor?
- Is the donor tested for the AIDS virus, CMV, hepatitis, chlamydia, venereal disease, serum karotyping and blood type and day 3 FSH? Is a drug screen done on the donor?
- Are eggs taken from infertility patients?
- How many times can a donor be used?
- Are all eggs from one donor used for one recipient or are the eggs split between recipients? If they are split how are they divided? Is there a primary and secondary recipient?
- Is the number of eggs guaranteed a recipient?
- Does the clinic freeze extra embryos?
- How long are medical records kept on the donor? Is the donor aware that, as in adoption, laws may change that could allow the child access to information about the donor at a specific age?
- Does the clinic maintain contact with the donor? This is important if you think you would want to use the donor again in the future. By maintaining contact, the clinic can monitor the health status of the donor as well.
- Does the clinic allow you to use the donor you bring into the program or do they require that you do a cross exchange (the eggs from the donor you bring in are put into the pool and you go to the top of the list to receive an anonymous egg)?

CHOOSING THE CLINIC

- If you are using ovum donation and IVF, ask if the IVF clinic you are considering is a member of the American Society for Reproductive Medicine's (formerly the American Fertility Society) Special Interest Group for Assisted Reproductive Technologies. (Consumer can call AFS at 205-978-5000 to find out.)
- Does the clinic have its own egg donor pool? What information is shared with the recipient about the donor?
- Do recipients have any choice about donor selection?
- Clarify what type of screening and counseling is done for egg donors.
- What are costs? Do you have to pay the full amount if the donor doesn't stimulate well or if the eggs obtained are few or fertilization is poor?
- What is covered by insurance?
- What are the viable pregnancies or live birth rates from the donor-egg program you are interested in?

15

Conceptual and Ethical Considerations in Medically Assisted Reproduction

MARY B. MAHOWALD, PH.D.

With each new medical advance, a troubling ethical question is raised: whether we *should* do what we *can* do. This question may be asked from the standpoint of society in general, through which its answer may be enacted into laws or policies, or it may be asked by individual practitioners and patients, who may make use of the advances regardless of whether laws or policies address them.

Some advances are more troubling than others because they involve basic understanding of who and what we are as human and sexual beings. Many techniques are available to prolong life, even when cortical function has ceased; behavioral and phenotypic characteristics may be altered through medical and surgical interventions. Perhaps most troubling, however, are the advances through which we can initiate new human lives in ways that had barely been imagined, let alone practiced, until a few decades ago. These involve not only in vitro fertilization and embryo transfer but also various forms of third-party involvement through gamete donation, embryo donation, and surrogate gestation.

This chapter provides an overview of conceptual and ethical considerations that relate to issues that arise in medically assisted reproduction. In the first part, two conceptual questions that are inseparable from the ethical issues are discussed:

1. What is a parent?
2. What, if any, are the morally relevant differences between gametes, embryos (in vitro or in vivo), and fetuses?

Elements that are morally relevant even to those who disagree in their positions about these issues are identified. In the second part, case-based and principle-based methods of dealing with ethical issues in assisted reproduction are presented. Common elements are again identified and are sorted into primary and secondary considerations for decision making. Finally, the ethical considerations are illustrated by examination of a specific issue, that of postmenopausal gestation.

WHAT IS A PARENT?

Parenthood is usually thought to begin with the birth of one's biologically related offspring. Although adoption is a legal means of becoming a parent in the absence of a biologic relationship, it is generally viewed as an exceptional route to parenthood, precipitated by the need for nurturance that some children cannot or will not obtain through their biologic parents. A distinction is sometimes drawn between "real" and adoptive parents, as if the biologic relationship is real and the adoptive relationship is not. Most parents would dispute this distinction because they experience the demands of child rearing as greater than those of childbearing. For some women, however, childbearing is not only painful but hazardous.

Since the advent of in vitro fertilization and embryo transfer, the genetic and gestational components of women's biological contribution to reproduction are separable. This has raised the question of whether a woman who gives birth to a child who is not genetically related to her should be considered the child's mother. It also introduces the possibility that some children have two biologically related mothers. Since adoption has already established a distinction between biologic parenthood and social parenthood, a child may in fact have five parents: three who are biologically related and two others who are their social parents.

Well before advanced methods of reproductive technology became available, some biologic fathers were not aware of their biologic progeny (Mahlstedt PP, Probasco KA, 1991). Among anonymous sperm donors, few think about the probability that they have biologic children who are being parented by others (Templeton A, 1991). With egg donation the same may be true for some women. In contrast, some women who gestate and give birth to children who are not genetically related to them regard themselves as mothers of those children. Anna Johnson, for example, who had agreed to accept payment for gestating a fetus conceived through in vitro fertilization of another woman's ovum, later changed her mind and sought parental status through the courts (*Anna J. v. Marc C. et al.*, 1991). Women or men who are genetically related to offspring borne by another may also regard themselves as parents of those children.

Consider the following definition of a parent as applicable to adoptive as well as biological parents of either sex: A parent is someone on whom another human being crucially depends for life or early nurturance. Gamete providers, gestators, and adoptive parents are all included in this definition. But within the context of health care, other parent figures emerge: the practitioners whose expertise and involvement facilitate the birth of children who would not otherwise be born. These include reproductive endocrinologists who successfully treat infertile patients, perinatologists who help women in high-risk pregnancies achieve live birth, and neonatologists who thwart the demise of very early and very ill newborns. This definition of parenthood would also include a group of women who historically nurtured newborns to whom they were not related either gestationally, genetically, or even socially: the "wet nurses" who literally fed the infants of others from their own bodies.

One factor that morally distinguishes some candidates for parenthood from others is that of intention (Mahowald MB, 1993). Sperm, egg, and embryo donors do not intend to be social parents of their biologically related offspring. Neither do practitioners who intervene to initiate life, preserve pregnancies, or save newborns; nor do women who agree to gestate fetuses or nurse infants for people who would be social parents, regardless of whether the social parents pay them for their crucial role. However, intention may shift during the course of gestation or even after birth. While its ethical significance is clear, the intention to rear a child is thus an inadequate criterion for determining who shall be the rearing parent in cases of conflict.

The interest of the child or potential child is another ethically significant feature for resolution of conflicts among would-be parents (Mahowald MB, 1993). This factor has been legally determinative in disputed cases such as that of Mary Beth Whitehead (*In re Baby M,*

1988). Accordingly, although the lack of intention to be a social parent is a legitimate reason for disclaiming responsibility for child rearing, it is not a sufficient reason for disclaiming any responsibility for other aspects of a child's or potential child's life. A prospective gamete donor, for example, is responsible for disclosing his or her known risk factors, such as genetic carrier status, to those for whom such risk is relevant.

Similarly, a gynecologist may be obligated to require evaluation of an individual's or a couple's competence for parenthood before performing in vitro fertilization and embryo transfer. Consistent with this sense of obligation, a physician in Michigan believes that he bears some responsibility for a child who would not be born without his assistance and knows that some people in society are credited with expertise for evaluation of competence for parenting (Mahowald MB, 1993). In circumstances in which competence for parenthood seems questionable, he asks the individual or couple requesting medical assistance to have their parental competence assessed by an appropriate expert, and he provides medical assistance only to individuals who are evaluated positively. Although some people view this practice as paternalistic, it is both logical and supportable. To the claim that couples who have children do not ordinarily have to pass an evaluative test of their parental competence, he can reply, "I am responsible only for that over which I have some control."

RESPONSIBILITIES FOR GAMETES, EMBRYOS, AND FETUSES

Some have claimed that responsibilities toward embryos are no greater than those toward gametes because both have the potential for full human development (Hare RM, 1975; Kuhse J, Singer P, 1984). Others deny that ga-

metes have a morally significant status but claim that embryos and fetuses are morally comparable to newborns or adults (Meehan M, 1984). Many authors distinguish sharply between gametes and embryos on the grounds that the embryo, unlike ova or sperm, constitutes a genetically complete and distinct individual (Noonan JT, 1970). They may also identify a morally relevant distinction between fetuses (even mature fetuses) and newborns: the fact that fetuses exist only within a woman's body, while newborns (some of whom are less mature than some fetuses) exist outside of her body and are directly accessible to others who may be responsible for their well-being.

It cannot be denied that the statistical probability of viable human birth increases during the course of human development (Grobstein, 1988). Nor can it be denied that at some point in the course of development, whether in utero or ex utero, the normal developing human organism achieves sentiency, that is, the ability to experience pain (Anand KJS, Hickey PR, 1987). Both of these features—life and sentiency—are ethically relevant considerations, regardless of whether they are imputed to persons as such. Thus the deliberate destruction of an individual human life and the deliberate infliction of pain on an individual are ethically justified actions only if some other ethical consideration, such as the welfare of another, is found to be overriding (Mahowald MB, 1993).

In contrast to human life and sentiency, personhood is not establishable by empirical criteria. People who impute full personhood to human zygotes or early embryos, whether in vitro or in vivo, subscribe to a minimal definition: A person is any distinct, living, human organism (Joyce RE, 1978; Noonan JT, 1970). Those who deny the personhood of fetuses have more demanding criteria, often including the requirement of self-consciousness (Warren MA, 1984). Those who are most demanding in their criteria maintain that human beings are persons only if they possess the capacity for moral agency or choice (Frankfurt HG, 1971; Engelhardt HT, 1988). This criterion eliminates from the ranks of personhood not only embryos and fetuses but newborns, the profoundly retarded, and unconscious or comatose individuals.

Even people who subscribe to minimal criteria for personhood acknowledge the controversiality of the concept and the fact that at some point in normal human development, personhood is uncontroversially achieved. I would propose, however, that the factors already mentioned—the probability of human live birth, the possibility of sentiency, and the potentiality for uncontroversial personhood—are morally relevant even to those who disagree about their implications. Together, these factors argue for increasing responsibility for a living human organism during the course of its development. Even if competing ethical considerations such as the preferences or welfare of a pregnant woman override these factors, their relevance must be taken into account in ethical decisions and policies about assisted reproduction.

PRINCIPLE-BASED AND CASE-BASED METHODS OF ETHICAL DECISION MAKING

Recent contributors to discussions of ethical issues in reproduction have proposed the principles of respect for autonomy and beneficence as the central considerations for resolution of dilemmas. Chervenak and McCullough, for example, distinguish between beneficence-based obligations toward the pregnant woman and toward her fetus and between autonomy-based obligations toward the pregnant woman and toward the practitioner (Chervenak FA, McCullough LB, 1985). Their model is a top-

down method of reasoning, matching particular cases to the basic ethical principles that philosophers have long sought to clarify and justify.

A number of problems arise from this model. First is the difficulty of explicating the meaning of autonomy, which, unlike beneficence, is not empirically describable or definable. Although clinicians can calculate the rations of burdens and benefits of alternative modes of treatment, they are at times uncertain about whether a particular patient, who may be distracted by pain or pressured by others, is truly exhibiting personal autonomy when she or he signs or refuses to sign a consent form. The legal requirement of obtaining informed consent may be met, but this is not necessarily equivalent to meeting the moral requirement of respect for autonomy.

An additional problem may bother philosophers but not others: the difficulty, if not impossibility, of demonstrating the validity of the basic principles. Various frameworks have been proposed. Some are based on appeal to a priori rules or laws, others on appeal to consequences, and still others on appeal to character or virtue. Religious traditions have often played a central role in identifying the basic principles and explaining their origin (Schenker JG, 1992). This is useful for adherents to those traditions but inadequate in a pluralistic society such as ours. The fact that philosophers themselves have not agreed on the adequacy of any single ethical theory strongly suggests that the foundations of the basic ethical principles that apply to reproductive decisions will continue to elude us.

A final problem associated with principle-based reasoning in reproductive ethics is that it represents a departure from the usual model of clinical reasoning, which is case-based. What typically drives clinical decisions is the set of symptoms observed in the patient. What one has learned in medical school, in scientific articles or books, and in medical conferences is useful and necessary but cannot provide adequate comprehension of the nuances of particular cases. The generalities that one has learned must be altered or interpreted to fit the case, not the other way around.

Obviously, the mere fact that practitioners are more accustomed to case-based reasoning than principle-based reasoning does not imply that either method is wrong. But a case-based method is more likely to be embraced by those whose ethical decisions take place in the clinical setting. Consider the case-based method of ethical reasoning recently elaborated by Jonsen and Toulmin (1988). These authors have attempted to revive the historically demeaned practice of casuistry by delineating its positive features and practical usefulness. Casuistry, as they describe it, starts with a particular case and compares the circumstances of that case with the circumstances of paradigmatic or analogous cases for which the issues raised have already been resolved. In the paradigmatic cases the issues were resolved through application of maxims that are generally accepted by the community. Whichever paradigmatic case best matches the present case is selected, and the same maxims are applied. The decision that is reached reflects the extent to which the present situation conforms to the paradigm.

Historically, one paradigm has been singularly influential in ethical assessment of assisted reproduction: voluntary intercourse between married partners as the normative means through which children are conceived. In that context the woman whose ovum was fertilized by her husband's sperm is also the one who gestates and gives birth to their offspring. The maxim provided by this paradigm may be formulated as follows: Children should be born to married women who conceive them through intercourse with their husbands. Justification for particular forms of medically assisted reproduction may be based on their proximity to this paradigm. For ex-

ample, in vitro fertilization for a married couple whose infertility is attributed to blockage of the fallopian tubes may be defended as a means by which an impediment to natural reproduction is facilitated. In vitro fertilization for an unmarried couple or for a single woman and fertilization involving gametes from third parties or another woman's uterus are more difficult to justify because they are greater departures from the normative paradigm.

Of course, the legitimacy of the paradigm is questionable in its own right. Why, for example, should marriage be a moral requisite for parenthood? Clearly, some married people are less competent parents than are some unmarried people, and some children are better raised by single parents than by couples or are better raised by adoptive parents than by biologically related parents (McGuire M, Alexander NJ, 1985). The requirement of conformity or proximity to the paradigm might exclude some individuals from parenthood who might be better parents than those who conform to it.

Further problems with casuistry include the legitimacy and adequacy of the maxims. These seem to function as general rules, raising some of the same questions that are associated with principle-based reasoning. Moreover, to the extent that general acceptance by the community is the means through which maxims are developed, the issue of relativism is raised. Ethical relativism involves denial of any universally applicable norms or standards by which human behavior can be assessed in a pluralist society such as ours. Racist, sexist, and classist standards that are generally accepted in a particular community could thereby be condoned.

A theoretical problem with case-based or casuistic reasoning is that the details of particular cases cannot be thought about except in general terms. Our knowledge of particulars derives from experience of unique events, but this knowledge is formulable only as concepts, whether articulated or not. Accordingly, there is no such thing as purely case-based knowledge. The case-based knowledge that clinicians acquire through their involvement with specific patients in unique circumstances is necessarily enmeshed in generalizations or concepts that are applicable to new and different cases. Without those generalizations the knowledge would be useless.

Just as case-based reasoning necessarily involves use of generalizations, principle-based reasoning necessarily involves use of particulars. The meanings that individuals attach to terms such as "autonomy" or "beneficence" derive from their concrete experience or interactions with other individuals. Thus in thinking about autonomy, we may picture an individual who offers to be an egg donor or someone who declines to undergo another attempt at artificial insemination. When we think of beneficence, we may weigh the risk, cost, and possible success of ovulation induction, in vitro fertilization, and embryo transfer for a specific infertile couple.

MINGLING PRINCIPLES AND CASE-BASED REASONING IN CLINICAL ETHICS

If the preceding analysis is correct, neither case-based nor principle-based ethical reasoning occurs in any pure sense in the clinical setting. What does occur is a mingling of particular and general considerations that are rarely articulated in philosophical terms such as autonomy and beneficence. The clinical calculus that is common to clinicians who assist in reproduction involves a weighing of risks and costs against the expectation of achieving the outcome desired by the individual woman or couple. Ordinarily, the desired outcome is a healthy newborn.

Further ethical considerations are articulated in terms of the woman's or couple's pref-

TABLE 15.1. Ethical Considerations Associated with Assisted Reproduction

Woman's preference
Woman's welfare
Partner's preference
Fetal welfare
Practitioner's preferences
Societal interests

erences. Occasionally, concerns about societal costs and whether the practitioner is willing to perform a particular procedure are discussed (Table 15.1). Preferences are expressions of autonomy, and welfare is another name for the good promoted through beneficence. Societal interests involve fairness or justice. The language in which the above considerations are articulated assumes some understanding of the principles of respect for autonomy, beneficence, and justice. But how the principles are to be interpreted and applied and how competing preferences and interests are to be handled can be determined only by examining the nuances of cases.

When third parties are involved in procedures, the women whose preferences and welfare are relevant may be surrogates or egg donors or both. The term "partner" may refer not only to the sexual partner of a woman undergoing infertility treatment, but also to the partner of a surrogate or egg donor or to a sperm donor. Clearly, the various individuals who are involved in assisted reproduction are affected differently. The biological contribution of men is always essential, and the expertise of clinicians is essential in most cases. But women who undergo ova stimulation, egg retrieval, pregnancy, and childbirth and embryos or fetuses whose survival and health status are directly affected by interventions are more drastically affected than are the men or practitioners who are involved in these processes.

TABLE 15.2. Primary and Secondary Ethical Considerations Associated with Assisted Reproduction

Primary Considerations:

    Woman's preference

    Woman's welfare

    Fetal welfare

Secondary Considerations:

    Partner's preference

    Practitioner's preference

    Societal interests

On the basis of the differing impact on individuals of various types of medical assistance in reproduction, the preceding factors may be sorted into those that are primary and those that are secondary (Table 15.2). All of the above factors are relevant to ethical analysis of questions raised in medically assisted reproduction. Beyond the ordering of the two sets of factors, the primary considerations are not always equally compatible, nor are the secondary considerations.

As used in Tables 15.1 and 15.2, the term "fetal" refers to any stage of development, including embryonic or pre-embryonic stage. Proximity to birth may strengthen the moral standing of the developing organism. However, the concept of fetal welfare does not apply to separate ova or sperm except in connection with their possible use in reproduction. Concerns about gametes and in vitro embryos typically have to do with the welfare or preferences of others who may be affected by their disposition.

The women whose preferences and welfare are relevant may be related genetically or gestationally to the potential offspring. Alternatively, their involvement may be based solely on their relationship to the man whose sperm is used in the procedure, as occurs, for example, in "surrogate" gestation through artificial insemination. Occasionally, the welfare and preferences of women who occupy different roles regarding gestation, genetics, and intended social motherhood may be at odds.

Among secondary ethical considerations in assisted reproduction, the "partner" may be the sexual partner and/or the married partner of any of the women mentioned above. The partner of the woman who wishes to have a child may be another woman, but few reproductive centers offer services beyond artificial insemination to single women, let alone women who are known to be living in a lesbian relationship. Although an anonymous sperm donor is not a "partner" in the usual sense of the term, he is obviously related to his potential offspring genetically and is thus a genetic partner in the process of assisted reproduction.

Practitioner preferences are ethically relevant in assisted reproduction, just as they are in cases of elective termination of pregnancy, because infertility treatment is not equivalent to treatment required for preservation of life or health. For this reason, practitioners are not obliged to participate in procedures that they regard as ethically inappropriate. However, they are obliged to care for infertility patients who need further care. For example, although an individual physician may decline to inseminate a single woman, once the woman becomes pregnant and needs assistance in delivery, such assistance should not be denied on grounds of moral objection to the insemination.

Societal interests include those of the potential child or children as well as the costs of infertility treatment and its aftermath. Disputes among claimants to parental rights are sometimes resolved on grounds of the best interests of the potential child or children. Moreover, obligations of gamete providers as well as gestational surrogates may also be imputed on this basis. Gamete donors, for example, would be expected to disclose any known genetic abnormality, such as carrier status, and gestational surrogates would be expected to refrain from behaviors that might endanger the fetus. It is questionable, however, whether these ethical obligations are legally or practically enforceable.

Costs of infertility treatment have been a subject of criticism by those who recognize the socioeconomic discrepancies between people who seek and obtain medical assistance for reproduction and those who do not do so or who serve only as gamete providers or gestational surrogates. Although infertility affects the poor as well as the affluent, it is hardly a treatable condition for the poor. If societal interests are defined in terms of providing equal opportunity to all, infertility treatment should be provided regardless of ability to pay. The current situation is consistent with a utilitarian rather than egalitarian interpretation of societal interests.

Recurrent issues of assisted reproduction may be examined in light of the preceding ethical considerations. These include disposition of extra embryos, fetal reduction in multiple gestation, gamete donation, surrogate gestation, and infertility treatment for single women. As long as all of the parties who are directly involved in any of these procedures agree to the arrangement, the preferences of women, their partners, and practitioners have been adequately addressed. Consideration of fetal welfare implies responsibility of gamete donors and potential surrogates to be forthcoming about any known medically relevant conditions that could affect their gametes. It also suggests an ethical rationale for fetal reduction in cases of multiple gestation that threaten fetal survival or welfare: If no fetuses are likely to survive, saving some through reduction seems justified. Retrieval and fertilization of extra ova are generally justified on grounds of women's welfare as well as preferences, but freezing, disposal, and donation of extra embryos raise other concerns. Since fetal welfare is threatened through freezing or dis-

posal, the question of the moral status of the early embryo or pre-embryo is inseparable from these decisions. For some people, including some practitioners, disposal of human embryos, whether in vitro or in vivo, is equivalent to abortion (Noonan JT, 1970; Johnstone B, 1984).

Women's welfare is particularly important in cases of surrogacy. The woman who gestates an embryo fertilized in vitro from others' gametes is fully a patient, even though she is not necessarily the person who initiated the relationship or the payer for her care. Partner preferences are generally less compelling because the partner is less affected by the process. Societal interests come into play in determining whether it is just that some individuals or couples have access to surrogacy or gamete donation while others do not. Society is also interested in the outcome of such pregnancies, that is, in the welfare of the children they produce.

AN ILLUSTRATIVE ISSUE: POSTMENOPAUSAL GESTATION

To illustrate in more detail how the primary and secondary ethical considerations outlined above are applicable to medically assisted reproduction, consider the issue of postmenopausal gestation. Of two cases recently reported in the media, the first involved a 59-year-old woman who gave birth to twins in a London hospital (Schmidt WE, 1993). The woman, described as wealthy, was not identified. Her physicians in London declined to provide medical assistance to achieve a pregnancy, allegedly because "they believed she was too old to face the emotional stress of being a mother." The woman and her 45-year-old husband went to a private infertility clinic in Rome, where eggs were retrieved from a younger woman, fertilized in vitro with the sperm of the older woman's husband, and transferred to the older woman's uterus. The second case involved a 61-year-old woman who was three months pregnant through the same procedures as described above. Her husband's age was not reported.

Since the first case involves a postmenopausal woman who has already given birth and the second case involves one who is three months pregnant, consider also a third scenario: that of a prematurely postmenopausal woman seeking medical assistance so that she can become pregnant. The third scenario is familiar enough to reproductive endocrinologists and unlikely to be reported by the media because of the ordinariness of pregnancy for a woman of normal reproductive age. Note, however, that the women who wish to be pregnant in all three cases are differently situated with regard to gestation: one has just delivered twins, another is pregnant, and the third is not yet pregnant. Ethical obligations to women may be different before fertilization, during gestation, and postnatally. They may also be different with regard to fetuses, potential fathers, and practitioners.

Primary Considerations

The preferences of the postmenopausal women in the above cases are clear, but the risks of pregnancy in women as old as 60 years of age are not clear. The medical complications of pregnancy for healthy postmenopausal women over 50 may not be significantly greater than those of their younger premenopausal counterparts (Sauer M, et al., 1992; Navot D, et al., 1994). Moreover, women in their sixties commonly undergo procedures, such as cosmetic surgery, that involve medical risk with no expected medical benefit. The birth of a child may, of course, be a benefit to the postmenopausal woman who wishes to be pregnant. Even without that benefit, however,

individuals should be free to obtain medical services as long as they are knowledgeable about the risks. A comparable argument applies to those who wish to undergo medical procedures for personal profit, for example, through blood or tissue donation, including egg donation.

Unfortunately, case reports of pregnancy in postmenopausal women have provided no details about the egg donors. Clearly, they undergo risks as well, and whether they do so with full voluntariness is a complex question, regardless of whether they are related to the recipients or remunerated for their risks. If people who serve as gamete donors are generally in socioeconomically less advantageous positions than those to whom they provide them, questions arise about justice as well as autonomy. These questions have already been addressed in the context of commercial surrogacy without producing social agreement about its legitimacy. In general, ethical concerns have been greater in situations in which money is exchanged than in situations in which third-party participants are not remunerated.

Ethical concerns have also been greater when the rationale for involvement of an egg donor or gestator is not medical. (Few questions have arisen regarding nonmedical reasons for sperm donation, probably because of the significant differences in remuneration and risks between sperm donation and egg donation or surrogacy.) Treatment of a woman of normal reproductive age who has no ovaries or no uterus through retrieval of another's ova or implantation of her ova in another's uterus is comparable to treatment for a disease or disability that interferes with functions that are typically associated with one's age and gender. Gestation beyond the natural occurrence of menopause is a departure from this paradigm. Medical assistance to extend the normal human reproductive life cycle is comparable to elective cosmetic surgery or prenatal interventions for gender selection of offspring in that all three are selling elective health services rather than treating a medical problem.

Beyond women's preferences and welfare, fetal welfare is a primary ethical consideration. Arguments in support of fetal welfare are often based on obligations to ensure the health of the children they are expected to become. As potential children, fetuses are imputed by some to have rights of their own, independent of the women in whom they develop, of those who provided the gametes from which they developed, and of those who wish to be their parents. But fetal welfare, in situations of postmenopausal women, might best be ensured through artificial insemination of the woman who provides the ova rather than through ova retrieval, in vitro fertilization, and embryo transfer to the postmenopausal woman. A surrogate gestation arrangement would produce a child who was genetically identical to a child produced by inducing gestation in a postmenopausal woman, with potentially less medical risk and lower medical costs. Admittedly, a surrogacy arrangement would introduce further complications, such as legal risks and costs, along with compensation for the surrogate. One would hope, nonetheless, that the postmenopausal women involved in the cases described above were apprised of this alternative.

Because of the tie between fetal welfare and child welfare, some have argued against postmenopausal gestation on grounds that the older woman is unlikely to have the stamina, health, or lifespan to care adequately for her child until his or her adulthood (Chira S, 1994). The physicians in London framed their objection paternalistically in saying that their patient "was too old to face the emotional stress of being a mother" (Schmidt WE, 1993). This argument is sexist as well as ageist in light of the fact that older men become biological fathers in greater number than women, typically evoking congratulations rather than criticism.

The argument that no one should become a parent beyond a certain age on grounds of

obligations to children is more prohibitive of men than of women because women generally live longer than men (Chira S, 1994). In the first case described by the media, the fact that the father of the twins is 45 years old suggests a high likelihood that at least one parent will be available throughout the child's childhood. If the ages of the couple had been reversed, even with the same medical circumstances, the case might have elicited no attention (Seibel MM, et al., 1994). A final factor favoring the potential child's welfare is the socioeconomic status of the couple in the first case and probably in the second. Even if both parents' ability to care for their children were compromised, economic resources would apparently be available to ensure that the needs of their children were adequately addressed.

Secondary Considerations

Both cases of postmenopausal gestation reported by the media involve married couples. Although the husband in each case is the genetic parent of the potential child, his wife, who is not genetically related, has been the focus of attention. Those who place great stock in genetic ties to offspring might deny that the postmenopausal woman is the child's mother. Others would claim that regardless of whether she is genetically related to her offspring, a woman who gestates and gives birth has a more compelling claim to parenthood than one who only provides the genetic material. Moreover, the partner of the woman who gestates is ordinarily not only genetically related to the fetus, but intends to be a rearing parent also. Accordingly, the partner's wishes or preferences about the pregnancy are ethically relevant, even though they do not weigh as heavily as the wishes of those who undergo health risks through ova retrieval or gestation and childbirth.

The third scenario does not stipulate whether the prematurely postmenopausal woman is married. She might, of course, have a male partner to whom she is not married; she might also be living alone or living with a partner of the same sex. If she has no male partner, she might request that sperm from an anonymous donor be used for in vitro fertilization. If she has a female partner, she might even ask that her partner's ova be fertilized in vitro, and the resultant embryos implanted in her for gestation. While the latter scenarios are unlikely, their unlikelihood is probably influenced by practitioner preference for dealing with heterosexual couples rather than with single women.

Practitioner preference obviously influenced the couple in the first case to go to Rome for medical assistance. This ethical consideration is most compelling when elective procedures are sought. When patients are in need of urgent treatment to prolong their lives or preserve their health, physicians are bound to provide it. Increasingly, however, treatments that are medically indicated for some are desired by others for nonmedical reasons. Respect for practitioner preference applies not only to refusals to provide treatment to patients requesting elective procedures but also to decisions to provide treatment to such patients. The willingness of the clinicians at the private fertility clinic in Rome to perform the procedures necessary for their postmenopausal patients to become pregnant is also an ethically relevant consideration.

Finally, societal interests are ethically relevant to the issue of postmenopausal gestation. Why, one might ask, in a world where the population may already be overreaching the limits of its resources, should we facilitate the reproduction of more children than unassisted nature can produce? Among health needs and social needs of all of our citizens, clearly this is not foremost. But, it may be retorted, consider the suffering of childlessness for those who wish to be parents, and consider the fact, in most cases of infertility treatment, that those who seek to have children do so at their own expense. As long as others are not required to pay for the required medical assistance or for the rearing of the children who are born through that assistance, societal interests are not compelling.

While the above retort may be satisfactory to some, it does not address the lack of access to fertility treatment that faces people who are unable to pay for it. It is doubtful, for example, that the physicians at the Rome clinic would have provided their services to postmenopausal patients if the women could not afford the treatment. For less affluent women who are childless but postmenopausal, such treatment is not an available option

CONCLUSION

The preceding considerations do not lead to a definitive answer to the question of whether medical assistance should be provided to achieve postmenopausal gestation. They do, however, suggest certain provisional conclusions about the issue. First, the practice should not be permitted unless the welfare and autonomy of the women who provide ova in such situations are protected. Second, women who are prematurely postmenopausal are more deserving of medical assistance for gestation than are those who are postmenopausal at the expected age. Third, the welfare of postmenopausal women and fetuses could be better served through artificial insemination and surrogacy than through the medical assistance required for postmenopausal gestation. Fourth, the autonomy of practitioners who decline or agree to provide medical assistance should be respected. Fifth, society should not be obliged to pay for medical treatment to achieve gestation in women who are normally postmenopausal.

These conclusions are supported by the principles of respect for autonomy, beneficence, and justice as delineated in the ethical considerations outlined above. They are also supported through casuistic reasoning based on proximity to the normative means of human reproduction and norms for provision of health services unrelated to medical need.

REFERENCES

1. Anand KJS, Hickey PR. (1987) Pain and its effects in the human neonate and fetus. New Eng J Med 317(21):1321–1329.
2. *Anna J.* v. *Mark C. et al.* (1991) 234 Cal. App 3d 1557.
3. Chervenak FA, McCullough LB. (1985) Prenatal ethics: A practical method of analysis of obligations to mother and fetus." Obstet Gynecol 66(3):442–446.
4. Chira S. (1994) Of a certain age, and in a family way: What's wrong with that? New York Times (Jan. 2, 1994), sect. 4:6.
5. Engelhardt HT. (1988) Medicine and the concept of person. In: M.F. Goodman, ed. What Is a Person? Clifton, N.J.: Humana Press, pp. 169–184.
6. Frankfurt HG. (1971) Freedom of the will and the concept of a person. J. Philosophy 68(January):5–20.
7. Grobstein C. (1988) Science and the Unborn. New York. Basic Books.
8. Hare RM. (1975) Abortion and the Golden Rule. Phil. & Public Affairs 4(3):201–222.
9. *In re Baby M.* (Feb. 3, 1988) NJ SupCt, No A-39-87, 14 FLR.
10. Johnstone B. (1984) The moral status of the embryo. In: W. Walters and P. Singer, eds. Test-Tube Babies. Melbourne Australia: Oxford University Press, pp. 49–56.
11. Jonsen A, Toulmin S. (1988) The Abuse of Casuistry. Berkeley: University of California Press.
12. Joyce RE. (1978) Personhood and the conception event. New Scholasticism 52(Winter):97–109.
13. Kuhse H, Singer P. (1984) The moral status of the embryo. In: W. Walters and P. Singer, eds. Test-Tube Babies. Melbourne Australia: Oxford University Press, pp. 57–63.
14. Mahlstedt PP, Probasco KA. (1991) Sperm donors: Their attitudes toward providing medical and psychosocial information for recipient couples and donor offspring. Fertil Steril 56:747–753.
15. Mahowald MB. (1993) Women and Children in Health Care: An Unequal Majority. New York: Oxford University Press.
16. McGuire M, Alexander NJ. (1985) Artificial insemination of single women. Fertil Steril 43:182–184.
17. Meehan M. (1984) More trouble than they're worth? Children and abortion. In: S. Callahan and D. Callahan, eds. Abortion: Understanding the Differences. New York: Plenum Press, pp. 145–170.
18. Navot D, Drews MR, Bergh PA, Guzman I, Karstaedt A, Scott RT, Jr., Garrisi GJ, Hofmann GE. (1994) Age-related decline in female fertility is not due to diminished capacity of the uterus to sustain embryo implantation. Fertil Steril 61(1):97–101.
19. Noonan JT, Jr. (1970) An almost absolute value in history. In: J.T. Noonan, ed. The Morality of Abortion. Cambridge, Mass.: Harvard University Press, pp. 51–59.
20. Sauer MV, Paulson RJ, Lobo RA. (1992) Reversing the natural decline in human fertility: An extended clinical trial of oocyte donation to women of advanced reproductive age. JAMA 268(10):1275–1279.
21. Schenker JG. (1992) Religious Views Regarding Treatment by Assisted Reproductive Technologies. J Asst Reprod Genet 9(1):3–8.
22. Schmidt WE. (1993) Birth to a 59-year-old generates an ethical controversy in Britain. New York Times, Dec. 29, 1993, pp. A1 and A6.
23. Seibel MM, Zilberstein M, Seibel SG. (1994) Becoming parents after 100? Lancet 343:603.
24. Templeton A. (1991) Gamete donation and anonymity. Brit J Obstet Gynaecol 98:343–350.
25. Warren MA. (1984) On the moral and legal status of abortion. In: J. Feinberg, ed. The Problem of Abortion, 2nd ed. Belmont, Calif.: Wadsworth, pp. 102–119.

16

Explaining Gamete Donation to Children

S. NORMAN SHERRY, M.D.
MOLLIE SHERRY, LICSW

Macbeth: Thou losest labour. As easily mayst thou the intrenchant air with thy keen sword impress as make me bleed. . . . I bear a charmed life, which must not yield to one of woman born.

Macduff: Despair thy charm, and let the angel whom thou still has served tell thee Macduff was from his mother's womb untimely ripped. (Shakespeare, 1606)

Although in Shakespeare's time, cesarean birth was considered unusual and extraordinary, today it is a common occurrence. Similarly, a decade ago, gamete donation was viewed as an unusual and extraordinary method of conception. However, the use of gamete donation has greatly increased over the last decade. In the United States alone, an estimated 15,000–20,000 infants per year are born through therapeutic donor insemination (TDI) (Bernstein J, 1993). Although children conceived by egg donation are currently considerably fewer than those conceived by sperm donation, as treatment is extended to perimenopausal and natural menopausal women, the number of births following this procedure is rising rapidly. Despite the growth of gamete donation, there is little information to guide parents in methods of explaining to the resulting children their origins.

A number of studies have suggested that few parents who conceive through gamete donation plan to disclose their children's genetic origins to them (Bernstein J, 1993; Daniels KR, 1986; Sokoloff BZ, 1987). Only 5% of interviewed American couples who received TDI planned to tell their offspring (Reading AE, et al., 1982; Amuzu B, et al., 1990). Even in France, where public information concerning TDI is widespread, only half of couples inform their offspring that they were conceived through donor insemination (Chevret M, 1977).

The reluctance to explain to children their genetic origins is unclear, especially in TDI, since the rearing father is considered the legal father. Although the legal rights of the rearing mother following egg donation are less clear, they will likely follow this example. Nevertheless, the Roman Catholic Church has considered gamete donation equivalent to adultery.

It appears that society has encouraged keeping a child's genetic origins a secret, and secret keeping can have negative consequences for family relationships, particularly in the areas of basic trust and identity formation for the child and guilt and anxiety for the parents. Daniels states that family relationships that are based on deception may be damaged (Daniels KR, 1987).

Brodzinsky's thoughts about revelation of the truth in the adoption situation are relevant here: "At the very least (telling) promises the foundation for an honest and trusting relationship between parents and children and it relieves the parents of the burden of deception, a burden that can weigh heavily on the parent-child relationship" (Brodzinsky DM, 1984). Secrecy also makes it difficult to take full advantage of support in critical times. Openness in the family about the child's biological origins generates trusting relationships, reduces unhealthy psychological defenses, and encourages the creation and use of support networks. Support networks should include both personal ties, such as friends and family, and professionals, such as the family pediatrician and, if necessary, an appropriate mental health advisor. An agency is often available for long-term support of an adoptive family. A similar long-term relationship with an agency may be beneficial in gamete donation as well.

PSYCHOLOGICAL READINESS

Intrapersonal and interpersonal conflicts may exist around infertility. Several studies show that secrecy around the child's genetic origins is employed to prevent parents' feelings of shame and guilt (Baran A, Pannor R, 1989; Daniels KR, 1988). Resolving these conflicts before conception will create an honest emotional base from which successful telling can grow. Parents' ability to accept and acknowledge the differences between conception by gamete donation and conception by the more usual method is key in the development of a healthy parent-child relationship throughout the child-rearing years.

Unlike adults, children have no psychological understanding of relationship by blood tie until they are well into latency. From children's perspective the adults who raise them are their psychologic parents, whether fully biologic, by gamete donation, by adoption, or even by foster ties. The physical reali-

ties of conception and birth are not the direct causes of emotional attachment of the child to the parent (Goldstein J, et al., 1973).

TELLING

Whether or not to tell a child of his or her genetic origins is a complex issue. These authors recommend that children be told about their biologic origins. Telling of conception by gamete donation is a process; it involves the gradual revelation of information over time. Information about origins should be imparted in an honest, open, respectful manner. The disclosure process may cover a span of several years.

Today, many possibilities of conceiving and carrying a pregnancy exist. To fully understand the process and implications of gamete donation, donor insemination, surrogacy, or in vitro fertilization, children need to be familiar with a number of concepts. At the very least, they need to understand reproduction, sexuality, anatomy, love, permanency, and parenting. Much of this information will be learned at school; some will be learned at home. Throughout, it is important to remember that children grow at different rates cognitively, physically, and emotionally. Parents should answer a child's questions honestly, imparting as much of the information as is necessary without overwhelming the child with facts he or she is unprepared for. Parents must consider their child's age and individual capabilities and should readily consult with their pediatrician or mental health advisor. We encourage parents to begin with the simplest facts and gradually add information appropriate to the child's growing cognitive abilities. In the following vignette, Amy was conceived by gamete donation.

Four-year-old Amy came home from a long day at her child daycare center and appeared tired and preoccupied. She had been picked up by her father but waited until both parents were with her at the dinner table before she asked, "Are you my mommy and daddy?" At school, an African American child who had white parents used show and tell time to announce that he was adopted. A discussion ensued at school. Amy's parents listened to her recital of the day's events and answered, "We are your parents, we are your mommy and daddy." Off Amy skipped to play with her dolls. When Amy's mother called her pediatrician to ask what else to say, he noted that the parents' reassurance seemed to have been successful. He suggested that as they tuck her into bed that night they say, "Good night, our lovely daughter."

At Amy's age she needed reassurance that her parents would always be there for her four-year-old needs. Because of Amy's age, it is unlikely that she can accurately grasp any of the concepts needed to understand gamete donation. Thus it is not suggested that her parents tell Amy of her biological origins at this time. Instead, they should file the conversation away for future reference.

If no special circumstances are present that necessitate telling at an earlier age, we believe that early adolescence (age ten to fourteen) is the best time for full disclosure. Early adolescence is a time of biologic and psychologic maturation. Cognitively, the stage of formal thought operations is achieved during these years. Most children in this stage can reason abstractly, have begun to use logic, and have become sophisticated in moral reasoning. Although normal adolescent turmoil and rebellion are on the horizon, they may not yet be in full bloom. Disclosure before the commencement of the adolescent struggle for identity and independence is suggested.

Diverse family makeups can affect how and when the child is given information. There are a number of situations in which it would be necessary to begin disclosure at a younger age. A single woman may use TDI if she is concerned about her fertility and she does not wish to marry. A lesbian couple may want children and opt for TDI. A 1979 study by Curie-Cohen et al. stated that almost 10% of all physicians responding to their survey performed artificial insemination on single women. In these two family circumstances the child may notice the lack of a father and question the parent, thus precipitating a premature onset of the process of disclosure. In a two-parent, heterosexual family the telling time is more likely to be governed by the parents' choosing.

Special circumstances require flexible and prepared parents. The five-year-old who arrives from school asking one of her two mothers why she does not have a daddy should be answered in an honest, nondefensive manner with information commensurate with her developmental stage and individual capabilities.

A number of books have been written for parents to read to children to explain various reproductive methods (University Department of OB/GYN, Jessop Hospital for Women, 1991; Gordon ER, 1992). These books both provide an explanation of the biologic concepts and articulate the parents' desire to have and raise a child.

REFERENCES

1. Amuzu B, Laxova R, Shapiro S. (1990) Pregnancy outcome, health of children and family adjustment after donor insemination. Obstet Gynecology 75(6):889–905.
2. Baran A, Pannor R. (1989) Lethal Secrets: The Psychology of Donor Insemination, Problems and Solutions. New York: Warner.
3. Bernstein J. (1993) The long-term psychologic effects of gamete donation. In: M Seibel, A Kiessling, J Bernstein, S Levin, eds. Technology and Infertility. New York: Springer-Verlag.
4. Brodzinsky DM. (1984) New perspectives on

adoption revelation. Early Child Development and Care 18:105–118.

5. Chevret M. (1977) Leveçu de l'insemination artificielle. Thèse de Médecine, Lyon.

6. Curie-Cohen M, Luttrell L, Shapiro S. (1979) Current practice of artificial insemination by donor in the United States. New Engl J Med 300:585–590.

7. Daniels KR. (1986) New birth technologies: A social work approach to researching the psychological factors. Social Work in Health Care 11(4):49–60.

8. Daniels KR. (1988) Artificial insemination using donor semen and the issue of secrecy: The views of donors and recipient couples. Soc Sci Med 27(4):377–383.

9. Goldstein J, Freud A, Solnit AJ. (1973) Beyond the Best Interests of the Child. New York: The Free Press.

10. Gordon ER. (1992) Mommy Did I Grow in Your Tummy? Santa Monica, Calif.: EM Greenberg Press.

11. Reading AE, Sledmere CM, Cox DN. (1982) A survey of patient attitudes toward artificial insemination by donor. J Psychosom Res 26:429.

12. Shakespeare W. (1606) Macbeth.

13. Sokoloff BZ. (1987) Alternative methods of reproduction: Effects on the child. Clinical Pediatrics. 26(1):11–17.

14. University Department of OB/GYN, Jessop Hospital for Women. (1991) My Story. Sheffield, England: Infertility Research Trust.

17

Egg Donation: Psychological and Counseling Issues Surrounding Disclosure versus Privacy

ANDREA M. BRAVERMAN, PH.D.

There is an ongoing and sometimes bitter debate about whether or not a couple should inform their child of his or her donor origins. Physicians are often on the front lines advising the couple about their choices. How the doctor or the nurse presents pertinent information to the patient may influence whether the woman will pursue egg donation as a viable option and whether she discloses their use to the child. Some physicians tend to suggest that the couple keep the use of a donor a secret. Other infertility specialists are conflicted about the advice they dispense to couples concerning disclosure.

In their survey of physicians, Leiblum and Hamkins found that 56% of doctors believed that the child did not need to be told, 21% were neutral, and 22% endorsed disclosing to the child (Leiblum SR, Hamkins SE, 1992). There is also an increasing body of anecdotal literature among mental health professionals to suggest that it is better for couples to disclose their use of a donor to any child conceived. Currently, there is no right answer to give patients and little empirical evidence on which to base a recommendation.

The source of the donated oocytes may influence a recipient's decision to disclose or not disclose the child's donor origins. For example, recipients who use family donors may feel that they are not depriving the child of any genetic information by not disclosing. On the other hand, a couple may feel very comfortable telling the child that a family member was a donor because they believe that the child will not feel "different" or excluded from the family tree by a different genetic history.

The search for a universal right or wrong answer for couples who are considering and using donor gametes may be irrelevant; there may not be a single right or wrong approach for a particular couple. Moreover, the right questions may not yet have been asked. In that regard, the issue of privacy and disclosure of donor gametes is similar to a three-dimensional puzzle. Depending on the angle from which a person views the configuration, certain truths appear to be self-evident. However, when the puzzle is viewed from a different angle, another image emerges.

It is helpful to reexamine the disclosure and privacy debate through five different areas of understanding donor gametes: (1) language, (2) medical, (3) sociological, (4) ethical, and (5) psychological. In examining each area, issues that may not have answers—and certainly have not been scientifically examined—will be raised. Defining the questions that must be asked will begin the journey toward helping each individual and couple make choices that will work for them.

LANGUAGE

The language that professionals are rapidly adopting to discuss these issues has already begun to influence patients and color thinking about the choices that these patients have made. For example, the language adopted in the abortion debate in the United States—for example, "pro-life" and "pro-choice"—has embedded in it the suggestion that to be "pro-choice" is to be "anti-life." Currently, the language that is used to discuss donor gametes employs the terminology "disclosure" versus "secrecy."

Language can play a critical role. Originally, the choices about whether or not to tell a child born through donor gametes were labeled "openness" and "secrecy." These terms were problematic because of the potential negative connotation of "secrecy" and positive connotation of "openness." Furthermore, the connotations of the term "secrecy" may prevent a couple from exploring all aspects of choosing not to disclose the donor's contribution. The negative personal and social values attached to the concept of secrecy may compel the couple to make a premature judgment.

Careful consideration must be given to whether the terminology of the choices being presented is biasing and complicating the decisions couples are making. In discussing the complexities of disclosure and nondisclosure, a more neutral use of language is to present the choices as being between "disclosure" and "privacy" to encourage the exploration process.

The issues introduced about whether to keep the use of the donor secret from the child must also be part of the counseling process because if the couple chooses not to tell the child, a secret is being kept. For some donor recipient parents, as will be outlined later, this secret will not be seen as burdensome because they will view withholding the information as being in the child's best interests. Other parents will see this as a fearful secret that could

destroy their relationship with the child. Couples must examine these issues carefully before engaging in treatment and must understand that this discussion will be protracted as the child grows.

MEDICAL

Part of the choice between disclosure and privacy must involve consideration of how the couple will deal with the oocyte donor's medical history. In anonymous donation situations the parents may have very limited information about the donor's history. The couple must decide how they will deal with this situation: (1) Disclose the donor's history or lack thereof, (2) represent the wife's medical history as that of the donor, or (3) incorporate the donor's medical history into the wife's.

Sometimes the only choice is to fully disclose the use of a donor to the child and/or his or her physician. For example, if the recipient has a medical condition that the child might inherit were egg donation not used, then full disclosure must be made because the child may be directly affected if the pediatrician has the impression that the child is at risk for a particular disorder. However, if there is no significant medical history on the wife's side, a couple could choose to incorporate the donor's history into the wife's history. If the couple edits the history under the supervision of a physician (such as the couple's gynecologist or reproductive endocrinologist), the child's medical care should remain unaffected.

SOCIOLOGICAL

Although no one paper can adequately address the myriad of sociological issues that are inherent in ovum donation, it is important to recognize that society does have an interest in how couples deal with their offspring concerning the information they receive about a donor. For example, consanguinity affects society. If offspring from the same genetic parent are raised in two different families and marry unknowingly, their child could potentially experience serious medical complications. Since there is the possibility of unintentional consanguinity as a result of gamete donation, society has a vested interest in how families handle the issue of privacy or disclosure. The fear of consanguinity has led to recommended guidelines regarding the number of offspring that should be allowed for each sperm donor.

The legal concept of "the best interests of the child" could also be applied in the donor gamete situation. Society does intervene in family situations when it is presumed that the parents are not acting in the child's best interests. If data emerges that demonstrates a medical or psychological harm due to either withholding or disclosing donor origins, then society may have a real moral responsibility to regulate the practice of donor gametes. In addition, the possibility (albeit remote) that society may suffer a financial burden in providing medical or mental health care beyond what the recipient would pay must also be addressed.

ETHICAL AND PSYCHOLOGICAL

The ethical and psychological issues related to gamete donation are controversial, and little research is available to lend clarification. As in all controversies, the issues are seen differently depending on whether the person espousing the views endorses the right to privacy or the right to knowledge, so examination of these issues should start with a look at the two "camps" of disclosure and privacy.

The disclosure camp gives four major arguments to support it's position that recipients should tell the child about his or her donor origins:

1. Individuals have a fundamental right to know the truth about their genetic origins.
2. Medical information is critical, and nondisclosure may limit the amount of information the child receives and/or may lead to wrong information being given about the recipient mother's genetic history.
3. Secrets are "lethal" and may permanently hurt the family and child.
4. Children born from donor gametes will sense that there is something different about themselves through subtle cues that will affect their sense of self and their relationship with their families.

Proponents of disclosure use the adoption model for guidance and feel that the adoption literature has shown definitively the adverse effects of secrets. Advocates believe that families and children do better when family origins are talked about openly.

Those who endorse recipient couples' right to choose privacy make five major arguments:

1. Individuals do not have a fundamental right to know the truth about their genetic origins.
2. Medical information can be incorporated into the child's and family's medical history to ensure accurate information.
3. All families have secrets (e.g., parents choose every day what is in the best interest of their child and do not tell their children everything), and we do not know that this is a "lethal" secret.
4. Children born from donor gametes will not sense anything different when they are raised in a home where the parents are loving and unconflicted about the use of a donor gamete.
5. Sperm donation has been done formally for decades, and less formally for centuries, under the restrictions of privacy, and these families appear to have managed well.

In other words, the absence of problems being presented to physicians or mental health professionals by these families indicates that privacy works for them.

This argument seems similar to the adoption argument made by advocates of disclosure. Both examples are compelling and suggestive, yet neither is conclusive. Just because not telling the child appears to have worked well does not prove that telling the child would not be more successful. Similarly, just because adoption works well with openness does not mean that gamete donation will. Adoption and gamete donation are not the same. In gamete donation the donor does not give up an unplanned child; the donor gives up a number of eggs or millions of sperm for a very much planned-for child. The psychological issues for the family and child could be very different.

The ethical debate about an individual's right to know about his or her genetic origins is heated. The fundamental question remains: Does a child have a right to know about his or her genetic origins? Furthermore, even if the argument that each person has a fundamental right to know about his or her genetic origins is held, the next ethical dilemma asks:

1. Does the parents' right to privacy supersede the child's right to know?
2. Does the parents' right to decide whether this knowledge would prove more harmful than helpful to their child supersede the child's right to know?

The psychological issues are both compelling and unresolved. The critical issue of whether knowing or not knowing is harmful to the emotional development of the child has not been addressed. Furthermore, the surrounding community, religious affiliation, and extended family contribute to the psychological adjustment of the child and of the immediate family. If these groups do not approve of the use of donor gametes, the child may experience prejudice, notoriety, or rejection

Little is known about the psychosocial issues of the donors themselves. Most studies have indicated that oocyte donors who have been psychologically screened respond well to the experience and feel positive about having tried to help another woman, and the majority would do so again (Schover LR, 1993; Schover LR, et al., 1991; Kirkland A, et al., 1992). Other studies have suggested that the medical treatment for donors is very stressful and difficult (Trounson A, et al., 1983; Raoul-Duval A, et al., 1992).

Less is known about follow-up with the families that are formed through egg donation. Again, sperm donation provides some analogous insight. Most studies on sperm donation have shown that marital satisfaction remains within the normal range during follow-up, and some suggest that the experience brings couples closer together (Klock SC, 1993; David A, Avidan D, 1976; Klock S, Maier D, 1991). It should be noted that these studies all included psychological screening or counseling as part of their protocol.

Recently, Weaver et al. looked at families formed through in vitro fertilization (IVF), therapeutic donor insemination (TDI), and unassisted conception (Weaver SM, et al., 1993). In measures of attachment, marital adjustment, and parental feelings, the donor insemination group measured as well or better on all dimensions. Furthermore, the fathers of the TDI children were unremarkable in comparison to their counterparts. The trend in the literature demonstrates that families formed through gamete donation may not have inherent issues. Perhaps these families have been overpathologized by an assumption that there has to be a disruption in intrafamilial relations based on genetic differences.

The psychological adjustment to parenting through donor gametes is probably evolutionary, just like adjustment to other life changes.

Parenting in general is thought to involve different stages, and the ability to parent effectively also changes with experience. The initial decision the couple makes to parent through donor oocytes takes place at the same time they are assimilating medical information, coping with the wife's loss of genetic contribution, and (often) the cumulative effects of undergoing infertility treatment. Any decisions about how they want to handle the information and specifically cope with the child may be subject to change once the crisis abates. Initially, the desire to become pregnant may loom larger than the hypothetical issues raised about parenting the child.

Potential parents must assimilate information on IVF, choices about whether to cryopreserve embryos, selecting a known or anonymous donor, issues of the cost of a donor ovum cycle, and concerns about a multiple pregnancy as well as whether they will even be successful. With all this information bombarding them, and with the emotional roller coaster ride of hope and loss, the initial stages of adjusting to donor oocytes may feel very different from later stages, when the information has been assimilated.

The tasks that are required at the beginning of the process are very different from those that arise after the pregnancy is established. Once the woman is pregnant, the high-tech aspect of the conception fades, and the couple is free to experience pregnancy like any other couple. It may be only then that the couple or one partner has the "luxury" of experiencing some of the feelings that were kept in check as a defense against the potentially crushing disappointment of a failed embryo transfer.

Initially, couples may feel a strong need to discuss their feelings and thoughts with others. As seen in Klock and Maier's study, 81% of subjects who had a child born through TDI and reported having told someone stated that if they could do it all over again, they would tell no one (Klock S, Maier D, 1991). This study suggests that the adjustment to using donor oocytes evolves over time and that feelings will probably change. In particular, the couple or one partner may feel that the process is strange or overwhelming at first. After they become comfortable with the concept and the process, there may be a stronger desire to feel "normal" and to be seen as a "normal" family. Regret about others knowing that a donor was involved may result because the couple does not wish to be seen as different or because they told others before resolving their issues. The issues of adjustment to new parenthood may be more immediate than the fact that an egg donor was involved.

Clinically, we have seen a heightened sense of anxiety just after birth because of concern that the baby's physical characteristics may be different from the parents' or visibly "stamped" with the donor's characteristics. In addition, many couples express an anxiety that they may not be able to love or attach to the child because he or she will be a genetic stranger.

Counseling is important in preparing the couple for a wide spectrum of feelings that can be considered normal. Recipients may feel that they need to eliminate any thoughts or feelings about the donor's involvement, but acknowledging these thoughts and feelings and putting them in perspective may provide an easier and less threatening transition. As new and different information emerges through experience in being a parent, understanding the personality and needs of their child, and clarifying their feelings about the donor's role, couples will need to anticipate that their emotions and reactions will shift over time. The goal is not to work on forgetting about the donor's contribution but to allow honest feelings and the opportunity to acknowledge that these feelings may change as the child grows.

Because data is lacking to support a recommendation of either privacy or disclosure, it is essential to be very cautious in discussing these options with patients. Medical and mental health professionals must recognize and acknowledge whether they bring any biases to the recipient's counseling. The questions in Table 17.1 are helpful in identifying any inherent assumptions and biases before conducting any patient counseling.

It is important that patients receive counseling that helps them to consider all aspects of choosing to form a family through gamete donation. The best tool is education. The physician can help to educate and support patients by gathering a library of articles for their patients that present different aspects of all these issues. Physicians can encourage the couple to continue their discussion about the role of donor gametes throughout the pregnancy and child's life. At the same time, physicians can reassure the couple that, as long as the donor is not a forbidden subject, they are probably well-equipped to cope with the feelings and issues.

It is also important for the physician, mental health counselor, or both to educate the couple that the impact of using a donor will likely vary throughout their child's life. For example, if a child unexpectedly begins to play virtuoso violin at age three, thoughts and feelings about using a donor may arise. Similarly, if the child is diagnosed with a learning disability, the couple may wonder about any genetic loading from the donor. Again, the ability to talk about using a donor allows the couple to experience their own particular feelings, both sad and happy, about making this choice in their lives.

Professionals can acknowledge that any decision the couple may make, or has made, must be taken into consideration during their exploration about disclosure. In other words, if the couple has already told all their friends and family members that they intend to use a donor, they may already have made a de facto decision to tell their child.

CONCLUSION

The choice to use donor oocytes involves many complex feelings and issues. There is an ongoing debate about whether couples should disclose the use of donor egg or sperm to the child. The language adopted in discussing gamete donation can influence patients' feelings and color their thinking about the choices made. Although there is no conclusive data to suggest whether or not parents should disclose, there is a clear need for thorough counseling to explore both the choice and the potential psychosocial consequences. Women and their partners who choose gamete donation will experience different stages of adjustment: during the treatment phase, pregnancy, and immediate postpartum, different issues unfold. For any family the choice to use donor gametes must include careful exploration and education to build a positive and healthy future.

TABLE 17.1. Questions That Are Helpful in Identifying Inherent Assumptions and Biases Held by Egg Donation Counselors

1. What role do you believe genetics plays in a person's personality, sense of humor, values, goals, etc.?
2. Are secrets necessarily "lethal"?
3. Do parents have a right to keep any information private?
4. Does a child have an inalienable right to know about his or her genetic origins?
5. Would you want to know if your parents used a gamete donor?
6. Can you live with a secret?
7. When are the parents' right to privacy superseded by a child's right to know?
8. Are feelings about disclosure or privacy entangled with the husband or wife recipient's feelings of shame or worthlessness?
9. How will the child's family and community react to the child's donor origins?

REFERENCES

1. David A, Avidan D. (1976) Artificial insemination by donor: Clinical and psychological aspects. Fertil Steril 27:528–532.

2. Kirkland A, Power M, Burton G, et al. (1992) Comparison of attitudes of donors and recipients to oocyte donation. Hum Reprod 7:355–357.

3. Klock SC. (1993) Psychological aspects of donor insemination. In: DA Greenfeld, ed. Infertility and Reproductive Medicine Clinics of North America. Philadelphia: W.B. Saunders, pp. 483–497.

4. Klock S, Maier D. (1991) Psychological factors related to donor insemination. Fertil Steril 56:489–495.

5. Leiblum SR, Hamins SE. (1992) To tell or not to tell: Attitudes of reproductive endocrinologists concerning disclosure to offspring of conception via assisted insemination by donor. J Psychosomatic Obstet Gynaecol 13:267–275.

6. Raoul-Duval A, Letur-Konirsch H, Frydman R. (1992) Anonymous oocyte donation: A psychological study of recipients, donors and children. Hum Reprod 7:51–54.

7. Schover LR. (1993) Psychological aspects of oocyte donation. In: DA Greenfeld, ed. Infertility and Reproductive Medicine Clinics of North America. Philadelphia: W.B. Saunders, pp. 483–497.

8. Schover LR, Collins RI, Quigley MM, et al. (1991) Psychological follow-up of women evaluated as oocyte donors. Hum Reprod 6:1487–1491.

9. Trounson A, Leeton J, Bosanka M, et al. (1983) Pregnancy established in an infertile patient after transfer of a donated embryo fertilized in vitro. Br Med J 286:835–838.

10. Weaver SM, Clifford E, Gordon AG, et al. (1993) A follow-up study of "successful" IVF/GIFT couples: Social-emotional well-being and adjustment to parenthood. J Psychosomatic Obstet and Gynaecol 14:5–16.

18

Conceiving the Future: The Impact of the Human Genome Project on Gamete Donation

ROBIN J.R. BLATT, MPH

Scientific developments in genetic research and testing have expanded so rapidly during the last two decades that they resemble science fiction. The resulting potential impact could affect individuals at all ages of life. Emerging scenarios that individuals may in the foreseeable future grapple with include:

- Preimplantation genetic screening tests are performed on a newly fertilized embryo following in vitro fertilization to determine the genetic constitution of potential offspring before pregnancy. Multiplex analysis enables numerous genes to be identified. "Imperfect" embryos are not transferred. Normal embryos are transferred. Amniocentesis and the need for abortion of abnormal fetuses are avoided.
- Newborns have a sample of genetic material obtained at birth. Genetic conditions or traits may be identified. The sample is stored in a DNA data bank for an unspecified future use such as a perfectly matched bone marrow transplant if the newborn should ever need one.
- Adolescents undergo a battery of genetic screening tests to determine susceptibility to breast and ovarian cancer, heart disease, mental illness, and other major illnesses for future health and family decisions.

- Upon applying for a job, a woman is queried about her personal health and genetic family history. She is expected to have tests to determine whether she may be at risk of genetic damage from substances in the workplace or where in the organization she ought to be placed.
- As part of obtaining a marriage license, a woman and her partner are required to have premarital genetic testing and counseling to determine genetic compatibility problems, such as both individuals being a carrier for Tay Sachs disease, that would create a serious problem for future children.
- A woman learns during pregnancy that the developing baby has a disability. She chooses to carry the pregnancy to term, but her child is denied health insurance because of a "preexisting condition."
- To avoid making child care payments, a husband claims that he is not the biologic father of his wife's child. After an interrogation, paternity testing is ordered prior to the resolution of divorce arrangements.
- A woman with a family history of breast cancer undergoes genetic screening to identify the presence or absence of the gene associated with the condition. The report comes back "positive," indicating an 85% probability that the gene is present.

The doctor schedules the woman to have both of her breasts and ovaries removed to reduce the chances of cancer occurring in later life. During the procedure, slices of her ovaries are preserved for a future pregnancy in the patient's uterus or in a gestational carrier.

- A new company developed by government-supported researchers has completed a market survey that reveals that the quickest and most profitable route for capturing the genetic service market in the next century is to develop proprietary, over-the-counter genetic technology that will sit prominently on drugstore shelves. The results are to be a new line of products that will include a gender test to determine fetal sex during pregnancy and other specialized kits designed to indicate predisposition to a variety of health conditions that occur in later life.

While these scenarios may appear wildly imaginative, they are not as farfetched as they seem. Genetic research is having a profound impact on all members of society, physically, emotionally, spiritually and financially. Current trends in molecular biology, the commercialization of science, and the launching of the Human Genome Project (HGP) are stimulating novel genetic research protocols and technologies directed toward individuals at all stages of the life cycle. What is being experienced at the end of this century is only an inkling of what is to come.

At this time in history it is critical for medical professionals and consumers to become familiar with the national genetic research agenda and to further the analysis of the social, political, economic, and legal forces promoting applications of genetic research, screening and testing. Rarely is there such a clear view of emerging science and technology and the moral dilemmas posed by such progress, and rarely are members of society informed about the advent of programs for technological change or the development of new technology until it is firmly established. Medical professionals and consumers must work collectively to shape the destiny of genetic research and science policy because they will ultimately affect the future of the human species.

GENETIC MAPMAKING: THE HUMAN GENOME PROJECT

The Human Genome Project (HGP) is a U.S. government–sponsored international research and technology development effort designed to produce a variety of biological maps that reveal the location of all the genes in the human body and to determine the chemical sequence of human DNA. Like the development of an astronomical chart that documents the position of the sun, the moon, and the planets, genetic maps are an attempt to define the order and pattern of genetic substance. The biological maps and new technologies that emerge from the HGP are expected to provide basic information about the role of the genes in human development and differentiation and in the control of functions of the human body.

This initiative is a major program for technological change. It involves many research projects supported through peer-reviewed grants and carried out in public and private laboratories, universities, and government agencies.

However, this project is not simply a scientific quest for knowledge. It is a research and technology development effort that is attempting to build an infrastructure that will strategically position the United States in the global economic and health care market in the twenty-first century.

GOVERNMENT COORDINATION OF THE HUMAN GENOME PROJECT

Like many of the United States' mega-science projects—creating the atom bomb and sending a person to the moon—the HGP is sponsored and coordinated by the federal government. It is not just one project but many research projects being undertaken in public and private laboratories, universities, and government agencies. Activities are supported through competitive grants for basic scientific research and for surveys, sociologic studies, public and professional education, conferences, and ethical and policy analyses. The agencies that are primarily responsible for coordination of this effort include the newly established National Center for Human Genome Research (NCHGR) located within the National Institutes of Health (NIH) and the U.S. Department of Energy (DOE). In addition to stimulating scientific research, each agency has established an Ethical, Legal and Social Implications (ELSI) program to concurrently assess the societal implications of this initiative. The international component of the HGP is coordinated by the recently formed Human Genome Organization (HUGO). Other government agencies such as the National Science Foundation (NSF) and organizations such as the Howard Hughes Medical Institute (HHMI) are also collaborating on aspects of the HGP.

SOCIAL AND POLITICAL ORIGINS OF THE HUMAN GENOME PROJECT

To understand the history of the HGP, it is critical to look at its social and political origins. For decades, genetic research and mini–human genome projects have been conducted in individual government, academic, and commercial laboratories around the world. As new developments in biotechnology have made it possible to explore genetic material, efforts to isolate and understand genes have become highly focused with little collaboration among scientific researchers. Consequently, developments of technologies, treatments, and therapies for illnesses in which the genetic error is known have been remarkably slow. The HGP has been designed to provide a coordinated effort in which all data describing the human genome will be made available to researchers worldwide to foster scientific collaboration, facilitate technology development and transfer, and new treatments.

The original proposal for sequencing the human genome was initiated by the DOE in the mid-1980s. Deciphering the genetic code was envisioned as a high-technology project that could be undertaken at its national laboratories with the primary goal of studying the effect of radiation on DNA. Subsequently, the NIH became involved in the project, since future trends in health care were likely to involve locating genes that predispose to or cause diseases. Constructing genetic maps of the estimated 100,000 plus genes on all of the human chromosomes (22 pairs plus X and Y) and determining the sequence of all the DNA, would involve enormous funding requirements, and costs had to be shared. Several researchers proposed that the U.S. Congress appropriate new money specifically for the HGP project. In 1986 the National Academy of Sciences (NAS) appointed a special National Research Council (NAC) to consider whether or not the U.S. government should sponsor the HGP. This fifteen-member committee addressed the issue for over a year and decided unanimously in its favor. In 1988 the NAC released a report proposing that the project begin with gene mapping and with efforts to improve sequencing technology. Around the same time, scientific researchers and government spokespeople convinced politicians who were concerned with health, the economy, and technology transfer that the HGP would build the necessary infrastructure for the future of our society, leading us into the next century. The U.S. Congress subsequently commissioned the Office of Technology Assessment (OTA) to investigate the scientific, medical, and economic implications of a widescale genetic mapping and sequencing effort and its possible organizational structure. The U.S. Congress approved the development of the HGP, and in October 1988 the NIH and the DOE signed a memorandum of understanding outlining plans for cooperating on this genetic research endeavor. In 1989 the National Center for Human Genome Research (NCHGR) was established with an official commencement date for the HGP of October 1, 1990.

PURPOSE AND GOALS OF THE HUMAN GENOME PROJECT

In 1990 the NCHGR published a five-year plan with goals for the HGP for the fiscal years 1991–1995:

1. To assemble genetic maps of the entire human genome to identify the relative location in which genes, genetic markers, and other genetic "landmarks" are found along human chromosomes.
2. To sequence the order of the human genome to generate information about gene structure and function. Recent technological developments have made it possible to construct these maps, which are expected to be used in a range of biological research studies, including the search for genes associated with illness and the development of new drugs and therapies.
3. To map and sequence the genomes of model organisms, such as a mouse or bacterium, in an effort to make comparisons to humans and to develop and validate new technology.
4. To develop new computer informatics (software, hardware, databases, and analytic tools) that can be used to support large-scale projects and assist in the interpretation of the genetic information that is collected.
5. To support the research training programs for predoctoral and postdoctoral fellows to encourage careers in genome research and biomedical sciences.
6. To develop innovative technologies and facilitate technology transfer and spin-offs that will give the United States a competitive edge in the global marketplace.
7. To develop programs and policies that address the ethical, legal, and social implications associated with the HGP, such as issues related to privacy of genetic information, fairness of use, and potential for discrimination in insurance, employment, criminal justice, adoption, and the military; impact on the practice of medicine, genetic counseling, and reproductive decision making; and the introduction and safety of new genetic tests.

HUMAN GENOME PROJECT TIMELINE

A fifteen-year projection for the HGP was developed. It was expected that between the years 1990 and 1995, 40% of all genes would be mapped, and 10% of genes would be sequenced. During the years 1996 and 2000, 95% of all genes would be mapped, and 50% of genes would be sequenced. By the years 2001–2005, all genes was expected to be mapped, and the sequencing would be completed. As of this writing, there is no specific timeline for the completion of the study of the ethical, legal, and social implications of the HGP and the development of public policies for consumer protection. It remains unclear which organizations, on both federal and state levels, will assume responsibility for developing and implementing policies, regulations, and mechanisms for oversight in this new scientific world order. The House Committee on Government Operations has recommended the establishment of a federally chartered advisory committee to independently review the results of the ethical, legal, and social research and to design appropriate genetic related public policies.

COSTS OF THE HUMAN GENOME PROJECT

The HGP is a $3 billion initiative funded by the U.S. Congress and supported by taxpayers. Annual appropriations for genetic research are provided to the coordinating government agencies. Approximately 5% of the yearly budget for human genome research is now allocated to the Ethical, Legal and Social Implications (ELSI) Program, which is assuming a more prominent profile as discoveries in genetics begin to outpace our ability to process their implications.

POTENTIAL BENEFITS

The HGP is expected to result in fundamental scientific information about how genes affect the development, differentiation, and functions of the human body and model organisms. In addition, it is expected to stimulate the emergence of new scientific and medical instrumentation, genetic screening, and diagnostic tests as well as new products, careers,

and services. The HGP is also being hailed as having significant promise for economic advantages in domestic and international commerce. Above and beyond any societal changes the HGP is likely to generate, however, it has been touted for its capacity to revolutionize health care.

Genome research is shedding new light on conditions that have traditionally been viewed as genetic, such as sickle-cell disease, cystic fibrosis, and Huntington's disease. It is also providing insights into heart disease, breast and ovarian and other types of cancer, behavioral and neurological conditions, and even aging. In addition to producing a variety of biological maps that pinpoint the position of genes on chromosomes and reveal sequence information, the HGP is expected to spawn the development of new treatments for a variety of health conditions. Already, biopharmaceutical research and gene therapy experiments are in progress for the treatment of a number of conditions, such as adenosine deaminase deficiency, thalassemia, sickle-cell disease, hemophilia, cystic fibrosis and hypercholesterolemia, infectious disease (e.g., AIDS), cancer (brain, colon, skin, breast, and ovarian cancers), and certain vascular diseases.

CRITICISMS AND CONTROVERSIES

Many of the concerns about the HGP are similar to those discussed and debated over the past few decades relating to genetic research. The HGP magnifies these issues and provides a sense of urgency in the establishment of safeguards and social guidelines to prevent the misuse of genetic technology and information.

Critics of the HGP argue that the effort is a waste of national resources in a time of fiscal austerity when the most basic health, food, and housing needs of society remain unmet and, in some parts of the world, unavailable.

There is concern that nontraditional directed (noninvestigator-initiated) research provides a small group of scientists and companies with a large amount of money and takes away funding from other investigator-initiated biomedical research projects that may be of benefit. Debate continues about whether mapping and sequencing the entire genome are an appropriate approach or whether only those portions of the genome that have known biological significance (estimated to be 5% of the genome's DNA) ought to be studied. Those in favor of the grand initiative argue that the nonfunctional or "junk" DNA may have important functions that have yet to be discovered.

Controversy exists regarding the HGP's potential to diminish human beings to no more than a genetic sequence. The effort has been considered reductionist in its approach, perpetuating a myth of scientific neutrality when, in fact, developments in science and technology associated with the HGP occur within a social and political context involving human values. Questions surrounding sociobiology and genetic determinism are being raised once again. The increasing focus on the genes as a cause of disability is believed by some to divert attention from dealing directly with the impact of the physical environment on health and mutagenesis. Research attempting to establish new links between genes, behavior, and disease furthers the "nature versus nurture" debate—Is it genetic or is it environmental?—when human beings are products of both genetics and the environment.

Ethical issues related to confidentiality of genetic information and genetic discrimination in insurance, employment, adoption, learning institutions, and occupational settings are becoming an increasing area of concern with the numbers of reports of discrimination in these areas on the rise. The creation of a map of the human genome raises questions about the meaning of disability and "normalcy." The role of government support in genetics and the World Health Organization statement that the prevention and control of genetic disease are a significant goal for Health by All for the year 2000 raise concerns about eugenics and disability rights. It can be argued that the fundamental goal of the HGP—to map and sequence the human genome with the intention of developing new genetic screening, diagnostics, treatments, and therapies to prevent or cure genetic conditions—embodies elements of eugenics. Eugenics is the science of improving the qualities of the human race by deliberately selecting certain types of people and characteristics to perpetuate. "Negative" eugenics involves the development of policies and programs to reduce the occurrence of genetically determined disease. "Positive" eugenics involves systematic or planned genetic changes to improve individuals or their offspring. Extreme caution and careful consideration must be given to any form of eugenics.

As history reveals, scientific information can be terribly misused. A renewed analysis of the future of disability rights in light of the HGP is desperately needed to ensure that the scientific research and medical technologies that emerge from the HGP are not in conflict with the rights of both able-bodied and disabled persons.

Reproductive rights and the impact of the HGP on women's health are very much in the forefront of discussion. Genetic testing that emerges from the HGP is being applied at all stages of the life cycle. Newborn screening, carrier screening, premarital screening, preimplantation genetic diagnosis and prenatal genetic testing, presymptomatic genetic testing, and occupational screening are becoming increasingly popular.

It has been recognized for more than a decade that models that encourage citizen participation in discussions about genetic-related public policy are needed. However, there has been minimal public participation in the development of the HGP. The lack of information associated with genetic decision-making processes; risk perception; and physical, psychological, personal, and family outcomes raises significant concerns. While attempts are being undertaken to assess the implications of genetic research and new technologies, current analysis of the ethical, legal and social implications associated with the HGP, although admirable, is based on traditional bioethical analysis, when, in fact, many contend that there is a need for an alternative discourse. Using broader methods of feminist ethical analysis that stem from an experiential perspective might better cause the impact of genetic screening and testing to be fully understood.

Claims that the HGP will bring forth the dawn of genetic healing are also under scrutiny. While the development of biopharmaceuticals, gene therapy trials, and new services are underway, there is concern about the safety of such experimentation. Although genetic research has the potential to produce "healing technologies," it furthers the medical paradigm by defining health in terms of predisposition, susceptibility to disease, and genetic risk. As new genes for a variety of conditions are identified and new tests are developed, it will become increasingly challenging to find reasons not to test.

ISSUES OF ACCESSIBILITY

In addition, equity issues, such as geographic, cultural, linguistic, and financial access to genetic services and treatments, particularly among underserved populations, have yet to be addressed. The development of a highly technical special professional language is emerging. Particularly in the medical profession, this can serve both a social and a political function and may hinder communication and understanding.

IMPACT ON HEALTH POLICY

Technologies that have been developed as a result of genetic research and the HGP are assisting in redefining health in a medical paradigm, in terms of predisposition and susceptibility to disease. Issues regarding interpretation of risk and how risk rates are presented remain unknown. Most recommendations for genetic testing are currently based on statistical probabilities of risk. Once health is put into a risk model and individuals are categorized as having low, moderate, or high risk for a condition, it is hard not to find some reason to test. Although such risk rates are frequently presented as statements of certainty, many of the commonly accepted risk figures are based on limited or out-of-date research. There is currently no comprehensive assessment of the number, variety, and distribution of people who are "at risk" for genetic conditions or the number of babies born with a specific genetic trait or related disability. Furthermore, the way in which different people view concepts or quoted risk rates can vary. Definitions of risk depend on the bias of the world in which we live, and how each of us interprets our personal risk status is highly individual. Although probability statistics and predictions of chance can be influential, decisions about medical care are often based on personal factors, our view of health and disability, our level of social and political consciousness, morality, culture, religion, and existing social and financial support services.

Human experimentation, the role of consumers in clinical research protocols, and the lack of culturally and linguistically appropriate guidelines to ensure informed consent or compliance are of significant concern. Aggressive recruitment efforts are underway to recruit families' participation in research, although issues of human experimentation and informed consent have not been adequately addressed. At present, there are no formally accepted standards or guidelines tailored to genetics that indicate what information ought to be required in the informed consent process for participation in genetic research. In addition, issues related to voluntary versus mandatory genetic screening and genetic screening in the absence of treatments are also undergoing renewed analysis, discussion, and debate.

Education and training issues are paramount to discussions regarding the HGP. Courses on genetics and ethics are not typically integrated into the educational curriculum in high school, college, or medical and health training programs. The lack of a sufficient number of trained health professionals who are familiar with genetics and counseling raises concerns about the transfer of new genetic information to consumers. The lack of a trained work force that is competent in biotechnology is also of increasing concern to companies that are involved in production and manufacturing.

IMPACT OF THE HUMAN GENOME PROJECT ON GAMETE DONATION

Because the HGP is designed to generate knowledge and spin off new technologies, it is reasonable to anticipate pressures from the medical and patient communities to use the information in many aspects of medicine, including gamete donation programs. Already reproductive endocrinologists, fertility specialists, and other medical specialists are attempting to seize and use this information as it emerges.

Once a gene is identified and subsequently sequenced, it will be technically possible to assess the presence or absence of a particular gene or gene mutation in eggs, sperm, or an early embryo. As a result, gamete or embryo donors contributing to such programs may eventually have their sex cells analyzed before

their genetic material is accepted or used. This raises profound issues for donors and recipients alike, in addition to having an enormous societal impact.

For example, experimental genetic tests are being developed to predict health conditions that may appear in later life (such as cancer). These tests will involve analyzing DNA for specific changes or alterations in genetic material that are believed to increase a person's susceptibility, predisposing him or her to a disease. Although these tests are currently undergoing research in adult populations, they may potentially be part of the prenatal genetic testing package that will be used to assess the health of the developing baby in utero or even part of gamete donation programs to assess the donor. As an example of research in this area, predictive genetic testing to identify cancer predisposition is currently underway. Cancer is a common multifactorial condition that occurs when cells reproduce and proliferate uncontrollably, resulting in the growth of tumor and spread of abnormal cells. For example, knowing whether you or your child may be predisposed to cancer might influence approaches to medical care, diet, work, or other aspects of lifestyle in a particular way that might diminish potential health complications. As such, the relevance of knowing one's predisposition could have enormous impact on gamete donation.

Also, research is underway to develop a laboratory technology that would allow groups of genetic analyses to be performed on one sample. By batching the tests performed, scientists and industry hope to develop what will definitely be an easier, faster, more efficient method for predicting specific genetic traits and conditions. Multiplex testing is thought to be a more efficient use of laboratory time because the technology enables several different DNA segments to be pooled and processed together. This process differs from conventional methods that enable only one single-stranded DNA segment to be processed at a time. Depending on the reason for the analysis, information may be generated that one would prefer not to know. Furthermore, what is of significant concern with regard to multiplexing systems is that a generic form of informed consent is expected to occur. However, the individual may be told that the test can potentially identify "chromosome conditions" without a proper explanation of each condition, its range of expression, resources, and other information that may be helpful in the decision to test or not to test. These problems are magnified with multiplex testing. When multiple genetic data will be generated, the informed consent and counseling process will become very complex and impractical, resulting in less information provided to potential donors. Furthermore, donors may eventually have no choice about which genetic analyses to undergo, since they will all be done together as a panel of tests.

Already in recent years, preimplantation genetic diagnosis, sometimes referred to as "embryo genetic disorder analysis" or "blastomere analysis before implantation (BABI)," has been undertaken to detect genetic variations in gametes before fertilization or in embryos fertilized in vitro before implantation in the uterus. Preimplantation genetic diagnosis is intended to identify genetic conditions or to perform chromosomal or DNA analyses in a very early conceptus when it is at about the eight-cell stage. Preimplantation genetic testing, while highly experimental and controversial, is beginning to be offered primarily to women and couples who have a family history of a genetic condition or to women who are getting pregnant by using assisted reproductive technologies such as in vitro fertilization. If donated oocytes are obtained from women who are known to be predisposed to a particular genetic disorder, preimplantation genetic diagnosis may allow their oocytes to be used by manipulating potential adverse outcomes.

This may be particularly useful when the donor is a sister who is known to be a carrier for a specific disorder.

Preimplantation genetic diagnosis is highly invasive and sufficiently new to be considered investigational. Between 30% and 50% of embryos may be lost as a result of technical manipulations. Only limited data exists to deduce immediate or long-term risks. While most researchers promoting the field claim that the microsurgery performed on the embryo does not affect the potential development of the baby, one must recognize that damage to the embryo could occur, and there is the chance that the surviving embryo(s) could be comprised in ways we cannot yet determine.

There are monumental issues related to preimplantation genetic diagnosis and genetic screening of gametes, some of which are addressed elsewhere in this book and many that have yet to be explored. This type of testing involves preselection of characteristics and traits, as well as the fate of the human species, raising the most serious of issues for individuals and society. Through gamete donation, embryo research and the HGP will collide, making it technically possible to apply genetic tests in the earliest stages of human development. This will no doubt have enormous impact not only on gamete donation, but on reproduction and family building in general. Conceiving the future is now only a matter of moral imagination and conscience.

DEVELOPING RESPONSIBLE TECHNOLOGY

There is no doubt that the speed of scientific advance in genetics is exceeding that of public and professional knowledge. Like many scientific and technological advances, genetic research may hold the promise of benefit to humanity. But as we have learned over and over in this century and before, technological change often brings with it a host of unintended social and environmental consequences and new ethical problems before which traditional cultural norms may falter. With the HGP underway and the explosion of new information and tests, an entire new spectrum of medical and moral issues has emerged.

Women's health advocates have long argued that the safety of a new procedure must be evaluated before the procedure is routinely offered. Despite such beliefs, there is no formal paradigm for genetic technology assessment, and many genetic tests that are developed or used routinely in health care are insufficiently tested before being introduced into the marketplace, raising significant health and safety issues for women, men, and potential offspring.

It is essential for consumers and professionals to enter into discussion and debate about the HGP to assist in the information of policies for the use of new genetic information and techniques and to help usher in this new era of genetics in a socially responsible way. Rarely do consumers and professionals have the opportunity to influence and shape the destiny of science as we do now. In most areas of science and medicine, consumers and professionals are generally not informed about the advent of new research directions or the development of new tests until they are well-established. But the HGP is still in its embryonic form. This is a historical juncture. The public and professionals have a great opportunity to understand and anticipate future issues associated with the application of information generated by the HGP, to shape the course of science and technology policy to reflect societal needs, and to help to usher in this new era in genetics in a socially responsible way. Gamete donation is likely to provide the forum for many of the more pressing issues to be discussed.

Index

Note: The letter *t* after a page number designates *table*; the letter *f* designates *figure*.